Front Line Extremity and Orthopaedic Surgery

Lawrence B. Bone
Christiaan N. Mamczak
Editors

Front Line Extremity and Orthopaedic Surgery

A Practical Guide

Springer

Editors
Lawrence B. Bone
Department of Orthopaedic Surgery
State University of New York at Buffalo
Buffalo, NY
USA

Christiaan N. Mamczak
Department of Orthopaedic Surgery
Naval Medical Center Portsmouth
Portsmouth, VA
USA

ISBN 978-3-642-45336-6 ISBN 978-3-642-45337-3 (eBook)
DOI 10.1007/978-3-642-45337-3
Springer Heidelberg New York Dordrecht London

Library of Congress Control Number: 2014936854

Printed on acid-free paper

Springer is part of Springer Science+Business Media (www.springer.com)

Without the valor and sacrifice of the brave soldiers fighting in this war on terror, our freedom would be in jeopardy. Despite immense danger, these warriors stand against our enemies with an unflappable commitment to protect the ideals of democracy. Displaced from their loved ones and the comforts of home, they continue to defend our country and the world from tyranny. Thus, it is with great respect that I dedicate this orthopaedic combat text to all of the soldiers who have fought for our freedom. Thankfully, most have returned home, but many have suffered tremendous injury. Only the dead have seen the end of war, but their ultimate sacrifice should not go unrecognized. My life was forever changed during my service in Afghanistan. Fighting to save our soldiers on their worst day remains the most humbling and rewarding experience in my orthopaedic trauma career. I am forever grateful to the men and women who fought and were injured in war.

With modern advances in combat trauma, surgeons are pushing the limits of treating non-survivable injuries. During this conflict, the complexity of injury severity continues to rise, but our revised understanding of combat wounding patterns and surgical techniques defy the odds by saving horribly injured soldiers who would have died in years past (i.e., the Dismounted Complex Blast Injury). This success is a testament to the hundreds of military physicians and surgeons who have expanded the principles of trauma casualty care. There remains a wealth of knowledge accumulated by our military medical services over the last decade of war. Currently, there are no collective orthopaedic accounts of this valuable experience. Eventually, this conflict will end, but losing the lessons learned during this war would be unjustifiable. I credit my co-editor, mentor and friend, Larry Bone, with the inspiration for this textbook. With his insight and vision, we have composed a unique guide for current and future military combat orthopaedic surgeons. I thank my colleagues and friends who authored chapters in their individual areas of expertise. Together, we share the accounts of front line medical heroism and the pearls of orthopaedic wisdom that we learned during our deployments in Iraq and Afghanistan. We have all learned that there is nothing that prepares a surgeon for war except war. Nevertheless, I hope that this book serves as a template for the future military surgeons, who I imagine will push the limits even further.

Lastly, I would like to acknowledge and thank my family for the understanding and patience they have demonstrated in support of my career as an orthopaedic trauma surgeon. It has been a long and tedious road; with many call days and deployments away from the people dearest to me. Luckily, they embrace my passion for orthopaedic surgery and desire to publish. I have been blessed with unconditional love from my wife, Debbie, and children, Zac and Alexandra. Coming home to them after each long day of work makes my life complete.

Christiaan N. Mamczak, DO

I would like to echo Christiaan N. Mamczak's dedication of this book to all the wounded warriors of the Iraq and Afghanistan wars. A special dedication to my son SGT Christian Bone whose courage and patriotism showed me the way to serving my country.

I would also like to dedicate this book to the men and women of the 1st Forward Surgical Team that I had the privilege to lead for 9 months at FOB Shank, Afghanistan. Their dedication to our mission of life, limb, and eyesight saved lives and returned injured soldiers home to their loved ones. They never checked out.

An Appreciation

I want to thank Cathy Buyea, my research coordinator at the Department of Orthopaedics, SUNY Buffalo, School of Medicine, for her editorial help with this book. Without her expertise this book would not have been finished on time. The editors greatly appreciate all her time and effort in the editing process.

Thank you.

LTC Lawrence Bone, MD, USAR, MC

Foreword

US Navy Captain (retired) Michael Bosse and I had the privilege to co-chair the fifth international Symposium for Extremity War Injuries in 2010. At that meeting, I was approached by a very respectful and energetic man in his 60s who introduced himself as Dr. Larry Bone. He then asked how he could join the Army and go to war to care for the injured men and women in Iraq and Afghanistan. I listened to his compelling story; of his own son being injured while serving in Iraq a few years previously; of his admiration for those who volunteered to deploy into harm's way; and of us, the military surgeons whom he felt had a great privilege of caring for them.

Thus began a 2-year quest for his commissioning as the oldest orthopaedic surgeon to ever be commissioned, and his two subsequent deployments, the most recent of which LTC Lawrence Bone served as Commander of the 1st Forward Surgical Team in Afghanistan. He has become a close friend, and mentor, while demonstrating the true ideals of a Soldier Medic: leadership, integrity, selfless service, and personal courage. Before he spent this past year deployed, he began collecting a vast field of experts, every one of them with first hand combat orthopaedic surgery experience in order to assemble this work. He is passionate, but realistic, and self-aware that a work such as this requires a cohesive team.

In 2011, I was serving as the Chief of Staff for the Army Surgeon General's Task Force on Dismounted Complex Blast Injuries – charged with study of a sudden rapid increase in multiple amputees from Afghanistan in 2010. This group developed a detailed analysis of the mechanisms, contributing situations and tactics, and best practices for initial management, transportation and definitive care of these previously lethal injury patterns. While we at home studied the injury, a few intrepid surgeons were "in the trenches" managing them. One of these, in the midst of the busiest treatment facility in Afghanistan that year, was an inspiring Naval surgeon named Christian N. Mamczak. I came to know him, largely by reputation, and later personally through his continued contribution to the study and care of Warriors with these injuries. There is likely no better team of editors to organize a team, and to know the absolute best practices for far forward orthopaedic care as Dr. Mamczak and Dr. Bone.

In a career of military service, strong bonds and enduring relationships are forged out of the shared struggles of military and medical training, of hardship, and withstanding what often seems like miles of regulations and bureaucracy. However, these relationships, especially within a shared profession, are solid and lasting. Many of the authors in this text have deployed together, and nearly all know each other through that network. I have had the immense privilege to lead Army Orthopaedics throughout the past 7 years of this conflict, and consider most of these experts to be personal friends. A few of those friends have given all they could give in service for their fellow Warriors, and I would be incomplete if I did not take this opportunity to remember a few souls who dedicated their lives to military orthopaedics and leadership. One in particular, CDR Mike Mazurek, who deployed in 2005 in central Iraq, Taqqadem, returned safely to share all he had learned with other trauma surgeons, residents in training and many of us. His unfortunate death in 2009 was an incalculable loss to Navy Orthopaedic Surgery, and indeed military medical education. Another Soldier medic was COL Brian Allgood, a graduate of Brooke Army Medical Center orthopaedic residency and the highest ranking officer to be killed in action in Iraq. These and several other physicians served, and saved, and demonstrated the utmost in giving of themselves.

I have had the privilege to preview the following pages, and acknowledge that the experts who have contributed are certainly not all of the dedicated and highly talented surgeons who have deployed over the past 13 years. However, they *all* are committed, proven, and articulate in presenting an informative text with the purpose of "how-to" for any surgeons deploying for the first time. In fact, the knowledge within this book is extremely valuable for surgeons of all specialties – who will undoubtedly perform initial management, debridement and likely skeletal stabilization of open combat related fractures. The chapters are directed toward the "bottom line up front", straightforward and quickly assimilated. I am proud to have had the opportunity to serve the more than 500 military orthopaedic surgeons who have deployed into Iraq or Afghanistan and more than 50,000 American Warriors who are alive with wounds sustained in those remote nations.

Honored to serve!

James R. Ficke, Colonel (retired) United States Army,
Department of Orthopaedic Surgery,
Johns Hopkins Hospital,
Baltimore, MD,
USA

Preface

The flight into a combat theater is a lonely time. Seasoned veteran or novice, the mindset is the same: introspective thoughts on the comforts you leave back home and calculated *expectations* of the mission ahead. Everyone remembers their first time and fighting back the inevitable feelings of anxiety and maybe even fear. As a medical doctor and surgeon, this is no way to approach your profession. But the truth in the matter is, that we are never prepared (in civilian training) for the magnitude of pathology seen in combat injuries. The famed, ancient philosopher, Hippocrates, has said, "War is the only proper school for a surgeon." And so, like every *battle* we have faced before this moment, we apply the principles of our practice to tackle the complex changes ahead. "See one – do one – teach one" is the motto at hand in combat medicine. There is no time for practice; lives are at stake. Many successful surgeons have embraced the challenge before you and so will you, because the fear of losing a wounded soldier is motivation enough to bring out your best and skills you may never have imagined.

No one goes into battle without a plan. The same is true for a combat surgeon. Over a decade of war in Iraq and Afghanistan has lead to cutting edge surgical and critical care. A multitude of lessons have been learned the hard way. Clinical practice guidelines exist to direct the talented hands of novice surgeons. In the modern era, the most common battlefield injuries affect the musculoskeletal system making orthopaedic surgeons among the busiest working groups downrange. Wounding patterns have become more complex, but the advances of modern combat trauma surgery yield survival rates higher than any other war in history. The only thing missing from this momentum was a collection of surgical tactics developed over the recent years of war.

Nothing truly prepares you for the brutality of war. The kinetic energy imparted upon our wounded warriors is unrivaled when compared to our civilian training. The intensity of combat care is unlike anything that you have been exposed to in the past. Complex as it may be, the principles of combat surgery remain the same: resuscitate, stop hemorrhage and stabilize. The challenge is adapting to new wounding patterns, operating in an austere environment and saving lives with fewer supplies than you are accustomed.

This *Front Line Extremity and Orthopaedic Surgery* text was conceived in order to prepare future surgeons for the uncertainties ahead of them in combat. It stems from our own fears of the unknown when we first landed downrange and the desire to be prepared for a *fight*. A collaborative effort between some of the most skilled and knowledgeable modern combat surgeons, this book serves as a high-yield reference for the most challenging realities of battlefield care. Intended to prepare novice combat orthopaedic surgeons for their mission, we hope that the collective experience of our authors alleviates some of the anxieties we all had. The pearls of wisdom and lessons learned within celebrate the success of our profession and the survival of our brave soldiers.

Contents

Contributors

Joseph Alderete, MD LTC MC USA
Deployment: FOB Jalabad, Afghanistan 2010
FOB Sharana, Afghanistan 2012

Romney Anderson, MD COL MC USA
Deployment: Chief of Orthopaedics, 10th CSH, Baghdad, Iraq 2009

Robert Beer, MD CDR MC USN
Deployment: Combined Joint Special Operations Task Force, Afghanistan 2009

Rodd Benfield, MD CDR MC USN
Deployment: Chief of Trauma, Kandahar, Afghanistan 2010–2011

Donald Bittner, MD CAPT MC USN
Deployment: Kandahar, Afghanistan 2010–2011

Robert Blease, MD LTC MC USA
Deployment: Commander, 274th FST, Basra, Iraq 2009
Shindand and Bala-Mur-Ghab, Afghanistan 2009

Lawrence B. Bone, MD LTC MC USAR
Deployment: FOB Warrior, Afghanistan 2012
Commander, 1st FST, FOB Shank, Afghanistan 2013

Mathew Bradley, MD LCDR MC USN
Deployment: Ship's Surgeon, USS George H W Bush 2011–2012

Christina Cawley, MD LTC MC USAR
Deployment: FOB Ghazni, Afghanistan 2009–2010
FOB Asadabad, Afghanistan 2011
FOB Salerno, Afghanistan 2012

Jean-Claude G. D'Alleyrand, MD LTC MC USA
Deployment: 10th CSH, Helmand Province, Afghanistan 2011
67th FST, Bala-Mur-Ghab, Afghanistan 2012

David Dromsky, MD CDR MC USN
Deployment: Camp Fallujah, Iraq 2007
Kandahar, Afghanistan 2012

Garth Elias, MD COL MC USA
Deployment: 339th CSH, Bagram, Afghanistan
933rd FST, Baghdad, Iraq
945th FST, Alkut, Iraq
1980th FST Sharana, Afghanistan

Eric Elster, MD CAPT MC USN
Deployment: Chief Surgeon/DSS, KAF, Kandahar, Afghanistan 2011

Mark E. Fleming, MD CDR MC USN
Deployment: 1st Marine Expeditionary Force, FRSS, Ramadi, Iraq 2008

Robert Gaines, MD CDR MC USN
Deployment: Helmand Province, Afghanistan 2009

Donald Gajewski, MD COL MC USA
Deployment: 31st CSH, Balad, Iraq 2004
555th FST, Asadabad, Afghanistan 2010–2011

Wade Gordon, MD Lt COL MC USAF
Deployment: Al Udied, Qatar, Commander, MFST 2006–2007
Bagram AF, Afghanistan 2010–2011

Roman Hayda, MD COL MC USA (ret)
Deployment: 758th FST, Naray, Afghanistan 2006

Melvin D. Helgason, MD MAJ MC USA
Deployment: Camp Dwyer, Afghanistan 2012

Eric P. Hofmeister, MD CAPT MC USN
Deployment: Orthopaedic Hand Surgeon, Fleet Hospital 8, Iraq 2008
TQ Surgical Company, Al Taqaddum, Iraq 2008–2009

Derek Ipsen, MD LTC MC USA
Deployment: 772nd FST, FOB Fenty, Jalalabad, Afghanistan 2009

Leo Kroonen, MD CDR MC USN
Deployment: Kandahar, Afghanistan 2011–2012

Christiaan N. Mamczak, DO, LCDR MC USN (ret)
Deployment: Kandahar, Afghanistan 2010–2011

Patricia L. McKay, MD CAPT MC USN
Deployment: OIF, USNS Comfort 2003

George P. Nanos, MD CDR MC USN
Deployment: FRSS, 2nd Marine Expeditionary Force, FOB Edinburgh, Afghanistan 2011

Benjamin K. Potter, MD LTC USA
Deployment: TF 115th CSH, Camp Dwyer, Afghanistan 2011

Dennis Rivet, MD CDR MC USN
Deployment: Kandahar, Afghanistan 2011–2012

Jonathon Sexton, MD CPT MC USN

Christopher S. Smith, MD LCDR MC USN
Deployment: Helmand Province, Afghanistan 2013

Joseph E. Strauss, DO CDR MC USN
Deployment: Kandahar, Afghanistan 2010

Diego Vincente, MD LT MC USN

Gregory A. Watson, MD MAJ MC USA
Deployment: Ghazni, Afghanistan 2010
Sharana, Afghanistan 2012

David Whittaker, MD CDR MC USN
Deployment: USS Theodore Roosevelt, OIF 2002–2003

Jason Zook, MD CDR MC USN
Deployment: Kandahar, Afghanistan 2011–2012

Prehospital and Enroute Care 1

Joseph F. Alderete, Gregory A. Watson, and Garth A. Elias

Contents

BLUF (Bottom Line Up Front) Box

1. Prompt recognition of the pathophysiology of the "triad of death" of hypothermia, coagulopathy, and acidosis and initiating prehospital measures to mitigate this spectrum of physiology will get the patient, *alive*, to higher care.
2. Recognize the dearth of data that comes with a casualty. Document early interventions to facilitate the ability to study prehospital measures and improve lifesaving capacity.
3. Recognize the leading causes of death on the battlefield, i.e., hemorrhage from a compressible site, tension pneumothorax, and airway compromise.
4. Master Tactical Combat Casualty Care recommendations and interventions for these leading causes of battlefield death.
5. Tourniquets save lives but one must obliterate the pulse. Do not be shy… control the hemorrhage!
6. Hemostatic dressings are a good tool but continued bleeding is optimized by applying compression in all wounds and rigidly immobilizing extremity wounds. Do not forget to compress bleeders!
7. Get an airway! Learning to perform rapid sequence intubation is sexy but impractical in some battlefield settings.

J.F. Alderete, MD (✉)
Department of Orthopaedic Oncology, Orthopaedic Surgery Residency, San Antonio Military Medical Center, San Antonio, TX, USA
e-mail: snjalderete@gmail.com

G.A. Watson, MD, FACS • G.A. Elias, MD
Department of Critical Care Medicine, University of Pittsburgh, Pittsburgh, PA, USA

L.B. Bone, C.N. Mamczak (eds.), *Front Line Extremity and Orthopaedic Surgery*, DOI 10.1007/978-3-642-45337-3_1, © Springer-Verlag Berlin Heidelberg 2014

Fig. 1.1 The soldier above all other prays for peace, for it is the soldier who must suffer and bear the deepest wounds and scars of war (Douglas Macarthur)

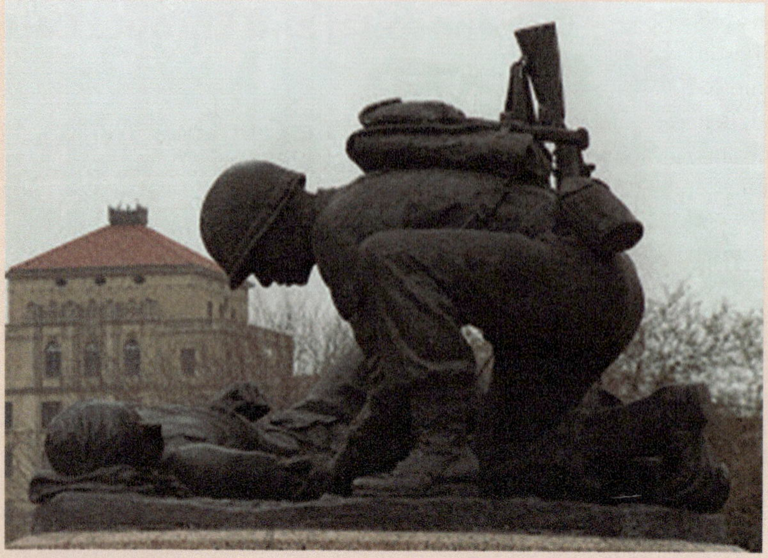

TCCC teaches cricothyroidotomy for a reason; master the anatomy and skills of a vertical incision cricothyroidotomy.

8. Blunt trauma + trouble breathing = chest tube. Persistent trouble breathing in the above setting = bilateral chest tubes. Penetrating chest trauma = immediate needle decompression followed by chest tube when timing permits (Fig. 1.1). Do not fail this intervention!

1.1 Introduction to Tactical Combat Casualty Care (TCCC)

We have seen many advances in combat casualty care in the last 12 or so years but none so dramatic as the revision in battlefield trauma as a concept. Tourniquet use, advanced IV fluids, and even some of our hemostatic dressings are improvements upon earlier models. It has been modifications in many of our tools combined with a better understanding of what kills soldiers on the battlefield and how to prioritize care that is the quantum leap forward. The break from civilian trauma concepts reflects the recognition that most of how we manage a trauma patient in the civilian setting is predicated on blunt trauma physiology. Blast trauma, penetrating injuries, massive extremity damage, and loss have necessitated an examination of battlefield mortality and a focus on interventions that manage the causes of the main battlefield killers, i.e., hemorrhage from a compressible site, tension pneumothorax, and airway compromise. The TC3 principles reflect that the medic, and sometimes physician, providing care on the battlefield must first neutralize the enemy and remember that the mission is still developing around him or her. Thus, one must think about providing care from a covered position realizing that he or she cannot engage so blindly as to become quickly overwhelmed. Once the enemy threat has quieted to a dull roar, then Tactical Field Care can take place and one can focus on more than just managing massive hemorrhage under fire.

Most physicians have little exposure to the TC3 concepts and algorithm because it is not an emphasis in our professional development. If you are reading this and find yourself nervous about one's familiarity with TCCC, do not despair. Simply Internet search "MHS Tactical Combat Casualty Care" and you will be directed to the Military Health System's webpage with a special section on combat casualty care. Print out the course slides and instructor guide, both published in PowerPoint and pdf, and commit them to memory. Finally, ask questions of your primary battlefield responders (medics, PJs, physician assistants) on some of the practical points of integrating unit and battlespace realities with the TC3 concepts. You'll be amazed by how much more prepared you feel.

1.2 Measures to Thwart the Trauma Triad: Acidosis, Coagulopathy, and Hypothermia

Despite the conceptualization of battlefield mortality, we health care providers must not forget that TCCC and its revisions or spin-offs are all designed to mitigate against trauma physiology. If one has this goal in mind, then the algorithmic approach to combat casualty care can evolve, and a medic or physician can move from one facet to the other (once massive hemorrhage controlled) and back again with ease and deliberate focus. Once acidosis, coagulopathy, and hypothermia reach a threshold, arrest and death are imminent.

Case Example: This is a dismounted casualty sustaining bilateral lower extremity traumatic amputations, scrotal and perineal wounds, several fragmentary wounds to the left chest, massive left forearm injuries, and a maxillofacial trauma with burns to the face and neck (Fig. 1.2).

This was a scenario reflecting one of the worst survivable injury spectrums imaginable. Advances in torso body armor have decreased the mortality from this spectrum of injury from 100 %; however, it still takes a talented first responder to get this soldier to higher care alive. Lairet and colleagues (2012) examined 1,003 combat-wounded records and described the incidence and efficacy of specific prehospital lifesaving interventions, or LSIs, and noted a much

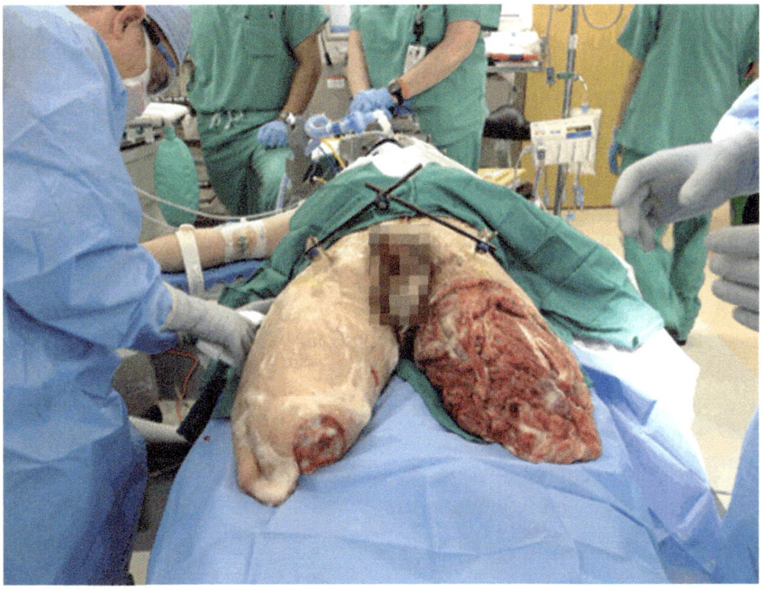

Fig. 1.2 The very astute medic on the scene first compressed Kerlex gauze into the lower extremities and placed tourniquets high bilaterally. He saw that the jaw was mangled and face burned and decisively performed a cricothyroidotomy for surgical airway and placed one of the combat lifesavers on the Ambu bag. He saw that the junctional wound on the right was unresponsive to tourniquet and placed the Combat Ready Clamp, or CRoC. Once this slowed the bleeding, he needle-decompressed both lungs and returned to the left upper extremity where another tourniquet was placed on the left brachium. The right upper arm was uninvolved, thus the medic placed an IO into the right proximal humerus where he infused 1 L of Hextend. Finally, after stuffing his remaining combat gauze into the perineal wounds, he Ace-wrapped both legs together and placed the HPMK. Finally, as the MEDEVAC Blackhawk arrived, he switched the patient to LR after the 1 L Hextend infused

higher rate of missed interventions consistent with the TC3 paradigm, in the airway and chest LSIs. In other words, we missed the surgical airway and needle decompression performed above. Thus, like in the above example, if one rapidly moves back and forth among only a handful of interventions that we know are life saving, with deliberate priority, the Dismounted Complex Battle Injury patient depicted above can survive. The way to do this conceptually is through the MARCH algorithm: massive hemorrhage, airway, respiration, circulation, and head injury/hypothermia. All of these measures are designed to thwart the "swirling vortex of death" while enroute to the FST or CSH or death during subsequent role II/III resuscitation.

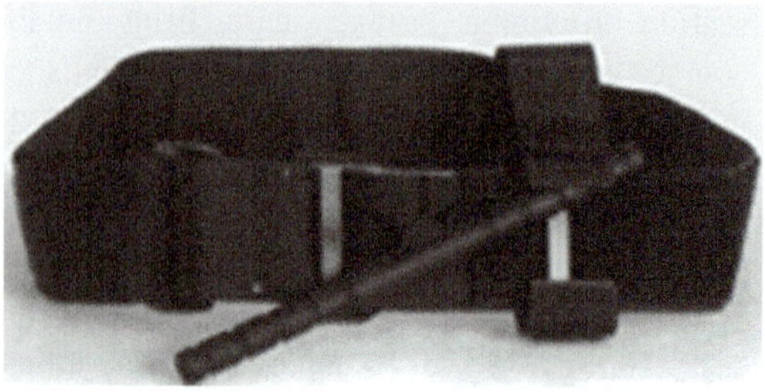

Fig. 1.3 The Combat Application Tourniquet® (C-A-T®) (Patent Pending) is a small and lightweight onehanded tourniquet that completely occludes arterial blood flow in an extremity. The C-A-T® uses a Self-Adhering Band and a Friction Adaptor Buckle to fit a wide range of extremities combined with a onehanded windlass system

1.3 Massive Hemorrhage

Hemorrhage is the cause of 83–87 % of all potentially survivable battlefield deaths. Fifty percent will be due to non-compressible truncal injury and the other half from compressible extremity injury (Kelly et al. 2008; Holcomb et al. 2007). We continue to see improvements in the management of massive hemorrhage due to penetrating injury, specifically in reference to the combat tourniquet, candidate solutions for junctional hemorrhage, and hemostatic dressings. Early interventions to mitigate the effects of tissue trauma and hemorrhagic shock are the most effective methods to avoid the trauma triad.

Tourniquets have been employed on the battlefield since 1674. Since then there have not been many advances in the concept or design. The modern tourniquet (Fig. 1.3) can be applied onehanded and by one's self or a buddy while under fire. Tourniquet use up to the most recent past has always been controversial owing to anecdotal reports of increased bleeding, nerve injury, or vascular injury. Its popularity substantiated by a number of papers that describe problems associated with application and the proper employment of the battlefield tourniquet use and how to take it off safely (Kragh et al. 2009; Mabry et al. 2000,'05 and'06). The bottom line is that tourniquets save lives and above all the mantra is *life over limb*. Where a combat gauze dressing cannot stop bleeding, a combat tourniquet should be applied, preferable directly on skin once garments have been cut away. A tourniquet should be applied as distal as practical to obliterate the pulse distal to the massive bleeding. One should get in the habit of doing pulse checks, either tightening the existing tourniquet or applying a second proximal to and directly adjoining the first. The only safe place for loosening or removing an effective tourniquet is the operating suite!

Junctional hemorrhage is a term coined to describe an injury to the regions where the neck and limbs join the torso. These are areas where body armor has practical weak points and thus vulnerable regions to penetrating trauma. Groin hemorrhage is the most common junctional hemorrhage and is usually refractory to standard tourniquet. Mabry and Eastridge publicized USAISR data demonstrating the most common cause of preventable death in the later years of OIF and OEF was from junctional hemorrhage of the proximal lower extremities and groin. Our previous solution popularized the MAST trouser to control hemorrhage about the pelvis but its effectiveness is poor and contraindications many (Roberts et al. 1999). Thus, we find a need for a device that can facilitate junctional control. Candidate devices take advantage of Poiseuille's law and the Bernoulli equation, where volumetric flow rate is controlled by applying direct compression. Our most recent fielded intervention is the Combat Ready Clamp, or CRoC (Fig. 1.4). It can be applied directly on the site of most massive

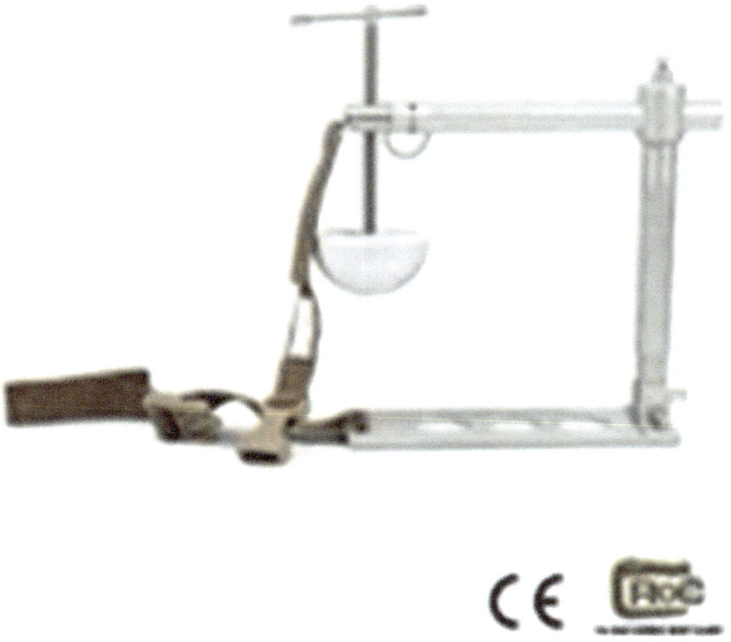

Fig. 1.4 The Combat Ready Clamp (CRoC) is a slip-proof expandable aluminum clamp tourniquet that works like a vise to maintain pressure on difficult bleeds when hemorrhage control in tactical environments is not possible with traditional methods and standard tourniquets. The most obvious example of CRoC application is the high femoral or inguinal wound

hemorrhage or proximally at the level of the inguinal ligament. When used in this fashion, the disc of the CRoC is placed just medial and distal to a line drawn from ASIS to pubic tubercle. The theory is to avoid placing the disc over the inguinal ligament impinging upon the superior pubic ramus; however, in practicality compression against a bony structure may be more efficacious. Although the device is rudimentary and application not yet widespread, it's development and fielding reflect a common-sense approach to a difficult problem.

Our final discussion point for hemorrhage control is the application of hemostatic agents. There are two methods by which topical hemostatic agents produce hemostasis: physically altering damaged tissues and sealing blood vessels, and accelerating/strengthening the body's clotting capacity. Arguably the most efficacious hemostatic dressing, fibrin sealant dressing/gauze was scrapped prior to widespread fielding because it is derived from plasma and is yet not FDA approved as a "biologic." The military needed industry to quickly produce other agents that were more effective than gauze, easy and cheap to produce, and did not need clinical trials for FDA approval. The answers were HemCon dressing and Quick Clot. HemCon was derived from chitosan with hemostatic properties. Quick Clot was designed to facilitate the rapid water absorption concentrating clotting proteins and cells in the wound. The problems with these candidate solutions were that HemCon did a poor job at controlling arterial hemorrhage and Quick Clot burned other tissue. Enter Combat Gauze, a mineral-based hemostatic dressing impregnated with kaolin. Kaolin is an important activator of the intrinsic clotting pathway, stabilizing the initial clot. This dressing is slower than many of the previous agents because it takes advantage of the host clotting response but has been shown to be effective in 80 % of catastrophic arterial injury (Kheirabadi et al. 2009). One must remember this last premise and measures to correct coagulopathy will increase the effectiveness of the now-deployed combat gauze.

1.4 Airway

As mentioned in the Lairet study, effective airway management continues to be an area we can improve on in combat casualty care. Lifesaving interventions in this category identified by this study as possible misses in the TCCC environment were nasal or oral airway insertion, endotracheal intubation, and surgical cricothyroidotomy. Missed LSIs, or life-saving interventions not performed but should have been, in this study within the airway category were 53 % endotracheal intubation, 27 % nasal or oral airway, and 12 % surgical cricothyroidotomy (Lairet et al. 2012). Most of the patients that had a missed intubation in this study were indicated for reasons other than neck or face airway compromise, which is where due to burns and trauma, the majority of true airway compromise arises from. Hence, be prepared to perform a cricothyroidotomy if the injury spectrum or local environment is too hostile for endotracheal intubation. We prefer a longitudinal incision over the cricothyroid membrane, as this can be extended easily and avascular planes taken advantage of. If the patient is unconscious but upper airway anatomy intact, simple nasal pharyngeal or oral pharyngeal airways will suffice.

1.5 Respiration

Tension pneumothorax is still the second leading cause of preventable death on the battlefield with an incidence of 3–4 % of all fatalities (McPherson 2006). Thus, current guidelines suggest needle decompression in casualties with chest trauma and progressing respiratory distress. Every effort should be made to seal the "sucking chest wound" with some sort of occlusive dressing. Many front-line providers are facile with rudimentary methods to achieve water seal, thus making a chest tube feasible if a prolonged evacuation is anticipated. Needle decompression can be achieved in the second intercostal space anteriorly at the midclavicular line or alternatively in the midaxillary line at the 5th intercostal space. Bottom line: don't point toward the heart or medial to nipple!

1.6 Circulation

Before OEF and OIF, medics carried as much as 25 lb of crystalloid into the field. Furthermore, many of the IV lines placed in casualties were done so for stable patients, rapidly depleting the supply and energy of the treating medics. Thus, current TCCC recommendations are to consider IV fluids only for patients in hemorrhagic shock. Also consider that fluids can hurt people. Bickell et al. in 1994 provided some compelling evidence for permissive hypotension when he demonstrated increased mortality in patients with penetrating torso injuries in whom IV fluids were given in the field than those who did not receive IV fluids. LR and NS administration has been shown in multiple studies to be pro-inflammatory and dilutes clotting factors. Furthermore, restoring a normal blood pressure is ludicrous as it disrupts the clot in many occasions. Therefore, we are proponents of permissive hypotension. What is the definition of "permissive hypotension" though, as some studies have demonstrated that a mean arterial pressure of 60–70 is inadequate to protect against cell death in traumatic shock and definitely deleterious in traumatic brain injury. Most studies have demonstrated that a MAP between 50 and 60 or SBP 80 and 90 is adequate for end-organ perfusion and actually associated with decreased transfusion requirements in trauma patients (Morrison 2011). 2012 TCCC recommendations also call for Hextend as the first line IV therapy for patients in hemorrhagic shock. Given the propensity for Hextend to hand around longer in the vascular tree and lack of immunomodulation, we support this recommendation. Hextend is administered first, to a volume of 1 L, then switched over to LR until the patient can receive massive transfusion of 1:1:1 product therapy or fresh whole blood. Be familiar with intraosseous catheter placement, especially sternal, proximal humerus, and iliac crest. In patients with massive dismounted trauma, the intraosseous line can be a valuable bridge to an extremity line for true resuscitation. We (JA) prefer the EZ IO for insertion and ease of transport. The robust venous circulation within the proximal humerus has been well studied in children and duplicated in adults. Where sometimes there is no conventional site, this is an incredibly powerful adjunct.

Finally, we are advocates of the use of TXA, or tranexamic acid, for use in massive hemorrhage given its ability to prevent clot breakdown and has been shown to have a significant survivor benefit in both the CRASH-2 (civilian) and MATTERS (military) trauma studies. This is administered within 3 h of injury and given as 1 g in 100 cc NS. Do not give in same line as Hextend!

1.7 Hypothermia Prevention

Hypothermia is defined as core body temp < 35 °C. Its presence adversely impacts on coagulopathy and acidosis and has been associated with increased mortality in combat-wounded patients (Wade et al. 2011). Therefore, prevention of heat loss is a cornerstone of *prehospital* combat casualty care and must not be overlooked in the chaos of treating a casualty's injuries.

For the most part keeping a wounded soldier warm involves common-sense maneuvers and the application of a *commercially available* hypothermia prevention device.

For example, a checklist which incorporates our experience with both the JTTS CPGs and the TCCC guidelines would include:

- Minimizing the patient's exposure to the elements
- Removing wet clothing
- Warming all IV fluids and blood products, if possible
- Protecting the casualty from wind during transport, if doors must be kept open
- Applying the Hypothermia Prevention and Management Kit (HPMK)

Just a word regarding the HPMK, this active warming system includes a skull cap, the Ready-Heat blanket (containing the exothermic chemical cells), and the Heat Reflective Shell (Older versions of the system use the Blizzard Blanket in lieu of the HRS). Used together, these three components have been shown to outperform other available systems (Allen et al. 2010). In, addition they can be used separately with reasonable effectiveness. Further refinement includes a water-resistant component, but we have no experience with this.

If the HPMK is not available, any material that will help maintain body temperature can be utilized. Possibilities include wool blankets, space blankets, poncho liners, sleeping bags, and even human remains pouches (HRP). Combining several of these passive items will increase efficacy. For example, the "Hot Pocket," consisting of a space blanket, two wool blankets, and inside an HRP, was shown to maintain core temperature at 120 min (Allen et al. 2010).

Finally, a couple of practical points. Use of the Blizzard Bag has been found cumbersome by some since it must be completely unwrapped to provide access to the casualty and has no apertures for IV tubing. The RH blanket will not heat if it becomes wet prior to activation. Also, the RH requires time to achieve maximal temperature and thus activation should be planned accordingly (Fig. 1.5).

1.8 Extremity Management

The bleeding near amputation can be a source of continued life-threatening hemorrhage. The main point here is to deploy the tourniquet where the combat gauze cannot control hemorrhage and find splint material. This can consist of anything from the patient's weapon to the pre-fab quick splints currently deployed. The limb should be secured to the splint with something elastic that will allow swelling, but should rigidly immobilize the wound to stabilize the clot. If the Hare traction femoral splints are used, pay special attention to the areas where the splint comes in contact with the patient, i.e., the ankle and ischial tuberosity. These are areas that can quickly break down if evacuation is prolonged. Finally, take advantage of the patient's torso with upper extremity injuries and sling them to their side if no evidence of chest trauma as it is stable, comfortable, and quick with any upper extremity injury.

1.9 Analgesia

Pain is a difficult symptom to treat in combat yet is one of the most common reasons soldiers seek medical attention in the combat environment. Early pain control is often overlooked as a potential point where intervention can decrease the inflammatory cascade and potentially decrease the incidence of PTSD. There are a number of available

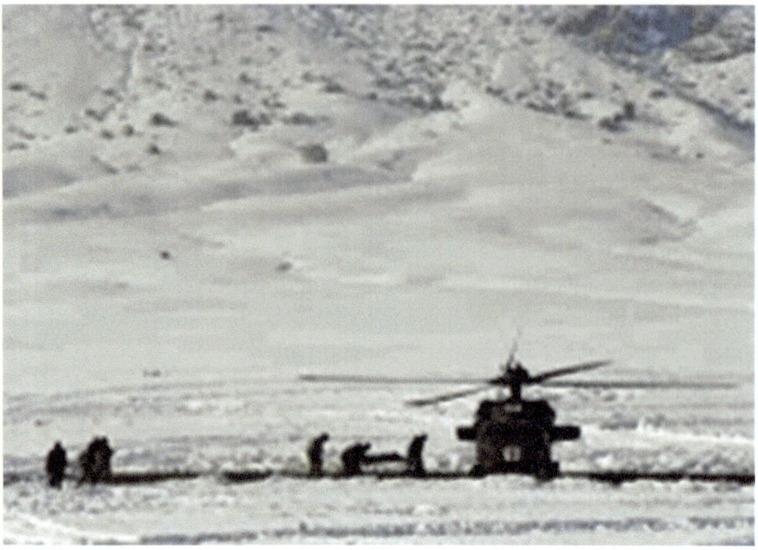

Fig. 1.5 Medical operations in extreme conditions. We must stand ready to provide decisive pre-hospital care under any condition. This requires constant training and research

analgesics in the deployed environment now, from meloxicam and Tylenol as the "Pill Pack" so the soldier can continue to fight to subanesthetic doses of ketamine. We recommend becoming an expert in just 2, morphine and ketamine.

1.9.1 Morphine: Does It Still Have a Place in TCCC Pain Management

In a review article describing pain management in operational settings, Wedmore et al. described opiate analgesia as the most effective drug class for severe pain. Morphine offers easy administration (via auto injector, intramuscularly) and a well-known side effect profile. A recent observational study involving 696 deployed US military casualties without serious TBI suggested that the early provision of IV morphine analgesia at Level I or Level 2 medical treatment facilities was associated with lower rates of post-traumatic stress disorder (PTSD).

Overdose and hypotension remain a concern with many front-line providers. Current opinion reflects that the IV administration of morphine is advantageous for relieving acute and severe pain as it provides quick relief and is easier to titrate, thus reducing the risk of overdose in individuals with severe pain. Its hypotensive potential is less than that of many available agents.

1.9.1.1 Mastering Ketamine

Ketamine hydrochloride was first used in humans as a dissociative anesthetic in 1965. Ketamine is highly lipid soluble; as such, clinical effects present within one minute of administration when given intravenously and within five minutes when given intramuscularly. Ketamine is known for its hemodynamic stability, advantageous airway and respiratory properties, low cost, broad range of clinical applications, ease of storage, and excellent therapeutic index. A particular benefit for the use of ketamine on the battlefield or in a TACEVAC setting is that when administered in small (analgesic) doses, it does not generally impair airway maintenance or spontaneous respirations and increases blood pressure and heart rate. Ketamine has a wide therapeutic window making it the anesthetic of choice in austere environments where monitoring equipment may be difficult at best. At higher doses, the utility of ketamine is limited by undesirable psychomimetic effects. These effects include excessive sedation, cognitive dysfunction, hallucinations, and nightmares.

Also, at higher doses ketamine may cause secretions, nausea/vomiting, headache, dizziness or blurred vision, a cataleptic state, and sedation with potential recall (memory loss) problems. Subanesthetic (low)-dose ketamine has demonstrated significant analgesic efficacy without these side effects. Master its use with an antisialagogue and Versed to reduce the potential for emergence psychosis.

Suggested Reading

Blackbourne et al. Prehospital combat casualty care: the starting point of battlefield survival. Eastridge, Brian J. 2011, p 11.

Lairet JR, et al. Prehospital interventions performed in a combat zone: a prospective study of 1,003 combat wounded. J Trauma Acute Care Surg. 2012;73:2.

Mabry R, McManus JG. Prehospital advances in the management of severe penetrating trauma. JSOM. 2009;9:2.

Combat Triage and Mass Casualty Management

2

Matthew Bradley, Diego Vicente, and Eric Elster

Contents

M. Bradley, MD, MS (✉)
Department of Regenerative Medicine, Naval Medical Research Center, Silver Springs, MD, USA

Department of Surgery, Uniformed Services University of the Health Sciences, Bethesda, MD, USA
e-mail: matthew.bradley@med.navy.mil

D. Vicente, MD
Department of Surgery, Walter Reed National Military Medical Center, Bethesda, MD, USA

E. Elster, MD
Norman M. Rich Department of Surgery, Uniformed Services University, Bethesda, MD, USA

BLUF (Bottom Line Up Front) Box

1. Triage involves rapid evaluation, prioritization, and continuous reevaluation of a casualty's status. Your facility's resources will also affect your triage of casualties.
2. Concerning triage criteria for major traumas include heart rate >120, systolic blood pressure <90 mmHg, respiratory rate <10 or >30, GCS score <13 or motor component <6, and penetrating injuries to the head, neck, torso, or proximal extremities.
3. A mass casualty is when the number of casualties overwhelms your facility's resources. Depending on your location, this could be as few as two patients.
4. The goal in a mass casualty event is to provide the greatest good to the greatest number of people, which means treating casualties with the highest probability of survival, not necessarily those needing the most urgent care.
5. It is important to know your role in a mass casualty event. You may be tasked as the triage officer or may be responsible for assisting the general surgeon in the operating room.
6. The principles of damage control surgery include rapid control of both hemorrhage and gross contamination as well as rapid stabilization of fractures during ongoing resuscitation.

L.B. Bone, C.N. Mamczak (eds.), *Front Line Extremity and Orthopaedic Surgery*,
DOI 10.1007/978-3-642-45337-3_2,

7. The tenants of damage control resuscitation include targeted resuscitation with 1:1:1 blood product transfusion ratio and minimal crystalloid infusion.
8. Tranexamic acid and recombinant factor VIIa are important adjuncts for hemostasis that should be used early, especially when blood product therapy is limited or unavailable.
9. Knowledge of your facility's massive transfusion and walking blood bank protocols is essential.

In this chapter we will introduce the reader to triage from a historical perspective as well as how it is applied on the modern battlefield. We will also introduce the concepts of damage control resuscitation, damage control surgery, and massive transfusion for initial management of combat casualties. Understanding the principles that guide triage and damage control described in this chapter will help physicians rapidly implement current guidelines to effectively treat even the most severely injured of casualties in austere environments.

2.1 Triage

Triage refers to the evaluation and prioritization of casualties based on each casualty's urgency for medical care and resources required for effective management of the casualty. It must be quick, accurate, and continuous. A casualty's clinical status can frequently change, often for the worse, so reevaluation and re-prioritization are necessary. Triaging patients in a US civilian emergency department, where supplies and staffing are regularly abundant, is usually not a significant issue on a routine day. However, the experiences of a forward-deployed medical team in an austere environment or of a medical center in a mass casualty situation in the United States are far from a typical day in the ED. In this setting, staff and material resources will be limited, and all deployed medical personnel must be up-to-date with their accessible resources so that a casualty's severity of injury can be matched to the capabilities of a facility. If a casualty's wounds are severe enough to rapidly exhaust the resources of a facility, then the patient needs to be rapidly stabilized and transported to a higher level of care. In the case of multiple casualties, triage can be an overwhelming task, especially when the provider may recognize the casualties.

2.1.1 History

Proper triage and evacuation of casualties has been a constant struggle throughout military history. Each new war has brought challenges to which our military and civilian trauma systems have had to adapt. During World War II, in an effort to cut down on evacuation time, Colonel DeBakey developed mobile surgical units termed Auxiliary Surgical Groups (ASGs) to maneuver with the troops. These ASGs were the precursor to the Mobile Army Surgical Hospital (MASH) units of the Korean War, which provided earlier resuscitation and stabilization of casualties prior to transport to distant field hospitals. The Korean War also saw the evolution of aeromedical evacuation with the use of a helicopter as an air ambulance, which significantly improved triage and evacuation times. In the early 1990s, Tactical Combat Casualty Care (TCCC), the military's version of Prehospital Trauma Life Support, was developed to address triage and care during the asymmetric, nonlinear, urban warfare in Somalia. TCCC prepares combat Navy corpsmen, Army combat medics, and Air Force pararescuemen to initiate triage and treatment on the battlefield. More recently, the Navy's Forward Resuscitative Surgical System (FRSS) and the Army's Forward Surgical Teams (FSTs) were designed to provide mobile damage control surgery (DCS) and damage control resuscitation (DCR) support for the advancing troops. All of these advancements have led to our current, highly integrated trauma system. This design for rapid triage with treatment and evacuation of the wounded to higher levels of care has significantly improved casualty care in the military. Similar systems incorporated into the civilian trauma setting have also led to improved patient care with appropriate resource utilization.

2.1.2 Triage Principles

Triage is based on a prompt clinical assessment of anatomic and physiologic criteria. The Glasgow Coma Scale (GCS) – an assessment of ocular, verbal, and motor responses – provides a quick and useful evaluation of overall neurologic function. The motor component is generally regarded as the most significant and predictive factor of the GCS exam in trauma and may be particularly useful in the case of an intubated patient or a patient with ocular injuries. Assessment should also involve a rapid interpretation of vital signs and anatomic areas of injury.

Concerning triage criteria for major traumas include heart rate >120 bpm, systolic blood pressure <90 mmHg, respiratory rate <10 or >30, GCS score <13 or motor component <6, and penetrating injuries to the head, neck, torso, or proximal extremities. If a GCS exam and vitals are not immediately available to the triage officer on the casualty's arrival, a rapid bedside assessment of pulse characteristic and motor component of GCS to evaluate for a weak or absent pulse (consistent with SBP ≤ 100 mmHg) and/or abnormal GCS motor (score less than 6) both of which are indicators of a high acuity patient who requires immediate attention.

Triage also includes identifying casualties that need surgical intervention and determining whether the appropriate resources are available at the current level of care. If resources do not meet the demand, rapid transport to the next level of care is required after stabilizing the casualty.

2.1.3 Echelons of Care

Triage starts on the battlefield and continues through several levels of care until patients reach the highest level, a major military treatment facility (MTF) in the continental United States (CONUS). There are five levels of care – referred to as "echelons" or "roles" by NATO – with each ascending level capable of providing more advanced support. Depending on the tactical situation, available aeromedical evacuation, and severity of injuries, a casualty may not be sequentially evacuated through each level. At each echelon though, casualties are reevaluated and prioritized so that the most appropriate care is given at all times.

Echelon I care begins in the field and is administered by self-aid, buddy-aid, or combat medical personnel trained in TCCC. These medical personnel are the first stage in the triage of casualties and often provide initial life-saving maneuvers such as airway management, needle decompression for tension pneumothorax, tourniquet application for compressible hemorrhage, application of topical hemostatics, and hypothermia prevention.

Following battlefield stabilization, casualties are often evacuated to an Echelon II facility. Examples of level II installations are Army battalion aid stations (BASs) and associated FSTs and Marine Corps shock trauma platoons (STPs) with collocated FRSS. The FSTs and FRSS are usually comprised of 10–20 service members, including one to two general surgeons and sometimes an orthopedic surgeon with the capacity to run one to two operating rooms. Basic laboratory and simple radiographic studies are often available, and they have the ability to carry and store blood products. Advanced trauma life support (ATLS) begins here, but, because of limited resources, patient support is typically limited to DCS.

The highest level of care within a combat zone is provided by an Echelon III treatment facility such as the Navy's hospital ships or the Army's Combat Support Hospitals. Additional resources and some subspecialty care, such as vascular surgery, may be rendered at these facilities.

Echelon IV is the first level of care outside the combat zone. Landstuhl Regional Medical Center in Germany is currently the major level IV installation. These facilities have blood banks, laboratories, and multiaxial imaging capabilities. Most surgical subspecialties and a multidisciplinary intensive care team are available at this level. Inpatient capacity can be up to 1,000 beds.

Echelon V care is provided in CONUS at such facilities as Walter Reed National Military Medical Center and San Antonio Military Medical Center. Definitive operations including complex general surgery, orthopedic surgery, neurosurgery, plastic surgery, and other subspecialty surgery can be done and initial physical rehabilitation take place at these institutions.

The development of the Critical Care Air Transport program by the US Air Force has allowed transport of critically injured patients from the combat zone thousands of miles away to Echelon IV and V facilities within a few days of injury.

2.2 Mass Casualty

A mass casualty is any situation that overwhelms a facility's resources. At an Echelon II installation, this may be as few as two patients. Triage priorities change during a mass casualty. Your goal is to provide the greatest good to the greatest number of people given your resources, which means treating casualties with the highest probability of survival, not necessarily those needing the most urgent care. This can be particularly challenging because it means potentially giving less attention to a casualty that may have received greater care under different circumstances. Ultimately, triage during a mass casualty involves identifying the hemorrhaging patients who will likely survive their injuries and getting them to the operating room as quickly as possible.

The color-coded system is the usual method for triaging in a mass casualty. Casualties will be assigned to one of four colors (green, yellow, red, or black) based on severity of injury. Patients "tagged" green have sustained minor injuries and are the "walking wounded"; they are treated last. Yellow-coded casualties are considered delayed, meaning they need an operation but not right away. An example is a casualty who has sustained a penetrating intestinal injury without an associated vascular injury; this patient needs an operation but will not die immediately. Patients listed as red require immediate surgical intervention. These are the patients that are likely hemorrhaging internally or need immediate airway management and need care within a few minutes. Black-coded patients are considered unsalvageable, such as a devastating head injury, or are deceased. In theater, this color-coded scheme may be replaced by a letter system (Alpha, highest priority; Charlie, lowest priority); however, the same triage principles apply.

Given the chaos surrounding a mass casualty event, as seen in Fig. 2.1, mistakes will be made. Casualties may be under- or over-triaged, so an error-tolerant environment must exist. Personnel will often have responsibilities outside their normal comfort zones, so rehearsals with mass casualty drills are essential. Although nothing can really prepare you for the real event, drills provide the groundwork for everyone to know his role during an actual mass casualty.

Among the various team players in a mass casualty, there is a designated triage officer responsible for the initial evaluation. This individual may be a physician (surgeon or nonsurgeon), a Medical Service Corps officer (i.e., psychologist), or a dental officer. This person should be the most experienced care giver on site and familiar with mass casualty triage to reduce errors during triage. Depending on *the situation, the triage* officer may make the sole decision as to who goes to the OR first, although if the triage officer is not a surgeon, then the surgeon will help with this decision. The surgeon's primary role in a mass casualty is control of both hemorrhage and contamination. The surgeon may also notify the blood bank personnel to have blood products ready in the likely event that transfusions are necessary. While there may be instances when an orthopedic surgeon needs to help triage, he is most often assisting the trauma surgeon in the OR with DCR and DCS. Since the majority of casualties are often hemorrhaging from extremity injuries, orthopedic surgeons should be familiar with damage control principles and massive transfusion (MT) protocols.

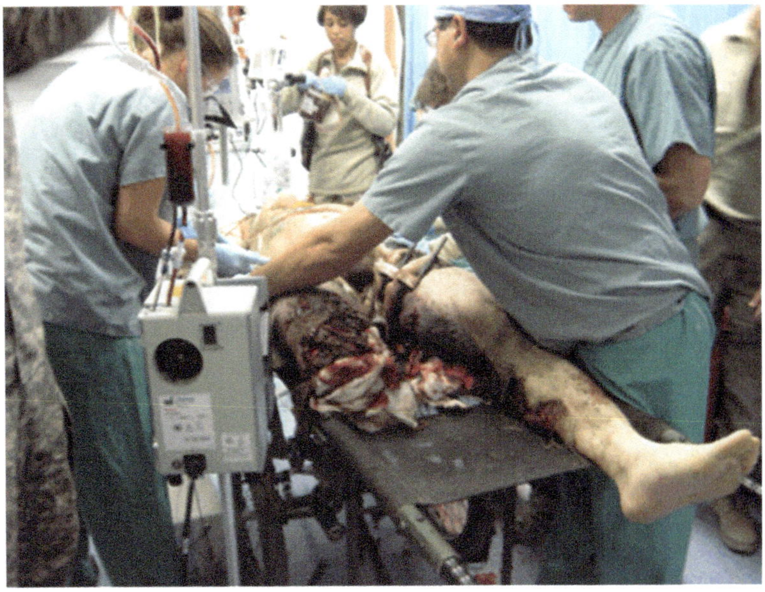

Fig. 2.1 Mass casualty event at role III in Afghanistan with multiple victims requiring extensive blood product and personnel resources

2.2.1 Massive Transfusions, Damage Control Resuscitation, and Damage Control Surgery

Damage control surgery and DCR (damage control resuscitation) are common principles of trauma management in the setting of hemorrhagic shock and are particularly useful for casualties requiring MT. Massive transfusion is defined as administration of ≥10 units of packed red blood cells (pRBCs) in a 24-h period. In general, patients who should be considered for MT include those with obvious ongoing hemorrhage and any combination of tachycardia (HR > 105), hypotension (SBP < 110), acidosis (pH < 7.25), anemia (HCT < 25 %), hypoxia (O_2 saturation <75 %), and coagulopathy (INR > 1.4). It is better to suspect a casualty will require MT and to initiate it early rather than delaying and trying to play catch up.

When an MT protocol is instituted, it is important to ensure that component therapies (pRBCs, fresh frozen plasma [FFP], platelets [plts]) are transfused as close as possible to 1:1:1 (pRBCs:FFP:plts) ratio. Communication with the blood bank is crucial to ensure the most recently collected or "youngest" blood be used during MT in order to minimize infusion of blood with storage lesions which can impede resuscitation efforts.

Damage control resuscitation, particularly in patients requiring MT, focuses on targeted resuscitation with blood products transfusion in order to restore tissue perfusion, resolve oxygen debt, and interrupt the lethal triad of acidosis, coagulopathy, and hypothermia. In hemorrhagic shock patients, the initial resuscitation should be based on the assessment of the casualty's prior and ongoing hemorrhage. Once hemorrhage is controlled, ongoing resuscitation efforts should be directed to ensuring tissue perfusion, resolving coagulopathy, and raising the core body temperature if needed. Resuscitation with crystalloid should be minimized throughout the resuscitation. Further information on DCR can be found in Chap. 3 as well in the US Army Institute of Surgical Research Clinical Practice Guidelines.

Damage control surgery principles are to save life over limb, control hemorrhage and gross contamination, and get in and out of the operating room as quickly as possible with minimal additional surgical trauma and minimal interruption to resuscitation. This often involves, among other management strategies, shunting vascular injuries, resecting gastrointestinal tract injuries without reanastomosis, and packing wounds. Specifically for the orthopedic surgeon, placement of external fixators and performing guillotine amputations will allow for quick control of injuries during ongoing DCR in order to get the casualty through the initial physiologic insult. The casualty can then be brought back to the OR for definitive surgical repairs after resuscitation and stabilization.

2.2.2 Tranexamic Acid, Recombinant Factor VIIa, and Whole Blood

Often situations arise in mass casualty events when component therapy is either limited or unavailable. This is when whole blood transfusions, obtained via a walking blood bank, and the use of tranexamic acid (TXA) or recombinant factor VIIa (rFVIIa) becomes critical to the resuscitation strategy.

All facilities should have a walking blood banks established, and all members of the trauma team should be familiar with its protocol so it can be initiated quickly if needed. It is important to note that despite the benefits of fresh whole blood (body temperature, appropriate pRBC:platelet:FFP ratio, and lack of storage lesions [i.e., loss of clotting factors and platelet activity]), component therapy carries the lowest risk of blood-borne infection transmission and hence remains the first line for blood product resuscitation in theater.

TXA, an antifibrinolytic agent, should be administered within 3 h of injury for maximal benefit in massive transfusion patients. As with TXA, the use of rFVIIa should be considered early to reverse or prevent coagulopathy.

2.3 Conclusion

Triage involves quickly evaluating, prioritizing, and reevaluating casualties. In the setting of a mass casualty event, triage should result in providing the greatest good to the greatest number of casualties, and stopping hemorrhage should be the number one priority. Since the majority of casualties present with extremity and other orthopedic injuries, it is mandatory that orthopedic surgeons be familiar with the principles of DCS and DCR, their facilities' MT protocol, and all available resources, including walking blood bank and adjunctive therapy.

2.4 Case Example

You are 1 week into your deployment to a level II facility in Afghanistan. You are deployed with two other general surgeons and an emergency room physician, who is assigned as the triage officer. Your facility has the capacity to run two ORs simultaneously. A report comes through of an IED blast with several casualties, and your facility is the closest to the scene. Initial triage in the field by the Navy corpsman identified seven total casualties. Approximate transport time to your facility is 15 min. The OR teams and blood bank are notified of the incoming casualties. There is enough blood for one MT, and TXA and FVIIa are also available. Casualties arrive in two waves by helicopter:

- Casualty #1 arrives with CPR in progress, which has been ongoing for at least a half hour. He has not had a pulse or any signs of life for the duration of the flight. Examination shows he sustained penetrating injuries to the head, chest, and abdomen.
- Casualty #2 is moaning and has bilateral thigh tourniquets in place. His left lower extremity has been traumatically amputated below the knee. Despite tourniquets, there is obvious ongoing hemorrhage. His vital signs reveal that he is tachycardic and hypotensive.
- Casualty #3 is also moaning of abdominal pain. He is slightly tachycardic, but his blood pressure is normal. Exam reveals a penetrating injury to his abdomen with significant tenderness.
- Casualty #4 walks over carrying all of the gear. His GCS is 15, and he has normal vital signs. On exam, he has some abrasions to the left side of his face and body.

- Casualty #5 arrives with a penetrating abdominal injury. He is also moaning and is tachycardic with a weak pulse. Exam demonstrates a distended and tender abdomen.
- Casualty #6 sustained some penetrating injuries to his right arm and leg. His neurologic status and vital signs are normal. On exam, he appears to have soft tissue injuries without vascular compromise.
- Casualty #7 limps over with his gear. His vital signs are normal, and his only complaint is left ankle pain.

The triage officer begins his evaluation. Given the injuries and absence of signs of life, he asks that CPR cease on casualty #1 and labels the casualty black. Casualties #2 and 5 are labeled red, and the triage officer alerts you and the nearby surgeons of their clinical status. Casualty #3 is considered yellow, and casualties #4, 6, and 7 are all labeled green. The MT and walking blood bank protocols are initiated, and each of the casualties heading to the OR is given a dose of TXA and FVIIa. You and one of the general surgeons take casualty #2 to the OR for DCR and DCS, while the other surgeon operates on casualty #5. You identify a transected femoral artery on the right and repair it with a temporizing shunt. Gross debridement of devitalized tissue is also performed. Following operative stabilization, the casualties are arranged for transport to the next level of care.

3 Initial Management and Damage Control Priorities

Robert Gaines and Christiaan N. Mamczak

Contents

BLUF (Bottom Line Up Front) Box

1. Combat orthopedic casualty care embraces a life and limb damage control surgery concept.
2. Polytrauma is the norm with multiple extremity and non-orthopedic injuries occurring in the same patient.
3. A multidisciplinary team approach expedites resuscitation and surgical interventions, thereby avoiding the dangers of prolonged operative time in critically injured patients.
4. The patient's hemodynamic status, your surgical environment, and command resources dictate the complexity of your operative treatment.
5. Downrange priorities are to correct ischemia and stop hemorrhage, decontaminate open fractures and blast wounds, stabilize long bone fractures and unstable pelvic injuries, span periarticular fractures, and, finally, care for small bone fractures.
6. Do not try to be a hero during the first surgery; this is a team project.
7. Combat wounds are both complex and contaminated. Multiple surgical debridements are necessary to decrease the risk of sepsis. Never definitively close combat wounds downrange.
8. Do not definitively fix US and coalition fractures downrange.

R. Gaines, MD
Department of Orthopaedic Surgery, Covenant Medical Center Lubbock, Lubbock, TX, USA

Naval Medical Center Portsmouth, Portsmouth, VA, USA

C.N. Mamczak, DO (✉)
Beacon Orthopaedic Trauma Surgery, Memorial Hospital, South Bend, IN, USA

Department of Orthopaedic Surgery, Naval Medical Center Portsmouth, Portsmouth, VA, USA
e-mail: dr_jibwex@yahoo.com

L.B. Bone, C.N. Mamczak (eds.), *Front Line Extremity and Orthopaedic Surgery*, DOI 10.1007/978-3-642-45337-3_3, © Springer-Verlag Berlin Heidelberg 2014

9. Read the CPGs prior to deployment. This is combat trauma not civilian trauma.
10. Use every opportunity to communicate injury patterns and treatment requirements with up-range surgeons.

3.1 Introduction

The initial management and prioritization of treatment for orthopedic combat trauma casualties embraces a multidisciplinary approach with damage control principles that focus on saving life and limb. The current echelons of care established within the downrange combat environment facilitate advancing patient stabilization along with expedited transfer out of theater. This system works to minimize the constraints of operating on complex injuries in an austere setting with limited resources. Deploying surgeons must understand and accept that definitive care for US and coalition casualties occurs out of the hostile combat region. Nevertheless, the most critical decisions pertaining to the salvage of life and limb begin with initial downrange care. Improper or hasty decision-making made by surgeons unfamiliar with combat orthopedic trauma care can lead to irreparable outcomes for wounded warriors that may affect their overall morbidity and mortality. Therefore, the deployed orthopedic surgeon should have an established knowledge of damage control priorities, the current military clinical practice guidelines (CPGs), and an understanding for musculoskeletal treatment pathways specific to combat blast injuries and wounding patterns.

3.2 Combat Wounding Patterns and Their Associated Pathophysiology

A historical analysis of battlefield casualties depicts a modern change in the number and location of bodily injuries. With the advent of contemporary body armor, helmets, and protective eyewear, extremity-wounding patterns have become far more common than thoracoabdominal or intracranial injuries. Blasting ordinance, most notably the improvised explosive device (IED), accounts for the majority (>80 %) of recent combat injuries. Penetrating trauma from gunshot wounds and blunt trauma from vehicular accidents, falls, or crush injuries should also be expected. A fourth, less familiar mode of injury surrounds the thermal effects of burns suffered from ordinance explosions.

The multitude of musculoskeletal (MSK) casualties places the deployed orthopedic surgeon at the forefront of combat casualty care. Although the treatment of wounded warriors is a multidisciplinary effort, the orthopedic surgeon consistently remains one of the busiest medical professionals regardless of their downrange location. Physical and emotional burnout is possible during a 6–12-month deployment, and the value of educating others to support the mission of MSK care is critical. A good working relationship with the general surgeon(s) and other subspecialty surgeons goes a long way. Despite body armor and protective troop vehicles, various polytrauma injury patterns do occur and often necessitate various surgeons working together to save a life or limb (i.e., a penetrating thigh wound with an open femur fracture and a dysvascular limb will require the skill set of orthopedic and general surgeons).

The kinetic energy imparted on the human body during battlefield injuries is unlike that typically seen in civilian trauma. Combat wounds from blasting ordinance and high-energy GSWs lead to greater soft tissue and bony destruction along with a much larger zone of injury (Figs. 3.1 and 3.2). The extent of the traumatized zone is not always evident to the naked eye during the initial clinical exam. Since most of these wounds come with inherent contamination from foreign debris and microorganisms, the index treatment is emergent surgical debridement with irrigation before the zone of necrosis evolves. If left untreated or improperly debrided, combat wounds can be life-threatening. Combat casualties typically have more than one extremity affected and often present with associated thoracoabdominal or head injuries. Injury severity scores have

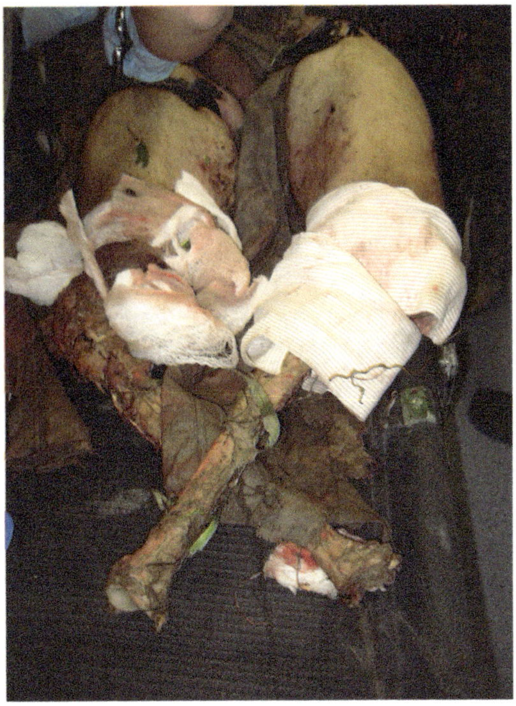

Fig. 3.1 Dismounted complex blast injury (DCBI) casualty with bilateral lower extremity incomplete, traumatic amputations depicted as it presents to the trauma bay. Field combat tourniquets play a critical role in early hemorrhage control and survival during medevac transport. Note the extent of soft tissue destruction caused by the blast and thermal effects of IEDs

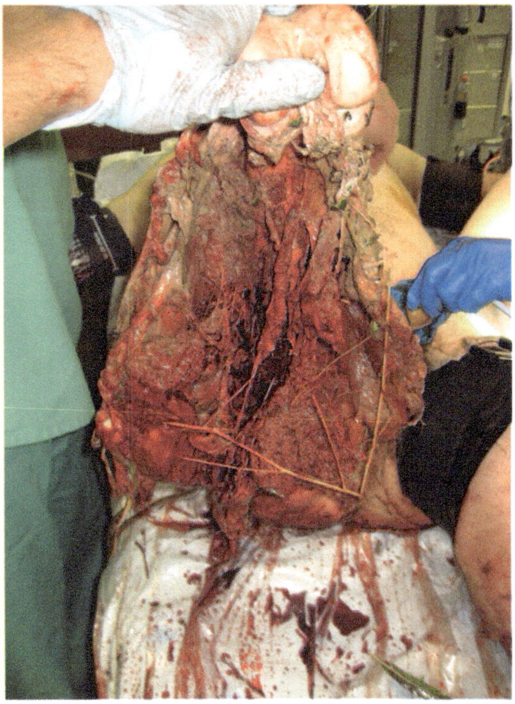

Fig. 3.2 Preoperative image of the same DCBI patient with illustration of the extensive posterior thigh soft tissue blast injury. Note that the nonviable tibia has been disarticulated and that the field tourniquets have been exchanged to pneumatic tourniquets for improved hemostatic control. This patient was revised to bilateral mid-transfemoral amputations using the intact anterior soft tissues as an atypical flap for coverage

continued to rise over the last decade of war. Life-threatening hemorrhage and under resuscitation are expected for urgent Alpha-level casualties medevac'd from the point of injury. The balance of necessary surgical care and adequate resuscitation walks a fine line, especially in the most critically injured where the upregulated systemic inflammatory response poses a significant risk for a secondary physiologic insult (i.e., surgery).

3.3 Prioritizing Combat Casualty Care

Index care for the multiply injured combat patient can be daunting, particularly for physicians experiencing this magnitude of trauma for the first time. No matter how significant the degree of injury, the principles of Advanced Trauma Life Support (ATLS) still guide the initial patient care and subsequent assessments. A medical team (critical care physician, general surgeon, orthopedic surgeon, nurses, and techs) should safely receive the casualty from the medevac and perform a timely but efficient primary survey. Large-bore and/or central intravenous access must be quickly established to begin volume replacement. Hemostatic resuscitation at a 1:1:1 ratio of packed RBCs or whole blood with FFP and platelets is now the standard of care for any complex open or closed injury presenting with significant blood loss (Fig. 3.3). The lethal triad of hypotension, hypothermia, and acidosis poses the greatest risk for death within the 24 h of injury. Despite complex injuries, most patients can be simultaneously treated with ongoing hemostatic resuscitation and lifesaving but time-sensitive surgical intervention. On rare occasions, patients must be further resuscitated in the ICU before they can survive an

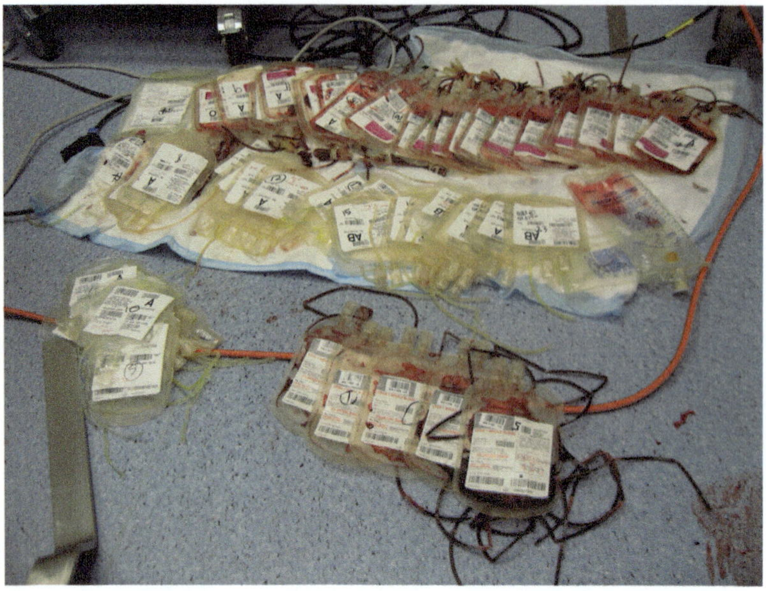

Fig. 3.3 Massive transfusion (>10 units of blood products within 24 h) is common in modern combat casualty care. CPGs exist to direct the 1:1:1 hemostatic resuscitation protocol and whole blood transfusions

index operation. Non-life-threatening orthopedic injuries must take a back seat to a more critical treatment measures and surgeries. Sometimes, the initial orthopedic intervention is a provisional splint or bedside washout before a critically ill patient is transported to a higher echelon of care.

The current military CPGs regulate that all downrange MSK surgical care follow the tenants of damage control orthopedics (DCO). Definitive fixation of fractures and definitive closure of combat wounds are highly discouraged because of the risk of infection. Therefore, the focus is on providing temporizing surgical measures to control fractures and soft tissue wounds without causing further harm to the already disrupted physiology. Although these procedures are not as gratifying as definitive care, they can be truly life and limb saving in a severely injured polytrauma patient. External fixation of femoral shaft fractures with associated head or chest trauma and temporary control of unstable pelvic ring injuries encompass the true doctrine of DCO. Although efforts should be made to salvage any viable extremity, a primary amputation for a crashing polytrauma patient with a reconstructable mangled limb can mean the difference between life and death. In contrast, limb damage control orthopedics (LDCO) entails the concept of temporizing control for extremity injuries where the sum of the patient's clinical picture is not immediately life-threatening (Figs. 3.4, 3.5, and 3.6). Thankfully, the majority of downrange orthopedic care falls into this category. Periarticular external fixation of a pilon fracture or I&D with external fixation of an open tibia fracture are common examples. Although definitive care can be performed, it is discouraged on US and coalition casualties despite what resources are available to downrange surgeons.

With CPGs and various limitations intrinsic to deployment in an austere setting, it is essential to establish a precedence for orthopedic injuries. The priorities for MSK combat casualty care include the following:

1. Correct limb ischemia with either field/pneumatic tourniquets, vessel ligation (irreparable or amputation), vessel shunting/repair, or extremity fasciotomy (when applicable).
2. Decontaminate open fractures and blast wounds with thorough surgical debridement and irrigation in order to lower the biologic burden.
3. Stabilize long bone fractures and unstable pelvic ring injuries with external fixation.
4. Span periarticular fractures with external fixation or splints to provide soft tissue rest and bony reduction using ligamentotaxis.
5. Care for small bone fractures and small wounds (<3 cm).

The details for treating various injury patterns will be discussed in later chapters. Deployed

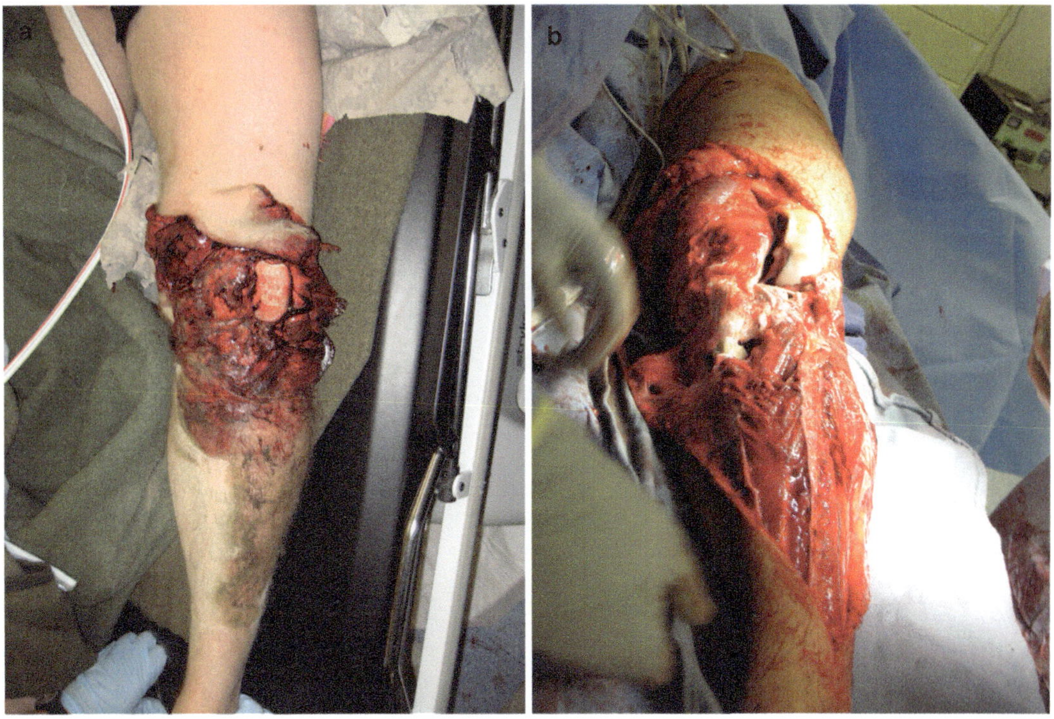

Fig 3.4 (**a**) Index presentation of complex, open intra-articular supracondylar femur and tibial plateau fractures sustained from a penetrating IED blast injury. A pneumatic tourniquet was applied after release of the field tourniquet, and vascular injury was ruled out with an ankle-brachial index (ABI) measurement. (**b**) Intraoperative image of the same injury after surgical debridement with irrigation. A lateral fasciotomy incision was utilized to release the anterior and lateral compartments prophylactically. This incision was strategically placed for future use in the tibial plateau ORIF up range

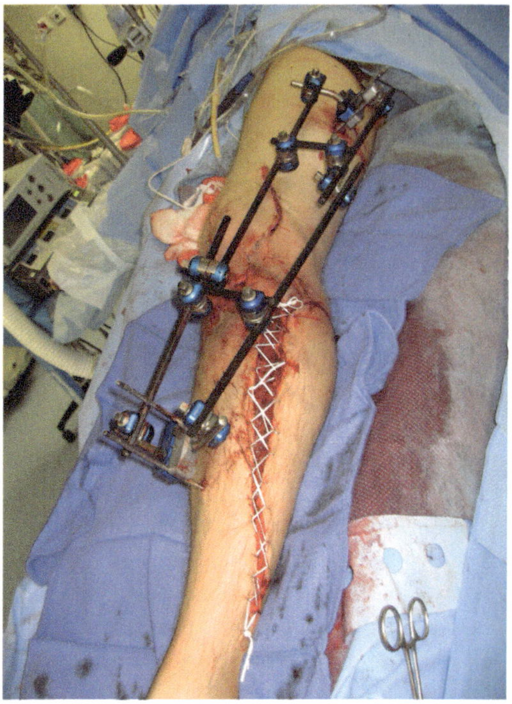

Fig. 3.5 Postoperative illustration after knee spanning external fixation, loose approximation of the traumatic stellate wound, and "Roman sandal" vessel loop approximation of the fasciotomy. Note the long working distance of the ex-fix is supported by a multiplanar construct that increases the stability and provides soft tissue rest and pain control through ligamentotaxis reduction

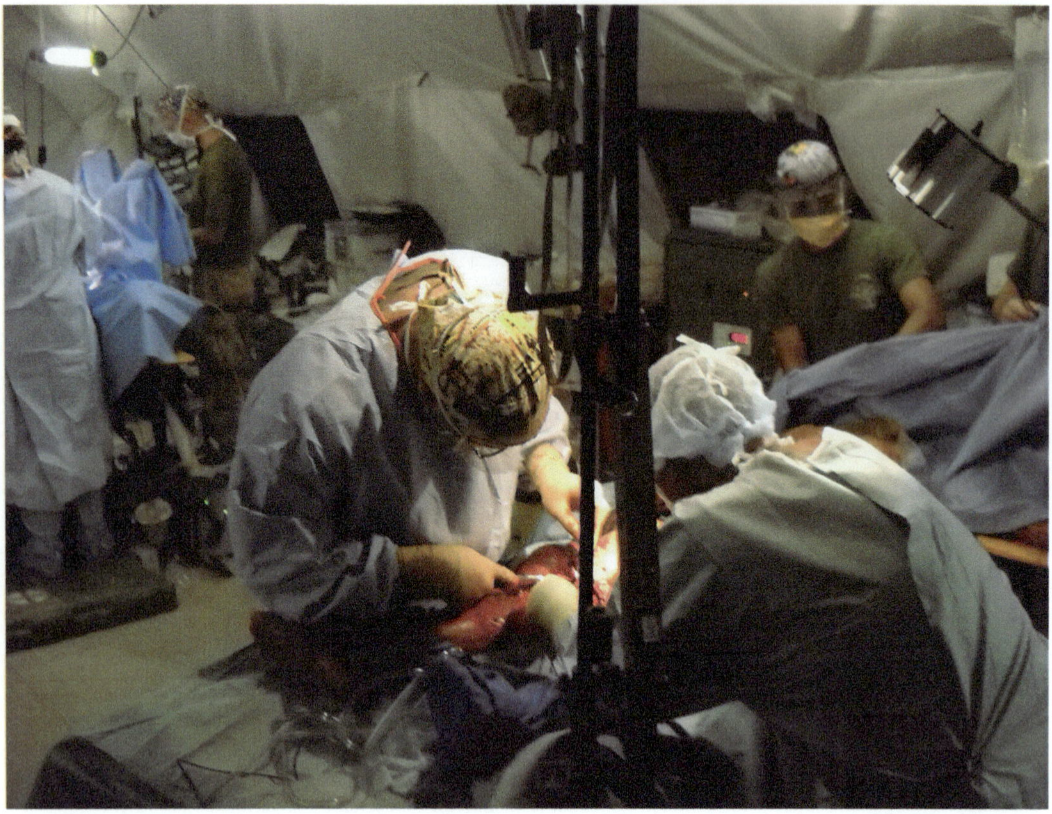

Fig. 3.6 Role-2 operating facilities depict the austere surgical environment with limited surgical resources, makeshift lighting, and the semi-sterile nature of operating in a tent

surgeons should commit to memory the hierarchy of care for orthopedic injuries and understand that it may be impractical to achieve all of these goals during the index surgical case. Variables such as facility resource constraints, hemodynamic instability, inadequate resuscitation, and insufficient time before patient transfers are all potentially limiting factors. The established echelons of care and rapid medevac transports create a unique system where a continuum of surgery, resuscitation, and reassessment occurs through the hands of many providers.

3.4 Echelon Resources Dictate the Level of Orthopedic Care

Knowledge of the combat tempo and your medical facility's resources or limitations will decipher the extent to which MSK injuries can be effectively treated. The descriptive means to describe the levels of care are now called Role 1, Role 2, and Role 3 for downrange casualty treatment (previously called Echelon 1, 2, etc.).

Role-1 care occurs at the point of injury and is referred to as "buddy aid." Critical lifesaving measures such as the application of field tourniquets and combat pressure dressings are employed here by fellow soldiers or medics. Often these devices may even be self-applied. Medevac teams are designed to quickly extract the wounded and continue the advancement of care with extremity splints and desperately needed IV fluids or blood products.

Role-2 care occurs at the field surgical team (FST) or forward resuscitative surgical system (FRSS). These medical treatment facilities (MTF) are mobile by design with rudimentary operating rooms, limited patient holding capacity, and minimal resources to handle more than

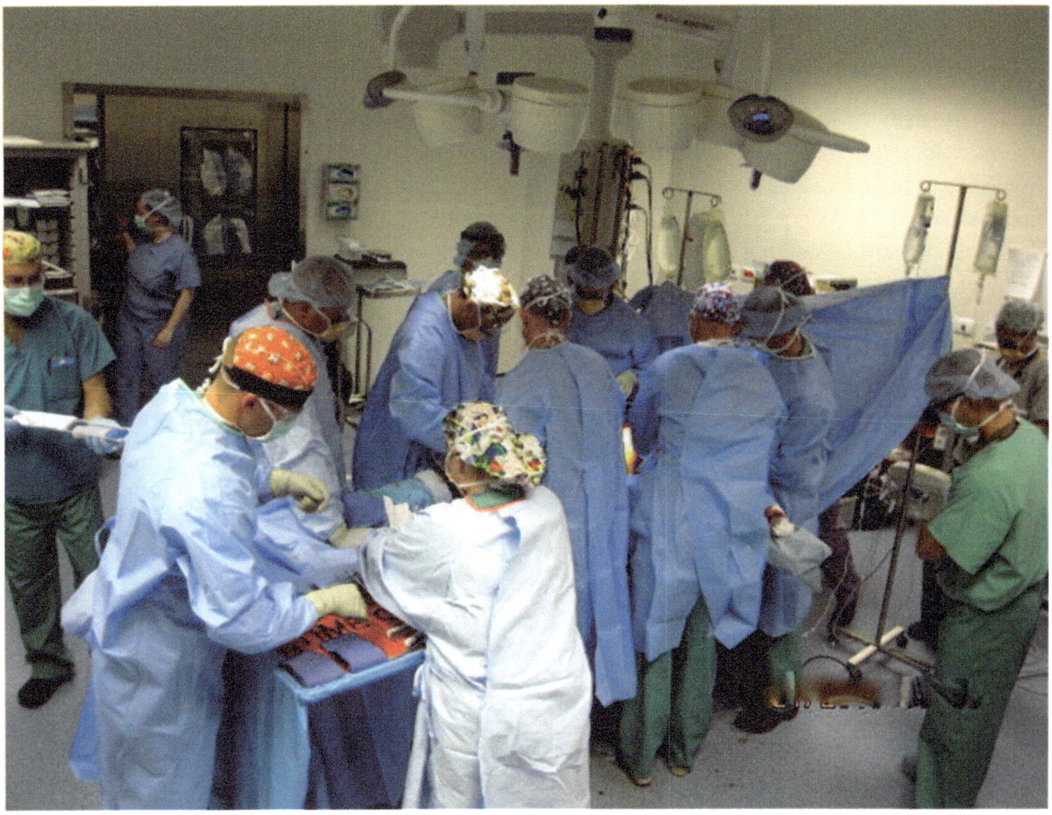

Fig. 3.7 In contrast the permanent Role 3 facilitates a sterile operating theater that is well resourced with support personnel, surgical equipment, and subspecialized surgeons

5–6 patients at a time (Fig. 3.7). Over the last decade of fighting, some Role 2s have been built up to include permanent facilities and increased medical supplies. Regardless of this fact, the DCO and LDCO concepts still apply. Most Role 2s have either limited radiographic imaging or no imaging at all. Fluoroscopy is essentially nonexistent and external fixation is dependent upon tactful surgical skill and anatomic landmarks. Orthopedic power drills and instruments are scarce. Salvageable vascular injuries are treated with shunts rather than repair. Blood products are significantly limited and walking blood banks are often critical to the survival of the combat casualties. Open wounds are covered more often with wet-to-dry or Dakin's dressings, and negative pressure wound therapy (NPWT) is rare at this level. The surgical treatment team generally consists of an anesthesiologist or CRNA, 1–2 general surgeons, 1 orthopedic surgeon, 1–2 OR nurses, and 1–2 techs. The mindset at Role 2s is to "stabilize, treat, and transfer."

Role-3 MTFs (Combat Surgical Hospital – CSH) offer the highest level of medical care within the combat zone. These are fixed hospitals with advanced resources that include multiple ORs, increased casualty holding capacity, abundant ICU care, routine use of standard radiography, fluoroscopy and CT imaging, a well-supplied blood bank, increased ortho supplies and instruments with power, and a larger team of providers to include subspecialties like urology, neurosurgery, vascular surgery, interventional radiology, and OMFS/ophthalmology. MSK care continues to escalate at Role 3s but still remains within the DCO and LDCO treatment guidelines for US and coalition casualties. Temporizing external fixation placed at Role 2s can be reinforced or revised with the assistance of numerous orthopedic surgeons and fluoroscopy. Local nationals and hostile troops may receive definitive MSK care at these facilities if it is "reasonable" and safe. Orthopedists should avoid the urge to place intramedullary nails or locking plates into fractures that may have complications surrounding infection, soft tissue coverage, or nonunion. Foreign national surgeons do not have the resources to deal with infectious complications and modern implants. Increased resources are available for vascular injuries to allow angiography and repair. Open fractures, extensive combat wounds, and soft tissue defects are routinely treated with NPWT. Role 3s represent the last chance for fracture reduction, wound washouts, final splinting, and soft tissue management before patients are transported out of the combat theater of operations to the Role-4 MTF in Landstuhl Regional Medical Center in Germany and then Role 5s in CONUS.

3.5 The Value of a Multidisciplinary Team

The injuries sustained by our fighting forces have evolved over the past decade of war. With IED encounters being the most common mechanism of injury, multiple casualties and polytrauma patients with numerous anatomic injuries is the norm. Because of this, it is vitally important for the forward surgical team to establish individual and team responsibilities early. Critically unstable patients and mass casualty situations are best dealt with a multidisciplinary approach. Every surgeon, medical provider, nurse, and tech should know their role and be comfortable in helping in their own capacity. Techs can be critically important in helping with tasks such as reconstituting blood products, activating the walking blood bank, applying pressure to multiple wounds, and splinting. Every asset must be actively employed in the treatment of the combat wounded. Injury patterns from IED blasts require surgical efficiency. General and orthopedic surgeons aggressively control hemorrhage, wound contamination, and fractures, while anesthesia providers monitor resuscitation. A multidisciplinary approach is invaluable in producing the best outcome for our wounded.

With each casualty, there should be a hierarchy of what needs to be accomplished. First and foremost is the abatement of ongoing hemorrhage and instituting hemostatic resuscitation to counter blood loss and coagulopathy. Then using a team approach, multiple anatomic sites can be addressed at the index surgical setting. When applicable, general surgeons can explore and control the abdomen or shunt vasculature while orthopedists are stabilizing long bone and pelvis injuries. This helps to lessen the physiologic stress of surgery and greatly decreases operative times (Fig. 3.8). Special attention should be paid to the resources in your role of care. Role-2 facilities are limited to resuscitation, hemorrhage control, and long bone/pelvic stabilization, where Role-3 centers are more robust and capable of performing procedures with increased complexity such as interventional angiography.

Keeping in mind the resources of each role of care, one should establish reasonable end points for the index surgery. The combat surgeon cannot expect to treat each injury as they would in a civilian setting. For instance, debridements at lower roles of care are often cursory giving way to hemorrhage control and long bone stabilization. These roles are limited and the focus should be on survivability of the war fighter with rapid transfer to a higher level of care when continued stabilization is accomplished. Even at higher roles of care, the operational tempo and number of casualties may dictate which lifesaving measures are taken on, leaving completion of debridement to the next available opportunity.

3.6 Critically Important Injury Patterns

It is important to understand the different combat injury patterns and the resources and efforts necessary to treat them. Several reviews of combat casualty care have outlined the Dismounted Complex Battle Injury (DCBI), where critically injured patients present with multiple extremity

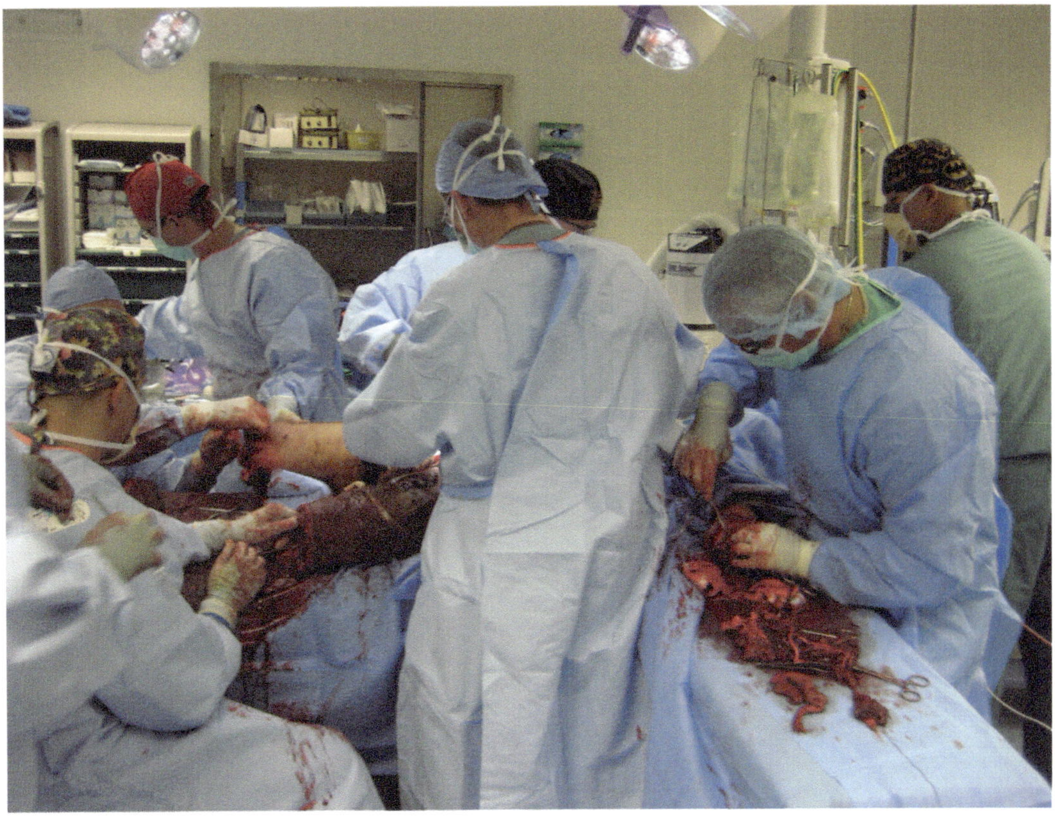

Fig. 3.8 The value of the multidisciplinary surgical team is epitomized in the case of the DCBI where numerous MSK and non-MSK injuries exist in patients presenting critically volume depleted, hypothermic, and acidotic. Here, the general surgeons have obtained proximal iliac vessel control, while orthopedic surgeons provide distal vessel ligation at the revision amputation levels. Concurrent surgery decreases OR time, blood loss, and the risk of a second physiologic insult

amputations and pelvic blast injuries. New CPGs highlight the necessary means to resuscitate and treat these devastating injury patterns. Damage control hemostatic resuscitation and massive transfusion protocols help to advance the treatment efficiency of injury patterns that include the multi-limb amputee with associated abdominal and perineal injuries. As previously mentioned, the improvement in personal protection of the thorax and head, combined with the use of potent IEDs by the enemy, has increased the number of multiple traumatic amputees surviving the initial treatment phase.

A recent review of injuries treated at the Role-3 hospital in Kandahar, Afghanistan, depicts several DCBI injury patterns and treatment strategies. Among the patients seen in this series, about half of the multiple amputees had an associated pelvic injury. Of these pelvic injuries, nearly 50 % were unstable ring patterns, which highlight the importance of pelvic stabilization to aid in hemorrhage control in this injury population. The authors also reported that half of these pelvic injuries were open. This further reinforces the concept of a surgical team approach. In this setting, the general surgeon can perform a diverting colostomy away from the contaminated wounds and definitive fracture incisions while the orthopedist stabilizes the pelvis via external fixation.

These unstable pelvic ring injuries require emergent surgical care to establish hemorrhage control. With the limited resources of the Role-2 facility, the pelvis can be provisionally stabilized with a poncho, blanket, or pelvic binder when they are available. External fixation is possible with the combat peel-pack external fixator components but note the limitations to this resource. First, multiple packs will be required for a sufficient frame; this may be limited by the overall supply. Secondly, without the use of fluoroscopy, multiple pins at each iliac crest are necessary rather than attempting single supra-acetabular pin placement. A small cutdown can be performed to indentify the inner and outer table of the pelvis to facilitate pin passage with the hand crank available in the combat, peel-pack external fixator set. In the Role-3 setting, fluoroscopy has the advantage of allowing visualization for supra-acetabular pin placement, improving control of the fractured pelvic ring and utilizing less pin and bar resources. In either setting, it is critical to provide stability to the pelvic ring prior to transport to the next level of care.

3.7 Packaging the Patient for Medevac

After the goal of resuscitative stabilization and surgical hemostasis has been met, the next priority is the expedited medevac of the wounded war fighter to the next higher level of care. An opportunity to transport a stable patient to the next level of care should not be squandered in an effort to surgically "improve" a stable patient. For the lower roles of care, expedient medevac of the stable patient is a must and clearly delineated in the CPGs. Forward surgical teams do not have the resources to manage a critically injured patient. Any "lift of opportunity" should be taken advantage of to get the wounded to facilities with more robust resources to manage their injuries. The Role-2 surgical team should focus on stabilization of the pelvis and long bone fractures to improve life and limb survivability. At this level of care, soft tissue wounds should be dressed with wet-to-dry dressings after focused surgical debridements. Extremity muscle compartments with acute swelling and concern for potential compartment syndrome should undergo fasciotomy, as transport can be unpredictable in a hostile kinetic environment and some injuries may not undergo a second-look evaluation in the short term. Although there is morbidity to a fascial release, catastrophic muscle death is avoided if untreated compartment syndrome occurs during transport.

The increased treatment capacity of the Role-3 MTF often allows for "controlled" casualty transfers. Here, a scheduled transport is more likely than at the lower levels of care. The receiving orthopedists should attend to optimizing the overall boney and soft tissue condition of the wounded. Repeat debridements should occur before transfer out of theater. Combat wounds should be serially debrided every 24–48 h, and communication between levels of care can appropriately direct soft tissue management. Repeat sharp excision of all nonviable tissue that has declared itself since the previous washout may pay dividends for the extremity by helping to decrease the risk of infection and improve the overall milieu of the soft tissue envelope. When there is opportunity and resources, long bone and pelvic external fixation should be reinforced and optimized for fracture stability utilizing fluoroscopy to achieve adequate reduction. Splints can also be used as adjuncts to external fixation to help maximize soft tissue rest and help with pain control during transport.

Dressing capabilities for soft tissue wounds also improve at the Role-3 facility. Wet-to-dry dressings are still appropriate and may be used in conjunction with Dakin's solution. Negative pressure wound therapy is often accessible at this level of care (Fig. 3.9). For American forces, the wound vac has been shown to be safe in transport even during longer flights out of theater to the Role-4 MTF in Landstuhl, Germany. The benefits of negative pressure therapy for previously decontaminated wounds are well described in the literature. The Role-3 facility is often a collection point for injured local nationals and may be the final facility utilized for the completion of their care. In this instance, NPWV can be used to help prepare soft tissue beds for final coverage procedures.

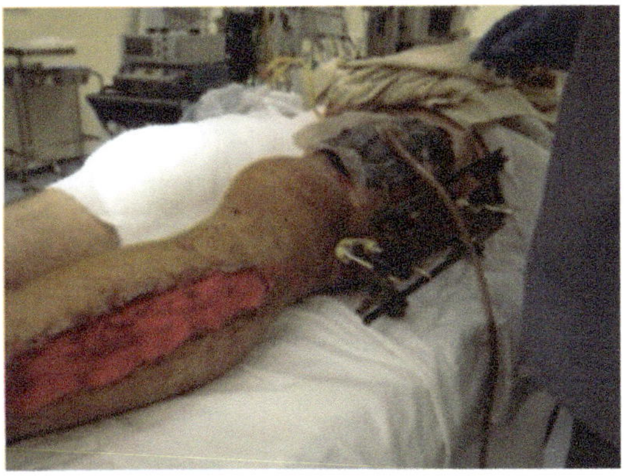

Fig. 3.9 Example of various wound dressing techniques, which include negative pressure wound therapy, "Roman sandal" fasciotomy approximation, and wet-to-dry dressing with gauze and kerlix

3.8 Communication Up Range

Communication between roles of care can be difficult and frustrating at times. In many Role-1 and Role-2 environments, direct electronic communication may be impossible due to the combat tempo or available resources. Casualties often arrive with little forewarning, and surgical teams must be ready to work at a moment's notice. To complicate matters, any paperwork sent with the injured war fighter may be damaged or lost all together during the pass off. In situations where direct communication with the next level of care is suboptimal, it is advisable to record pertinent treatment information on the casualties' dressings. Indelible marker can be used to communicate underlying injuries, procedures performed, and resuscitation efforts that the casualty has received on any available tape or splint material attached to the injury (Fig. 3.10).

When direct communications are possible, the surgical team should make every effort to contact the surgeons at the receiving location. Coordination of surgical interventions and allocations of resources can often be accomplished while the casualty is in transit. It is also important for the receiving team to understand the nature of the injuries and what interventions have already been accomplished to avoid the "undoing" of an effective measure like pelvic packing for hemostasis.

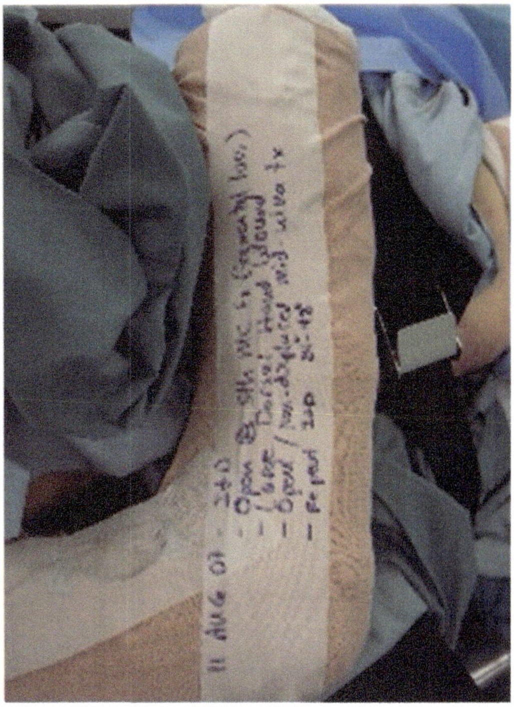

Fig. 3.10 Depiction of downrange communication techniques where the injury pattern and surgical treatments have been written on the specific extremity. This is a valuable means of documenting what has been done and what needs to be done

It is easy to be a Monday-morning quarterback, and up-range surgeons should remember the limitations of their peers downrange.

Just as higher levels of care have more medical resources, they also have improved and consistent communication systems. In the more controlled environment of the Role-3, time should be taken to package operative reports and laboratory and radiographic studies with the casualty before transport to the next level of care. Direct communication via phone and email helps to reduce confusion and facilitates advanced transfer to Role-4 and Role-5 MTFs out of the combat theater. Video teleconferencing has been established between military treatment facilities stateside, intermediaries like Germany, and larger role facilities in the combat theater to track patient status and further coordinate treatment protocols for the wounded warriors as they arrive back home for definitive care.

Conclusion

MSK combat casualty care is unlike civilian trauma, and a mindset focused on the principles of life and limb damage control surgery is paramount for early survival and the index care of the wounded. Due to the unique blast and penetrating mechanisms, combat wounds and fracture patterns tend to be more extensive often violating a larger zone of injury than expected. Knowledge of the military CPGs directing downrange orthopedic care can guide inexperienced combat surgeons. A multidisciplinary team approach is the best medicine for polytrauma patients with multiple extremity and non-orthopedic injuries, especially the DCBI where patients arrive in extremis and cannot tolerate prolonged individual procedures. The resources and limitations of your deployable MTF will dictate the surgical volume and complexity. Combat casualty care is a team project facilitated by multiple teams at different locations sharing the responsibility of care. Compliance with the CPGs and the priorities of MSK trauma consistently yields positive results and has lead to the highest survival rates of any war. Embracing the system (Roles 1–5), effectively communicating up range, and respecting the limitations of downrange teams lead to the greatest success.

Blast Trauma

4

Robert E. Blease and Christopher S. Smith

Contents

BLUF (Bottom Line Up Front) Box

1. The amount of energy, and thus soft tissue damage, imparted by a high-energy blast is an order of magnitude greater than almost any other known mechanism of injury.
2. There are four distinct components which comprise the blast injury mechanism: primary, secondary, tertiary, and quaternary.
3. The blast wave, which is responsible for the majority of imparted energy, exhibits its fluid-wavelike characteristics.
4. Massive soft tissue loss and damage is the sine qua non of blast trauma.
5. Understanding of the physiological requirements and stresses of the blast trauma patient and participation in its management is critical for the orthopedic provider.

R.E. Blease, MD (✉)
Department of the Army/Medical Corps US Army,
Army Trauma Training Center, Ryder Trauma Center,
1850 N.W. 10th Avenue, Miami, FL 33136, USA
e-mail: robert.blease@army.mil

C.S. Smith, MD
Department of Orthopaedic Surgery,
Medical Corps, U.S. Navy,
620 John Paul Jones Circle, Portsmouth,
VA 23708, USA

Orthopaedic Trauma, Orthopaedic Surgery
Department, Naval Medical Center Portsmouth,
Portsmouth, VA USA
e-mail: christopher.s.smith@med.navy.mil

L.B. Bone, C.N. Mamczak (eds.), *Front Line Extremity and Orthopaedic Surgery*,
DOI 10.1007/978-3-642-45337-3_4, © Springer-Verlag Berlin Heidelberg 2014

6. This is damage control surgery at its extreme!
7. Dismounted complex blast injury is a newly identified injury pattern that defines the current limits of blast trauma survivability based on current management strategies and preparedness.
8. In a blast trauma patient, the decision to perform limb salvage surgery vs. completion amputation need not necessarily be made early if the patient is physiologically stable and has viable distal tissues (Fig. 4.1).

During Operation Iraqi Freedom (OIF) and Operation Enduring Freedom (OEF), blast trauma has become the most common mechanism (78 %) of wounding among US and coalition troops, greatly outnumbering wounds from small arms fire (18 %) [1, 2]. Improvised explosive devices (IEDs) have increased in magnitude, frequency, and sophistication throughout the course of these conflicts. Enemy combatants have improved their techniques as the escalation of technology, tactics, and countermeasures have advanced. By far the most commonly deployed explosive device used by enemy combatants is the improvised explosive device (IED). IEDs constitute a broad range of devices, deployment methods, sizes, and levels of sophistication. Examples of the spectrum of deployed devices include everything from low-tech devices using common household items, to reutilized artillery shells with triggering devices, to Trojan Horse IEDs that are embedded in stolen US government property (i.e., handheld radios), to suicide/homicide bombers to massive and highly destructive vehicle born IEDs.

Reasons for the significant increase in the deployment and use of these destructive devices include:

1. The ready availability of materials
2. The massive amount of devastation that they are capable of unleashing
3. The relatively low risk that their use presents to the enemy vs. direct engagement with better equipped and trained coalition forces

The net effect of these attacks has been to:

1. Cause large-scale and frequently overwhelming soft tissue injuries (Fig. 4.2)
2. Inflict multiple fractures and amputations (Fig. 4.3)

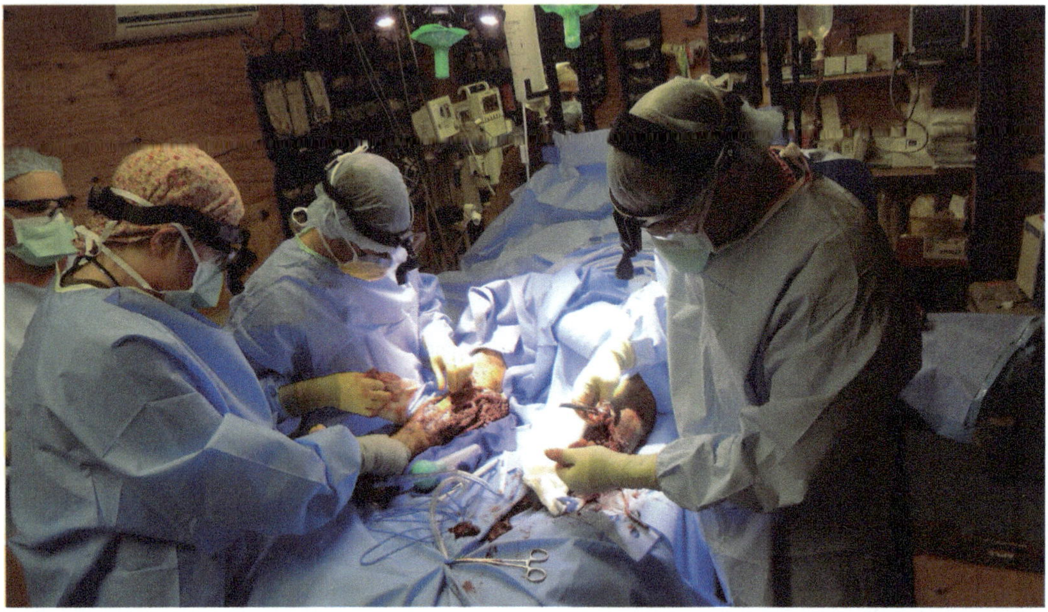

Fig. 4.1 IED blast involving bilateral lower extremities (Photo courtesy of Christopher S. Smith, M.D.)

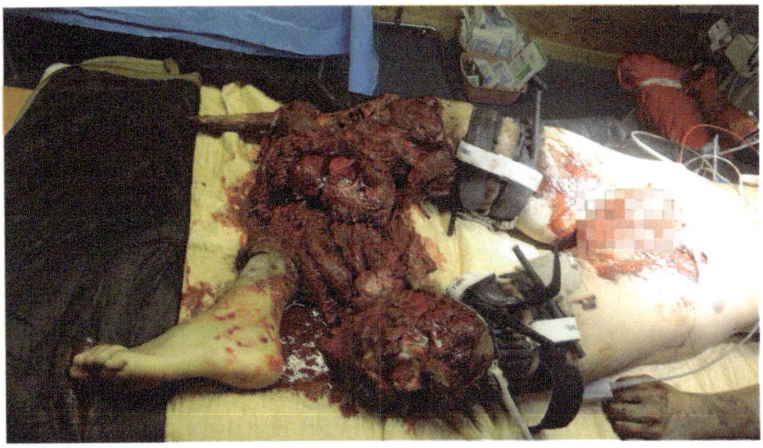

Fig. 4.2 IED blast involving a traumatic left through-knee amputation, traumatic right mangled extremity with near-complete amputation above the knee, and genital trauma (Photo courtesy of Christopher S. Smith, M.D.)

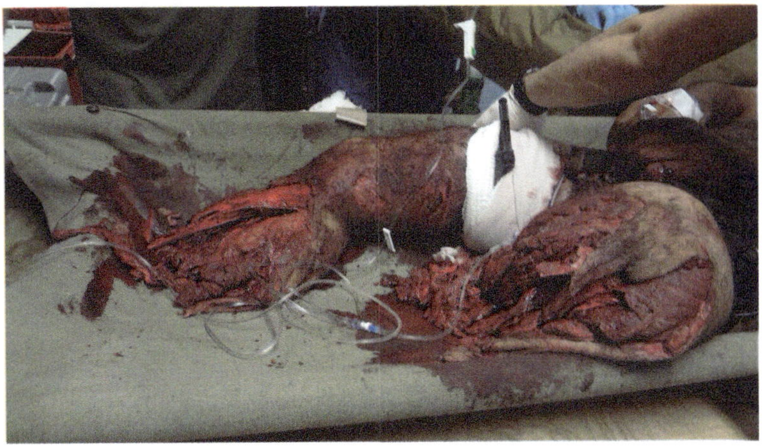

Fig. 4.3 IED blast injury with left traumatic above-the-knee amputation and right traumatic below-the-knee amputation (Photo courtesy of Christopher S. Smith, M.D.)

3. Create heavily contaminated wounds with both organic and nonorganic debris (Fig. 4.4)
4. Cause significant concurrent damage to multiple other organ systems to include the bowel, the middle ear, and the lungs

As our understanding and experience with these injuries has increased, so have our treatment techniques and strategies improved. Primarily, the importance of staged, multidisciplinary management of these complexly injured patients has been recognized and appropriate treatment algorithms implemented. Significant advances have been made in soft tissue debridement and coverage techniques. Additionally, great strides have also been made in the use of nontraditional, length/function preserving amputations, rehabilitation strategies, and prosthetics.

4.1 Blast Mechanics

Blast devices can be categorized into two broad categories based on the speed and magnitude of their energy dispersion. These categories are based on the speed at which the explosive burns:

1. Low-energy (LE) devices. An LE explosive burns, or deflagrates at a speed of 3,280 fps (feet per second) or less. Common examples include black gunpowder, smokeless gunpowder, and gasoline. They tend to produce large amounts of gas that explode only when confined, such as that which occurs in a common pipe bomb.
2. High-energy (HE) devices. Conversely, HE explosive burns at a speed in excess of 14,763 fps. This creates a supersonic blast wave (shock wave) even if the ignited explosive is unconfined. Typical examples include

TNT, dynamite, ammonium nitrate-fuel oil, and plastic explosives such as C4 and Semtex [3]. This category will be discussed throughout the remainder of this article. The net result of the detonation of HE devices is:

(a) The generation of a blast shock wave traveling at up to 6,000 fps (feet per second). (Note: a typical handgun projectile that is traveling at approximately 800 fps out of the barrel and an assault rifle bullet that leaves the barrel roughly 2,300 fps)
   (i) The initiation of an HE explosion creates an almost instantaneous, supersonic, circumferential shock wave of blast overpressure that, in an open environment, dissipates rapidly and at a predictable rate as it expands over time and distance. This is known as a Friedlander curve or wave [4] (Fig. 4.5a, b).
   (ii) At the point of detonation PSI may exceed 14 million PSI (pounds per square inch), with as little as 60–80 PSI being frequently fatal (Fig. 4.6).
   (iii) Individuals in closest proximity to the detonation have little chance of survival, although those standing as little as 10–20 ft away may sustain relatively minor blast wave injury.
(b) The disbursement of an enormous amount of injury to the soft tissues and skeletal system incorporates sufficient energy to create brisance, which is a shattering effect to the skeletal system.
(c) Soft tissue damage potentiation via primary and secondary projectiles will be discussed below.

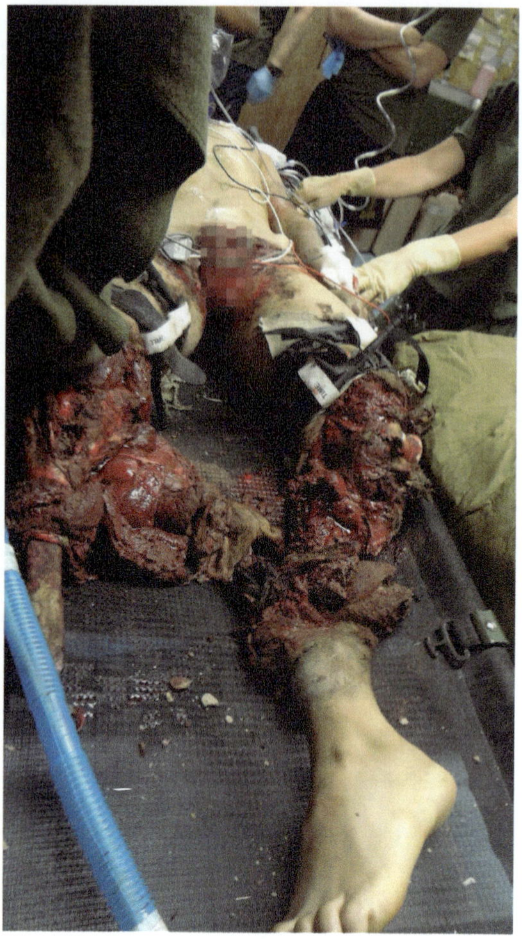

Fig. 4.4 IED blast with traumatic left near-complete amputation of the left lower extremity and traumatic right below-the-knee amputation (Photo courtesy of Christopher S. Smith, M.D.)

Blast waves follow a number of fluid-wavelike characteristics, awareness of which will aid in the understanding of the wounding patterns that they cause:

1. They can be deflected by large, fixed structures.
2. They will flow around obstacles, resulting in a concentration of forces.
3. They will deflect off of fixed structures, likewise causing a multifold increase in the concentration of force at the areas of deflection, much like a spring being compressed.
4. Individuals protected behind a fixed object, which is capable of deflecting the force of a blast wave, are subjected to an order of magnitude less energy.
5. Blast waves initiated within closed spaces do not exhibit a typical Friedlander wave pattern and will continue to bounce off opposing walls causing retention of energy, higher peak pressures, and a blast wave consisting of longer duration within that confined space.
6. A blast wave set off in a liquid medium, such as a body of water, tends to travel much more quickly and to dissipate energy much more slowly.

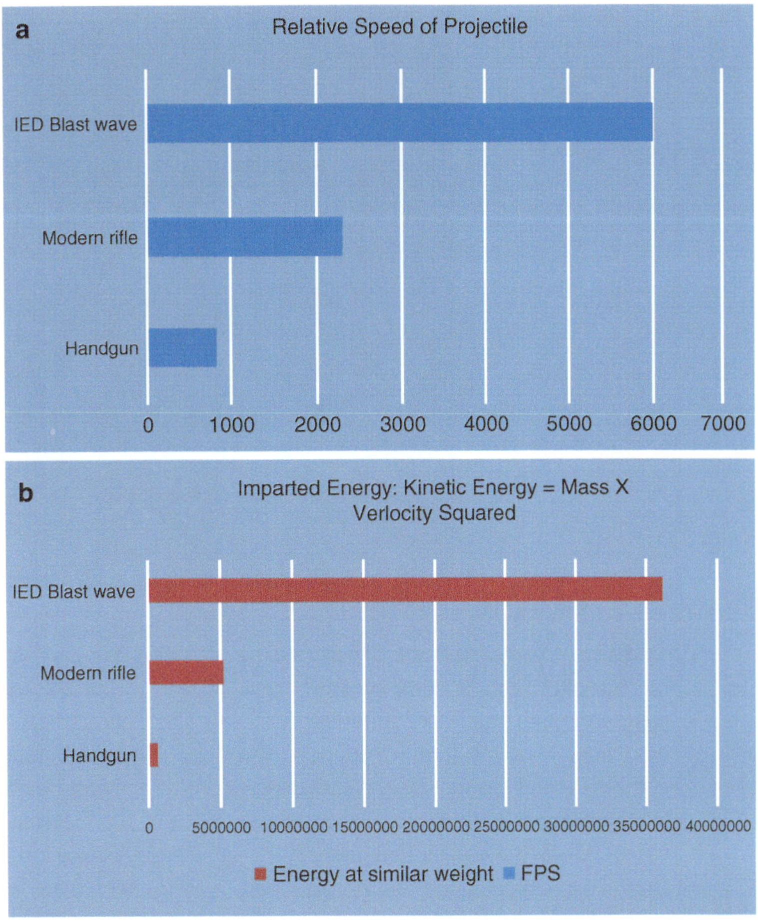

Fig. 4.5 (**a**) Graphic of relative velocity of three of the most common combat wounding mechanisms. (**b**) Per the ballistic formula $KE = MV^2$: The mechanisms noted in graph a, above translate to a logarithmic increase in imparted energy to blast victims

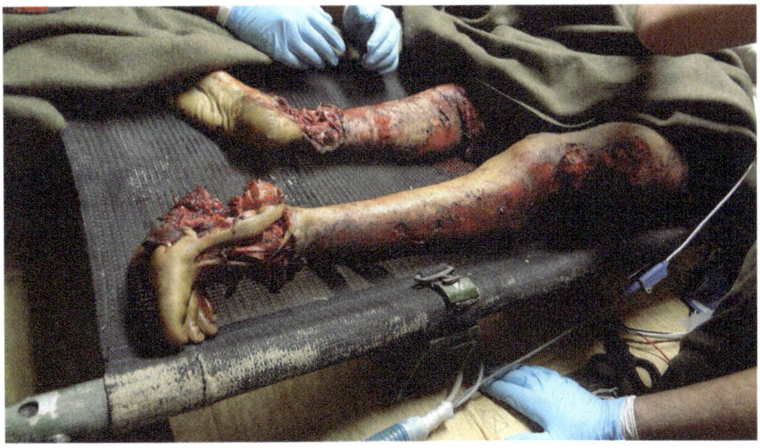

Fig. 4.6 IED blast with mangled bilateral lower extremities and fragmentation blast pattern of left lower extremity (Photo courtesy of Christopher S. Smith, M.D.)

High-energy blast waves create four distinct phases of injury. These have been well described by multiple authors as:

1. Primary blast injury – This is unique to HE and results from the impact of the overpressure wave with the body. Much of the devastating soft tissue trauma that occurs during a blast is due to the effects of this pressure wave as it passes through soft tissue. Several mechanisms have been postulated as causing these effects:

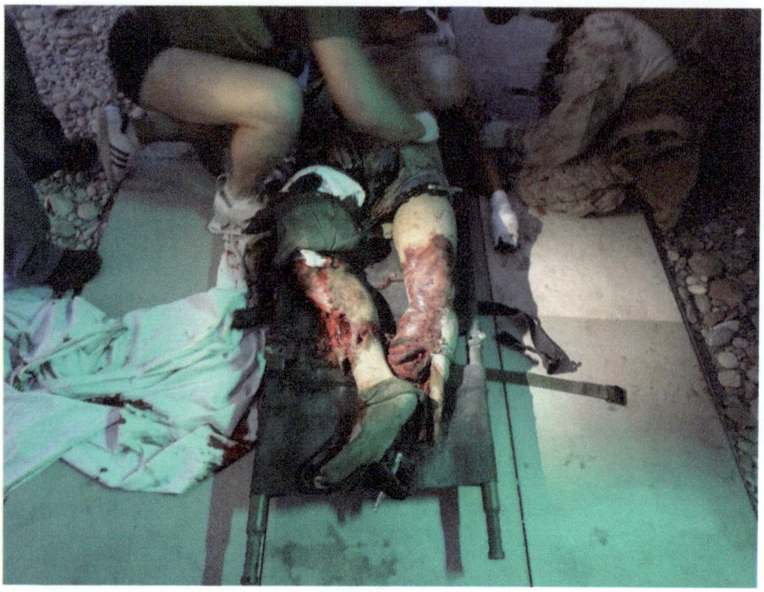

Fig. 4.7 IED blast with left traumatic below-the-knee amputation and mangled extremity of the right lower extremity (Photo courtesy of Christopher S. Smith, M.D.)

(a) Spalling – Covey and Born [5] describe the mechanism of injury as the pressure wave passes through tissues of different densities, notably at air/fluid interfaces as a combination of spalling (the forced, explosive movement of fluids from more dense to less dense tissues, i.e., lung tissue).

(b) Implosion – the sudden and forcible collapse of hollow organs, followed by rapid re-expansion and tissue injury after the pressure wave passes.

(c) Brisance – the shattering effect as the pressure wave passes through soft tissues has been well described. This can result in fractures throughout the skeleton system and when combined with shearing and stretching forces can result in partial or complete traumatic amputations [6].

  (i) Though a traumatic amputation by itself is rarely life-threatening, it does serve as an indicator to concomitant injury to the lungs and other hollow organs (Fig. 4.7).

  (ii) Survival of a victim who has sustained a blast injury amputation may be tenuous (Fig. 4.8).

2. Secondary blast injury – This results from flying debris and bomb fragments. Secondary blast injury is caused by several types of fragments acting under a spectrum of ballistic forces:

(a) Primary fragmentation (flying debris from the explosive device itself). In the case of the IED, this has been noted to include random household or industrial objects such as bolts, nuts, finishing nails, ball bearings, marbles, jacks, etc.

(b) Secondary fragmentation (those objects which are picked up by the blast wave and propelled in its wake – may be organic as well as inorganic in nature) (Fig. 4.9a, b). This is the most common cause of death from a blast [4] (Fig. 4.10).

In the case of the suicide/homicide bomber, this may include tissues from the bomber himself.

(c) Both primary and secondary projectiles will act somewhat in accordance with well-recognized ballistic characteristics as they penetrate soft tissues based upon both their mass and velocity at time of impact.

  (i) As opposed to regularly formed, aerodynamic rifle or handgun projectiles, these fragments will be more irregularly shaped.

  (ii) Are larger and may be flying in irregular patterns.

  (iii) This results in a host of bizarrely implanted projectiles, greater cavitation effect, and amputations from flying debris.

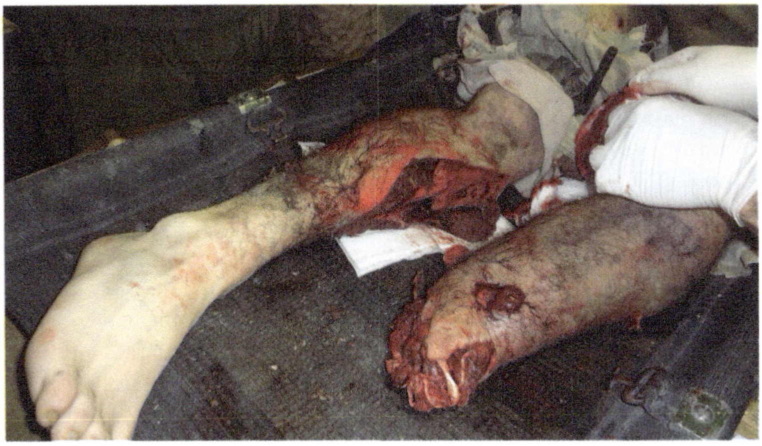

Fig. 4.8 IED blast with traumatic left below-the-knee amputation and open fracture of the right tibia (Photo courtesy of Christopher S. Smith, M.D.)

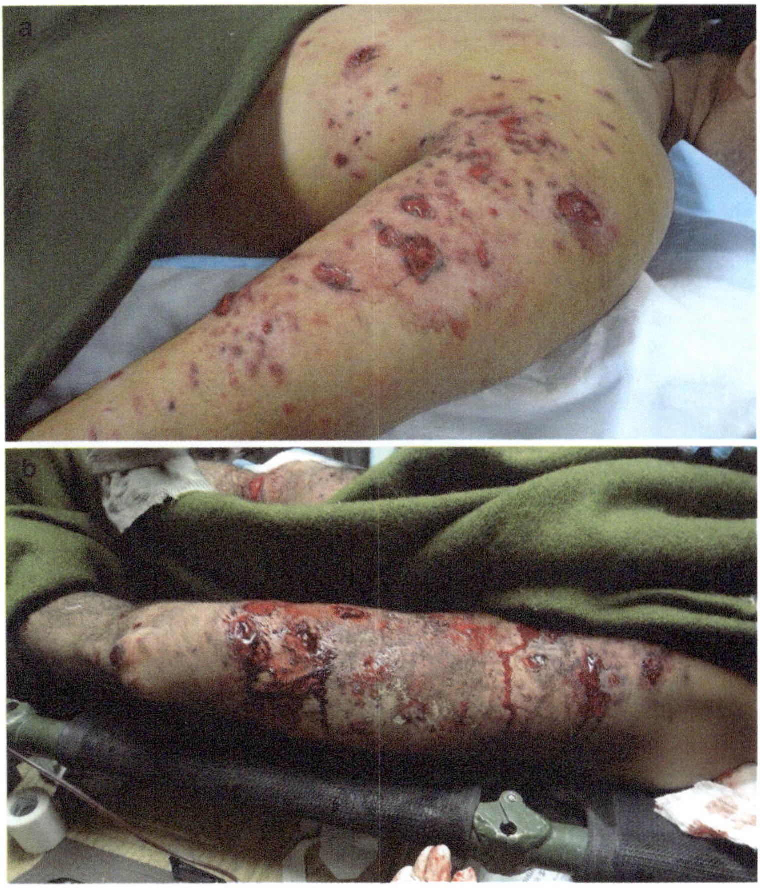

Fig. 4.9 (**a**, **b**) IED blast from a grape charge with a typical small fragmentation wounding pattern (Photo courtesy of Christopher S. Smith, M.D.)

3. Tertiary blast injury – This results from being thrown by the blast wind. This phase of blast injury consists of injuries sustained by victims as they are hurtled along with the blast wave, resulting in strikes against hard structures along their paths, and against fixed objects or the ground, resulting in a number of potential orthopedic injuries.
4. Quaternary blast injury – This encompasses all other injuries resulting from explosion, which

are not due to primary, secondary, or tertiary mechanisms. The phase of blast injury is less well described but constitutes the later effects of blast trauma and includes:

(a) Compartment syndromes
(b) Myonecrosis
(c) Burns

4.2 Medical Management System

Deployed coalition forces have developed a number of effective strategies for managing the medical aspects of the aftermath of an HE explosive. These include:

A. Expectation of mass blast trauma as a normal course of activities with logistical preparation and personnel deployment in expectation of this eventuality.
B. Having forward placed surgical assets within minutes of the point of injury with blood transfusion capabilities (Fig. 4.11).
   Having Medevac capability readily available and within close proximity to the point of injury.
C. Outfitting patrolling servicemen with advanced body armor and antiballistic helmets with resultant protection to the chest abdomen and head.
D. Placing medics ubiquitously within the maneuver units. The rapid application of tourniquets by these medics, as well as by the trained servicemen, has saved many lives, and nearly all deployed US servicemen are supplied with these and are instructed in their use. This advancement has brought tourniquet use from an indication of last resort to use as a frontline lifesaving device.
E. The deployment of a relatively young, motivated, and underlying disease-free population.

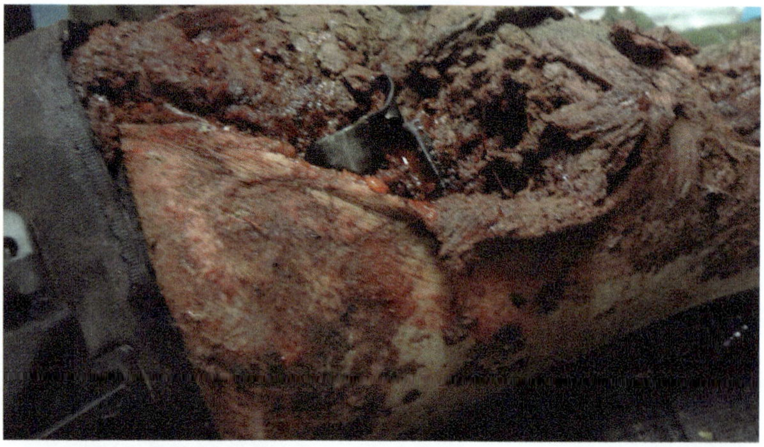

Fig. 4.10 IED blast wound with embedded dirt and secondary debris (Note the ammunition belt link which was hurtled by the blast wave into the injured tissues). (Photo courtesy of Christopher S. Smith, M.D.)

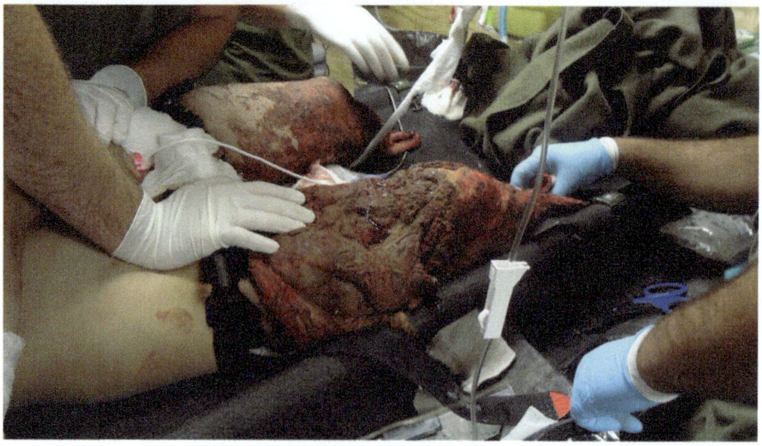

Fig. 4.11 IED blast with traumatic bilateral lower extremity amputations with retightening of the combat application tourniquet (Photo courtesy of Christopher S. Smith, M.D.)

4.3 Orthopedic Specific Issues

Advances in the medical management system have resulted in an unprecedented high survival rate among combat-injured US and coalition servicemen in the Iraqi and Afghan conflicts. This has led to increased recognition of injury patterns that may not have been significantly recognized during previous conflicts due to dismally poor survival rates. The result of dismounted troops who are subjected to massive IED blasts has been the recognition of a category of blast trauma patients that fit what is now recognized as dismounted complex blast injury (DCBI) [7–9]. Specifically, two patterns of injury have been described:

A. The first pattern has been well described by Mamczak et al. [9] and consists of bilateral (generally high above the knee) lower extremity amputations, frequently noted to be found in combination with open pelvic fractures, genitourinary injuries, and massive exsanguination. These patients present in extremis and require intensive, staged treatment efforts, both surgical and resuscitative, to offer even a chance of survival. Control of hemorrhage, up to and including cross-clamping of the descending aorta or proximal control of the iliac arteries and pelvic packing, in combination with pelvic ring external fixation and massive transfusion, is required during the initial resuscitation phase. The initial treatment is followed by staged washouts of extremity and soft tissue wounds, further resuscitation, and frequent amputation revision as the soft tissue wounds evolve. Those who survive the initial insult and resuscitation still sustain a high incidence of mortality secondary to multisystem organ failure or sepsis, or both. Mucor species fungal infections are reported with some frequency, with a resultant need for aggressive debridement.
B. The second category of DCBI patient, as described by Andersen et al. [7], has been the multiple major amputation patient. Concurrent with the increase in relative blast energy and imparted blast trauma noted above, a statistically significant increase in double, triple, and quadruple amputees has been noted. These patients likewise present in extremis; require an aggressive, team-oriented approach; and will have significant treatment, rehabilitation, and prosthetic challenges throughout the course of their recovery and remaining lives.

4.4 Key Learning Points

A. Effectively applied tourniquets save lives and result in the loss of relatively few limbs [10]. Currently, nearly every deployed serviceman is supplied with and trained on the use of these tourniquets.
B. Junctional bleeding (groin and axilla) is still a source of concern and has been a significant management problem outside of the operating room. Newer tourniquets are now available to assist with major groin vessel hemorrhage. However, significant further work remains in this realm.
C. Blood transfusion is critical [11]. Key issues:
   (a) Both the specific ratio of transfused components (a 1:1:1 ratio of PRBCs/plasma/platelets) and the rate and volume of transfusion have been described in the literature as saving lives.
   (b) Whole blood transfusion from a predesignated donor pool has also been noted to be significantly beneficial to the patient in extremis but is fraught with many potential complications.
D. Surgical care and skilled resuscitation prepositioned as close as possible to the point of injury saves lives if utilized effectively.
E. The blast trauma patient in extremis cannot tolerate extended time in the operating room. In this setting, damage control surgery is kept to 1 h or less. They are likely in or bordering the "triad of death" hypovolemia, hypothermia, and hypocoagulability.
   (a) As opposed to a typical civilian trauma where each surgical service operates in turn in a priority-based serial approach,

the blast trauma patient needs a prioritized yet parallel effort in order to maximize the benefit of physiologically limited surgical time.

(b) Once the initial evaluation is conducted by the trauma team, the principal surgical services must agree on, and execute, a coordinated resuscitation and surgical stabilization of the patient. Especially for the orthopedic surgeon, doing too much in this situation can jeopardize the patient's life.

(c) Due to the patient's tenuous physiological condition, further resuscitation frequently must be carried out in the ICU prior to a second or third round of surgery.

F. In blast trauma, the management of a relatively simple fracture is made significantly more complex due to the loss of skin, subcutaneous tissue, or muscle that can frequently be measured in square feet as opposed to square inches.

(a) These injuries are highly contaminated and continue to evolve for days to weeks.

(b) Early definitive fixation results in a high rate of infection, failure, and potential amputation.

(c) Multiple staged washouts, antibiotic management, antibiotic bead pouch placement, and wound vac therapy are required until the wounds are healthy and viable and ready for closure, flap closure, and/or definitive fixation.

G. Limb salvage vs. amputation continues to be a controversial issue in both military and civilian trauma settings [12].

(a) Amputation, in the blast trauma scenario, should be considered at the far end of the debridement spectrum and not separate from it (Fig. 4.12).

(b) The basic rule is to retain what appears viable and to discard anything that does not.

(c) Completion of a partial amputation can occur anywhere along the echelons of care and need not occur at the patient's initial interface with surgical care (Fig. 4.13).

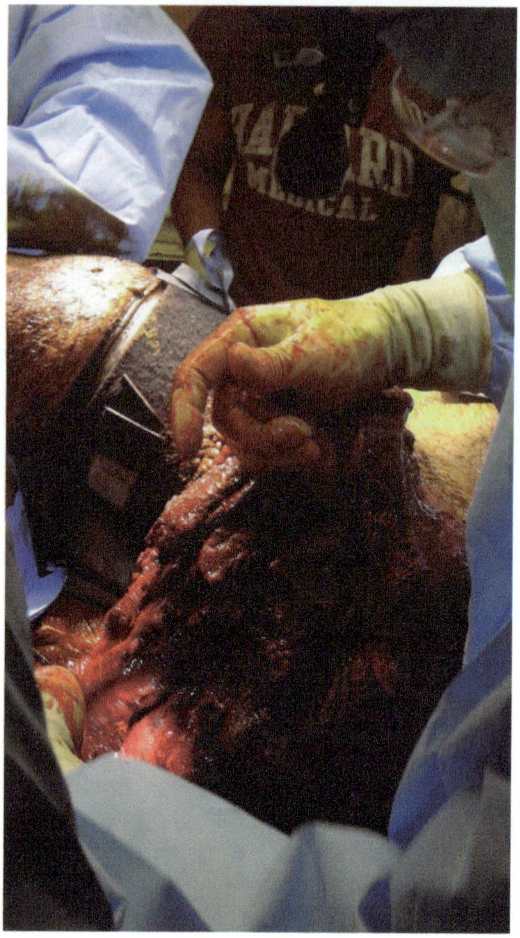

Fig. 4.12 Debridement of traumatic above the knee amputation with delivery of the bone end through the wound (Photo courtesy of Christopher S. Smith, M.D.)

Even though an extremity is likely headed toward eventual amputation, attempt to save any viable tissues, particularly skin and muscle that may be used in the coverage or reconstruction of other wounds.

(d) With advances in modern prosthetics, traumatic amputations should not be converted to standard level amputations (Fig. 4.14). A definitive level of amputation should not be committed to until the soft tissue envelope declares the limits of viability (Fig. 4.15).

(e) Completion of amputations should not necessarily occur through the sight of a

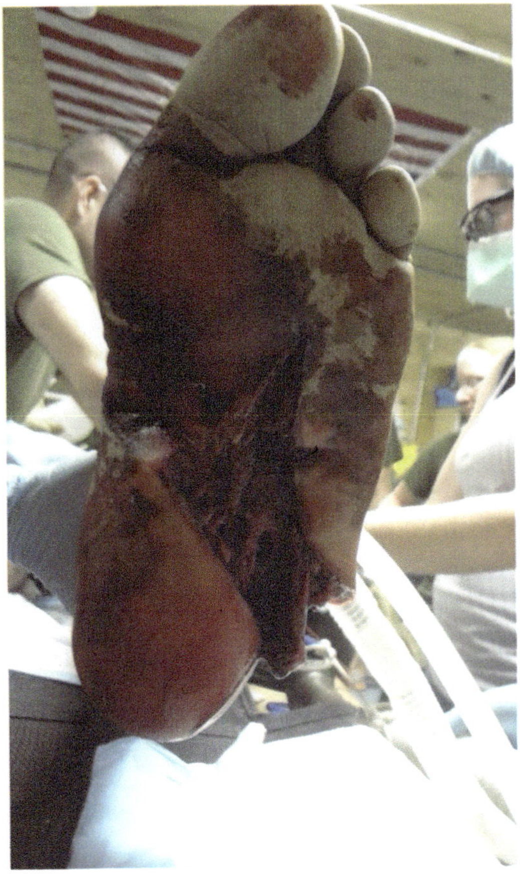

Fig. 4.13 IED blast involving typical wounding pattern of the foot with open fractures (Photo courtesy of Christopher S. Smith, M.D.)

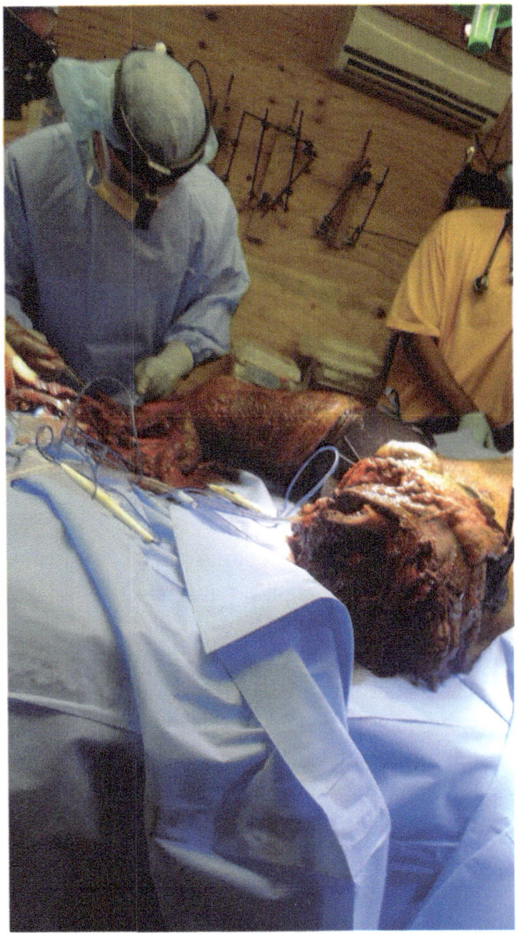

Fig. 4.14 IED blast with left traumatic above-the-knee amputation and right below-the-knee amputation (Photo courtesy of Christopher S. Smith, M.D.)

more proximal fracture. Fracture fixation can be performed above a traumatic amputation to conserve length as long as adequate soft tissue coverage exists distally [13]. Gordon et al. demonstrated a high complication rate to include infection and heterotopic ossification. However, fractures healed and the level of amputation salvage was successful in all patients. These patients had improved function secondary to preserved length. However, when treating local nationals in a third-world country, the orthopedist must be realistic about the standard of care the patient will receive once he or she enters the local healthcare system. Complex limb salvage or nonstandard amputation does not serve these patients well in most instances. These patients will also lack sophisticated prosthetics and rehabilitation support.

H. The energy imparted by blast trauma has a high propensity to stimulate heterotopic bone formation [8]. This often causes extreme discomfort and complications to the patient's rehabilitation course. This frequently results in the need for later surgical excision of the affected tissues and occasionally the need for a higher level of amputation.

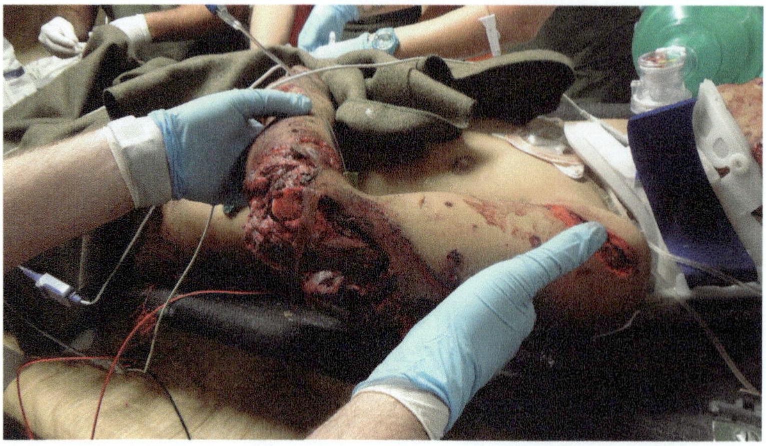

Fig. 4.15 IED blast with open upper extremity fractures (Photo courtesy of Christopher S. Smith, M.D.)

Conclusions

Blast trauma is ubiquitous in the theater of war. The force and devastation that is imparted to the victims of an HE explosion by the blast wave mechanism cannot be overemphasized. The amount of force imparted can be massive, is frequently fatal, and is responsible for a large percentage of the overwhelming injuries that are sustained during an IED attack. Understanding the mechanics of blast waves and their effects on physiology and soft tissues will help providers effectively manage these complex injuries [4]. Understanding of the secondary, tertiary, and quaternary mechanisms of blast injury trauma will aid in the evaluation and management of these patients throughout the spectrum of their initial care and through their often long and often complex rehabilitations.

References

1. Belmont Jr PJ, et al. Epidemiology of combat wounds in operation Iraqi freedom and operation enduring freedom: orthopaedic burden of disease. J Surg Orthop Adv. 2010;19(1):2–7.
2. Owens BD, Kragh JF, Wenke JD, et al. Combat wounds in operation Iraqi freedom and operation enduring freedom. J Trauma. 2008;64:295–9.
3. Ritenour AE, Baskin TW. Primary blast injury: update on diagnosis and treatment. Crit Care Med. 2008;36:S311–7.
4. Champion HR, Holcomb J, Young LA. Injuries from explosions: physics, biophysics, pathology, and required research focus. J Trauma. 2009;66:1468–77.
5. Covey DC, Born CT. Blast injuries: mechanics and wounding patterns. J Surg Orthop Adv. 2010;19(1): 8–12.
6. Hull JB, Cooper GJ. Pattern and mechanism of traumatic amputation by explosive blast. J Trauma. 1996;40(3):S198–205.
7. Andersen RC, et al. Dismounted complex blast injury. J Surg Orthop Adv. 2012;21(1):2–7.
8. Fleming M, et al. Dismounted complex blast injuries: patterns of injuries and resource utilization associated with the multiple extremity amputee. J Surg Orthop Adv. 2012;21(1):32–7.
9. Mamczak CN, Elster EA. Complex dismounted IED blast injuries: the initial management of bilateral lower extremity amputations with and without pelvic and perineal involvement. J Surg Orthop Adv. 2012; 21(1):8–14.
10. Kragh JF, et al. Practical use of emergency tourniquets to stop bleeding in major limb trauma. J Trauma. 2008;64:S38–50.
11. Alfieri KA, Elster EA, Dunne J. Resuscitation and blood utilization guidelines for the multiply injured, multiple amputee. J Surg Orthop Adv. 2012;21(1): 15–21.
12. Tintle SM, Keeling JJ, Shawen SB. Combat foot and ankle trauma. J Surg Orthop Adv. 2010;19(1):70–6.
13. Gordon WT, O'Brien FP, Strauss JE, Andersen RC, Potter BK. Outcomes associated with the internal fixation of long-bone fractures proximal to traumatic amputations. J Bone Joint Surg Am. 2010;92(13): 2312–8.

Foot and Ankle Injuries

5

Wade T. Gordon

Contents

BLUF (Bottom Line Up Front) Box

1. Combat-related foot and ankle injuries are typically high-energy injuries and are frequently open.
2. Wound debridement and temporizing stabilization, with fasciotomies as needed, are typically the extent of the frontline management of combat-related foot and ankle injuries.
3. Initial management should be performed with the ultimate reconstruction in mind and done in a manner as to not compromise that reconstruction.
4. With the exception of unreconstructible vascular injuries, sepsis, and obviously nonviable limbs, amputation should be deferred the patient arrives at a higher level of care.
5. When acute amputation is performed, length-preserving, open amputations are preferred, maintaining all tissue that would permit maintenance of the most distal functional final level of amputation.

5.1 Introduction

With the increasing use of ground-based explosive devices in the modern, complex combat environment, penetrating and high-energy injuries to the lower extremities have become

W.T. Gordon, MD
Department of Orthopaedic Surgery, Walter Reed National Military Medical Center, Bethesda, MD

Department of Surgery, Uniformed Services University of the Health Sciences, Bethesda, MD
e-mail: wade.t.gordon.mil@health.mil

L.B. Bone, C.N. Mamczak (eds.), *Front Line Extremity and Orthopaedic Surgery*,
DOI 10.1007/978-3-642-45337-3_5, © Springer-Verlag Berlin Heidelberg 2014

exceedingly common. These injuries often result either in the traumatic amputation of the distal portions of the lower limb or in severe, penetrating, or closed injury to the foot and ankle. Additionally, when structures collapse or large objects are displaced by blast injuries, crush injuries to the lower limb are common.

The principles guiding the initial management of severe combat-related foot and ankle injuries are similar to that in other regions of the appendicular skeleton. They do, however, present a very specific set of challenges worthy of independent discussion.

5.2 Principles of Initial Management

Foot and ankle injuries sustained in combat are likely to be just a part of a polytraumatic injury. Standard ATLS protocol should be followed, and addressing the extremity injury may initially be limited to hemorrhage control and revascularization of dysvascular limbs. The patient may present with tourniquets in place. Tourniquets should be removed in a controlled setting, with the required instruments and equipment necessary for the surgical control of any resulting hemorrhage.

Initial management should consist of debridement of open wounds, fasciotomies of the leg or foot as necessary, and temporizing stabilization with splint immobilization, external or percutaneous fixation as appropriate. The guiding principle in the early management is the understanding that the process of reconstruction starts immediately. Starting with the initial debridement, the surgeon should be mindful of the subsequent course of reconstruction of the injury and be careful not to "burn bridges" with respect to future surgical approaches, implant placement, or soft tissue coverage.

The standard principles for the debridement of traumatic, open wounds apply. Removal of gross contamination, followed by sharp, aggressive serial debridements of necrotic and devitalized tissue is performed, followed by wound irrigation. Tissue that is of questionable viability, but which would be potentially important in the future reconstruction of the limb, can be preserved and reevaluated at the time of the next debridement.

5.3 Fasciotomies

Fasciotomies of the leg are covered in detail separately in the text and should be performed when indicated. Fasciotomies of the foot are more controversial. Acute compartment syndrome of the foot is difficult to diagnose in the best circumstances, and the austere combat environment makes diagnosis even more difficult. Compartment pressure monitoring is not readily available, and pain out of proportion to that expected from an injury is difficult to assess in polytrauma from a blast injury. In the austere environment, the surgeon must rely on a high index of suspicion, along with the available clinical exam in the diagnosis of compartment syndrome of the foot.

The decision of whether or not to perform surgical releases of suspected compartment syndrome of the foot is controversial. Many surgeons believe that the sequelae of the surgical management of compartment syndromes of the foot are worse than the sequelae of a missed or intentionally neglected compartment syndrome. If surgical release is going to be performed, it should be done within the first 24 h. After this time, the benefits of release can be expected to be minimal and the likelihood of complications related to compartment release to be greater.

There are nine generally agreed upon compartments of the foot: the calcaneal, four interosseous, adductor, medial, lateral, and superficial compartments. Release of all nine compartments can be accomplished through three incisions: a medial plantar incision to release the medial, lateral, calcaneal, and superficial compartments. Two dorsal incisions are placed between the first and second metatarsals and between the fourth and fifth metatarsals. Through these incisions, the interosseous and adductor compartments are released (Fig. 5.1).

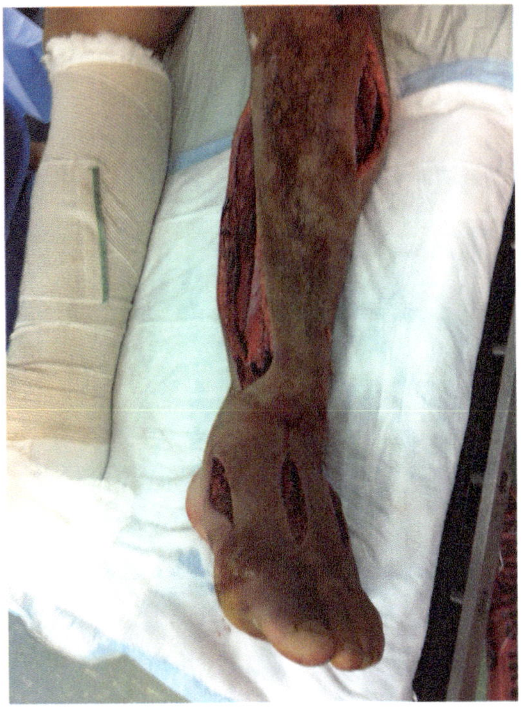

Fig. 5.1 Appropriate foot fasciotomies performed in conjunction with lower leg fasciotomies and debridement of an open tibia fracture. Note the location and extent of the two dorsal incisions, as well as the medial incision

5.4 Temporizing Stabilization

The choice of temporizing fixation depends not only on the injury pattern but also the time and resources available to the surgeon. External fixation provides optimum stability for the temporizing fixation of unstable fractures of the ankle, as well as the advantage of improved wound management. High-energy, axially unstable fractures of the ankle (such as pilon fractures) or unstable fracture-dislocations of the ankle are best managed initially with external fixation. In the mass casualty setting, however, or when external fixation is unavailable, these injuries can be initially managed with splint immobilization, while the patient is transported to a higher echelon of care.

Injuries of the foot are typically best managed with initial splinting, although percutaneous Kirschner wire fixation can be considered in certain fractures when resources permit.

5.5 Specific Injury Patterns

5.5.1 Pilon/Distal Tibia Fractures

High-energy fractures of the distal portion of the tibia are routinely associated with a compromised soft tissue envelope, prohibiting early, definitive fracture fixation. High rates of wound complications with early open reduction and internal fixation of pilon fractures have led to the mainstream adoption of a staged management protocol for these injuries. In addition to managing any associated wounds, initial temporizing external fixation should be performed with the goal of regaining the length and gross alignment of the limb.

Ankle-spanning external fixation is typically placed from the anteromedial tibia to the calcaneus in a "delta" frame configuration. Standard principles of external fixation stability apply, and temporizing fixation should be performed with the definitive reconstruction in mind – with respect to both the surgical approach and the implant placement. Whenever possible, pins should be placed avoiding open wounds. Two 5 mm half pins are sufficient in the tibia and are placed just off the medial side of the tibial crest. This avoids the problem of slipping off the crest during pin placement and also helps minimize the thermal injury to the tibia that can occur from placing the pins through the thick apex of the tibial crest. More than one point of fixation is required in the foot in order to provide the necessary control of the fracture in the anterior-posterior, as well as medial-lateral planes. A single calcaneal pin will tend to posteriorly displace the foot relative to the tibia along the vector of force application from the anterior aspect of the leg.

A transfixion or half pin is placed in the calcaneus. A second calcaneal pin, talar neck pin, or metatarsal pins can be placed. Talar neck pins should be discouraged in instances where fluoroscopy is not available or when the pin tract will interfere with the optimum surgical approach for definitive fracture fixation. First metatarsal pins are easily placed without fluoroscopy, and fifth metatarsal or third metatarsal pins can be added as necessary to adequately control the fracture (Fig. 5.2).

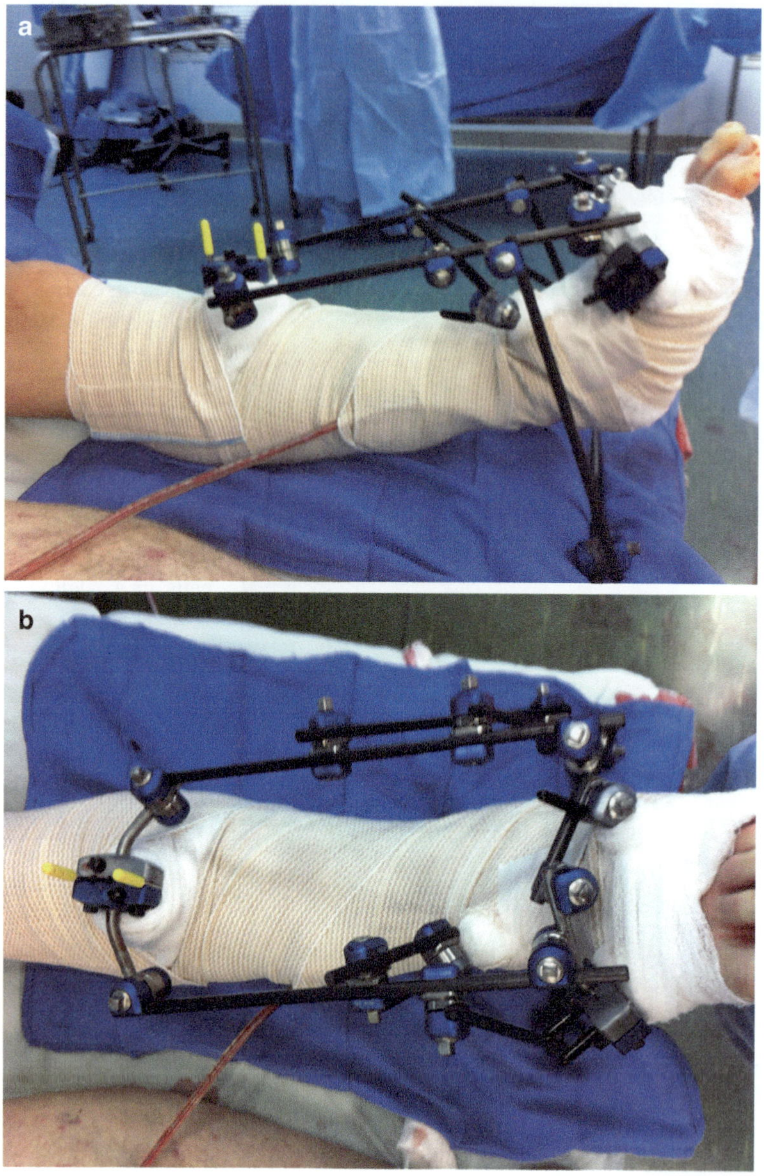

Fig. 5.2 (**a**, **b**) Example of an external fixator construct for a combined distal tibia and calcaneal fracture. Note the absence of a calcaneal pin secondary to fracture of the calcaneus. Stability is instead imparted through a pin in the talar neck and multiple metatarsal pins

5.5.2 Rotational Injuries of the Ankle

Lower energy ankle fractures and fracture-dislocations are common injuries in the combat environment. These injuries can also occur from a blunt mechanism as a patient is thrown or falls as the result of an explosion. Relatively stable, closed injuries can be treated with splint immobilization, and external fixation should be reserved for situations where wound management or gross instability makes splint immobilization less desirable. It should not be overlooked that ankle sprains also occur commonly during combat operations, as service members move with heavy loads, over uneven ground, and are often forced to do so quickly. These injuries should be treated in similar fashion to their civilian counterparts.

5.5.3 Crush Injuries to the Foot

Crush injuries to the foot often result in multiple fractures, open wounds, and foot compartment syndrome. Wound management and splinting of fractures are the normal treatment of these injuries in the austere combat environment. There should be a high index of suspicion for compartment syndrome of the foot, and compartment releases should be considered. The decision to perform compartment releases in the foot should be weighed against the risks of infection, wound closure/coverage difficulty, and future shoe wear difficulty that frequently complicate the surgical treatment of foot compartment syndrome.

5.5.4 Talus Fractures

Displaced fractures of the talar neck present a challenging problem in the austere combat setting. Non-displaced fractures should be treated with splint immobilization, with definitive surgical treatment deferred. With displaced talar neck fractures, the risks of open reduction and definitive fixation normally outweigh the risks of avascular necrosis and should be avoided. One exception would be an extruded talus causing skin compromise, though the surgeon must carefully consider the available resources, implants, and the degree of sterility possible in the surgical management of these injuries. If closed reduction is possible, percutaneous fixation and splinting can safely provide adequate stability as the patient is transferred to a higher echelon of care.

5.5.5 Calcaneus Fractures

Severely comminuted and open calcaneus fractures are a signature injury of service members sustaining a blast injury while seated in a vehicle. This occurs as a blast forces the floor of the vehicle up into the patient's foot, imparting a tremendous amount of energy to the heel in a very short time.

The reconstruction of these injuries is challenging, and many ultimately result in amputation. Combat-related calcaneus fractures are typically associated with severe soft tissue compromise precluding internal fixation. This is often the case with severe closed, as well as open, blast-related closed calcaneal fractures. In these cases, closed reduction and percutaneous fixation is the definitive management. The goal here is to restore the length, height, and alignment of the heel, while avoiding a prohibitively high rate of wound complications associated with a surgical approach through a severely damaged soft tissue envelope.

The earlier the correct length, height, and alignment of the heel can be achieved, the easier it will be and the better the chance of achieving a satisfactory reduction. It is appropriate in these complex calcaneal injuries to perform a closed reduction and percutaneous pinning of the fracture if it appears that a formal open reduction and internal fixation will either be substantially delayed or be even precluded altogether by the degree of compromise of the soft tissues of the heel. This is normally not possible until the patient has arrived at a level of care where surgical power instruments and fluoroscopy are available.

The patient should be placed in either the lateral or prone position, and an external fixator half pin can be placed in the tuberosity fragment of the calcaneus and used to reduce the tuberosity relative to the talus, as well as to the anterior process. Large diameter Kirschner wires (2.0–2.8 mm) can then be placed from the tuberosity fragment into the body and neck of the talus, as well as through the anterior process fragment into the cuboid (Fig. 5.3). In some cases, the talonavicular joint is also disrupted. This can make reduction of the calcaneus difficult, as the talus dorsiflexes unopposed with the reduction maneuver. In these instances, pinning the talonavicular joint will not only serve to stabilize that articulation but also help with reduction of the calcaneus.

In open calcaneus fractures, wound management is also a challenge. After a healthy soft tissue envelop is achieved, soft tissue coverage often presents a challenge. Free tissue transfer to the foot leads to problems related to flap bulk and difficulty with shoe wear. There are rotational flap options for some lateral wounds (extensor digitorum brevis rotational flap), but this flap is not routinely available. We must therefore balance the need for primary wound closure with the tenuous nature of the skin and subcutaneous tissue involved, as the soft tissues will retract very quickly, making future wound closure impossible. Even when future debridements are planned, making progress with skin approximation at each debridement is important. This should be done to the degree possible without putting the skin closure on so much tension that it creates more ischemia and necrosis (Fig. 5.4).

Conclusion

While the initial management of combat-related injuries to the foot and ankle is usually limited to debridement, wound management, and temporizing stabilization, it is a critically important step in the reconstruction of these challenging and severe injuries. The understanding that the reconstruction of the injury begins at the first debridement is of paramount importance and can make the difference between the success and failure of the course of limb reconstruction. Adhering to the principles of management for polytrauma patients, debridement, temporizing stabilization, and applying them to the patient's specific injury pattern, is the vital first step in that process.

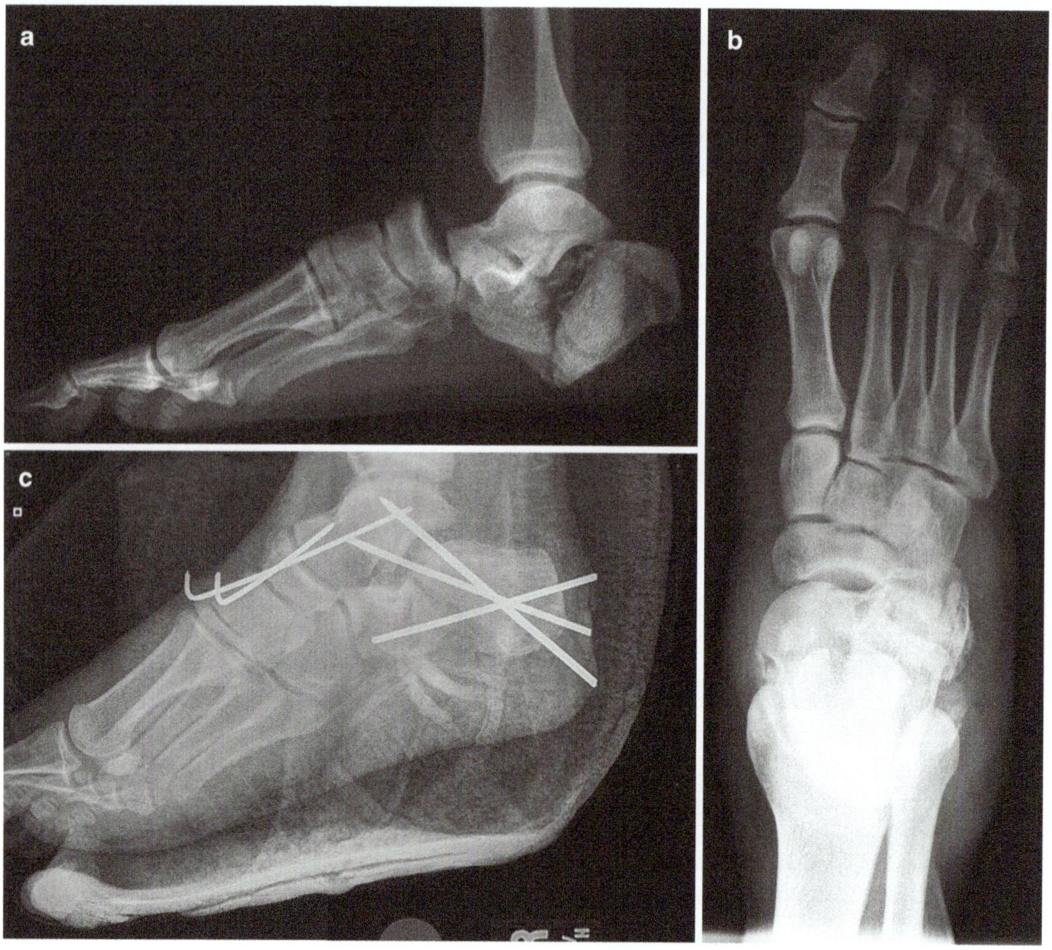

Fig. 5.3 (**a–d**) Open calcaneus fracture treated with primary closure of the plantar open wound, closed reduction, and percutaneous pinning. At 3 years post-injury, the patient has progressed to high-level competitive cycling, runs with the help of an AFO, and has not yet progressed to subtalar fusion

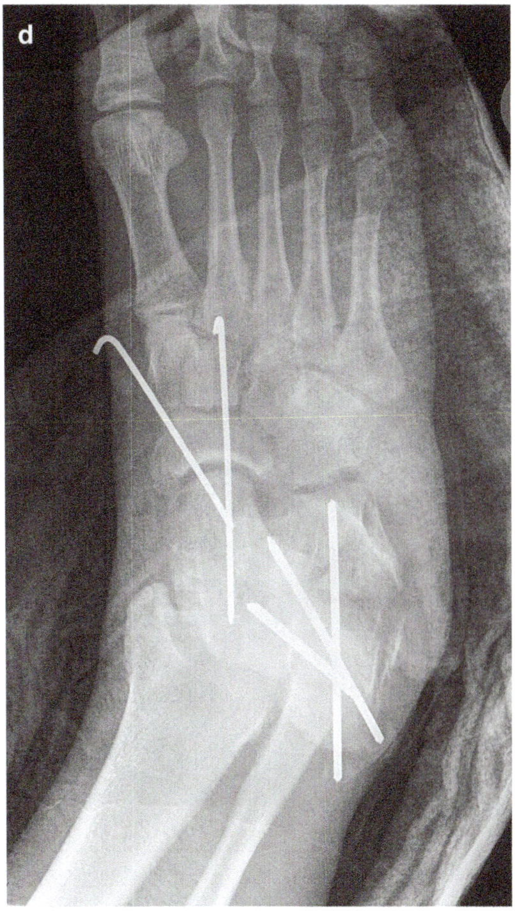

Fig. 5.3 (continued)

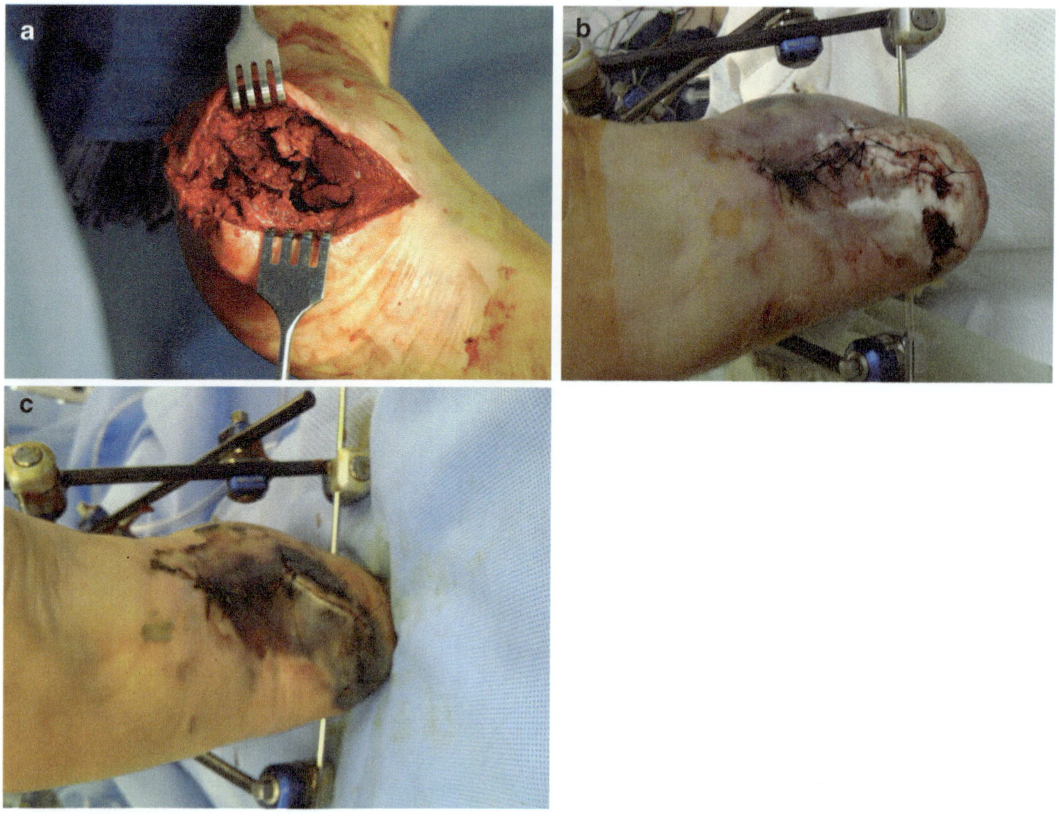

Fig. 5.4 (**a–c**) Plantar open wounds are most commonly encountered in the setting of mounted blast injuries. It is important to make progress with skin approximation before the retraction of the soft tissue makes primary wound closure impossible. This must be balanced against the tenuous nature of the soft tissues and the tendency to induce further ischemia and death of the skin flaps from excessive tension with primary wound closure

Tibia and Below-the-Knee Injuries and Fractures

6

Lawrence B. Bone and Robert E. Blease

Contents

BLUF (Bottom Line Up Front) Box

1. This is damage control surgery.
2. Know your anatomy; things are not always where they should be.
3. Irrigate, debride, and save any viable tissue in the OR.
4. Decisions about amputation rarely need to be done at the first operation; when in doubt, save and stabilize.
5. General surgeons should know how to place simple external fixator frames.
6. Tag nerve ends.
7. This is damage control; shunt vascular injuries.
8. When in doubt, do the fasciotomy.
9. Do not close wounds.

The highest percentage of injuries sustained by the soldiers in Afghanistan has been to the extremities. These injuries will be nothing like you have seen in civilian trauma, even if you worked in a level I trauma center (Fig. 6.1). The injuries are rarely isolated, so that you are managing a soft tissue and fracture of the tibia that is attached to a soldier with multiple other injuries. Whether you are in a role 2 or 3 medical treatment facility, this is damage control orthopaedics. Lessons learned over the past 12 years of this conflict are that these injuries are more extensive than initial impression with a greater risk for compartment syndrome, wound infection, and osteomyelitis than is seen in the

L.B. Bone, MD (✉)
Department of Orthopaedic Surgery,
SUNY at Buffalo, School of Medicine and
Biomedical Sciences, Buffalo, NY, USA
e-mail: bone@buffalo.edu

R.E. Blease, MD
Department of the Army, Medical Corps US Army,
Army Trauma Training Center, Ryder Trauma Center,
1850 N.W. 10th Avenue, Miami, FL 33136, USA

L.B. Bone, C.N. Mamczak (eds.), *Front Line Extremity and Orthopaedic Surgery*,
DOI 10.1007/978-3-642-45337-3_6, © Springer-Verlag Berlin Heidelberg 2014

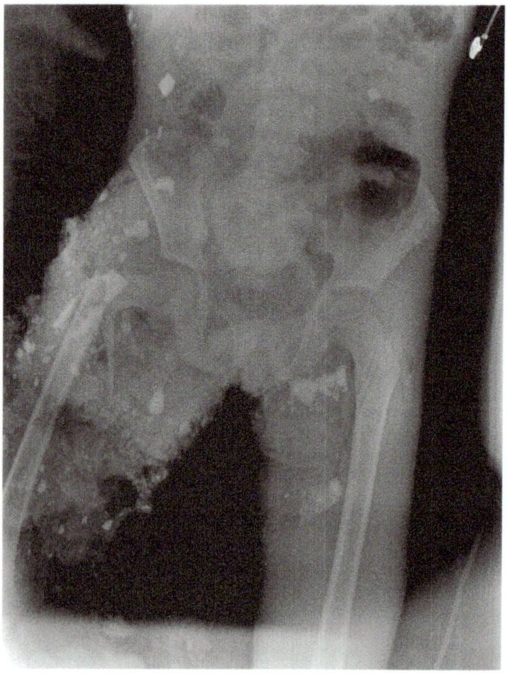

Fig. 6.1 IED blast, showing the upward energy and force that is created

civilian world. There is no place for definitive stabilization of these high-energy injuries at the time of initial treatment and debridement. Most, if not all, surgeons who routinely manage these injuries throughout the echelons of care have regularly experienced frustrations due to the prolonged period of wound evolution and the expanded zone of injury that is caused by high-energy blast trauma. Not infrequently have experienced surgeons agonizingly watched the soft tissue envelope die over well-placed internal fixation, even after the wound appeared to have stabilized and the soft tissue envelope begun to recover. Caution is critical to avoiding further salvage procedures, bailout strategies, and worse yet amputation or amputation to a higher level. Local national patients treated in a military level II or III facility likewise benefit from judicious management of their injuries. Sterility, surgical instruments, imaging, and technically qualified assistance are not often found at near the same level as we routinely expect in our regular practices. This limits what we can and should try to do in managing the injuries in this subset of our patients. A well-placed external fixator can be easily removed by local physicians, or auto mechanics, long after we have departed the area, whereas an intramedullary nail, plate, or especially a locking plate cannot be so easily removed. Cases have been reported of the need for amputation in order to remove an infected locking plate. Keep this in mind when considering primary management strategies and secondary implications for these patients. Further, external fixation imparts minimal further damage to the soft tissue envelope; allows for continued, staged wound management; and provides the least risk of catastrophic osteomyelitis.

6.1 Mechanism

While past wars and conflicts have seen the use of land mines and booby traps, the use of the improvised explosive device (IED) has been the signature injury for the Afghan and former Iraqi conflict (Fig. 6.2a–c). The wounds created by these high-energy explosive devices are much more extensive with damaged and devitalized soft tissue much higher in the extremity than one would initially think. Chapter 4 on blast injuries in this book goes into details of the mechanism of injury from the IED.

Gunshot injuries from high-powered military weapons still occur. The advanced body armor that the infantry soldier and marine wear helps protect the torso, but their extremities are still exposed. These fractures are therefore, by definition, high-energy open injuries.

While the dismounted infantryman is exposed to the IED, the mounted soldier is exposed to rollover and IED explosion of their vehicle which can result in open as well as closed lower extremity fractures.

6.2 Initial Management

These extremity injuries will almost certainly have tourniquets placed by the medic at the point of injury (Fig. 6.3). It is important to remember that the first responder soldier or field medic

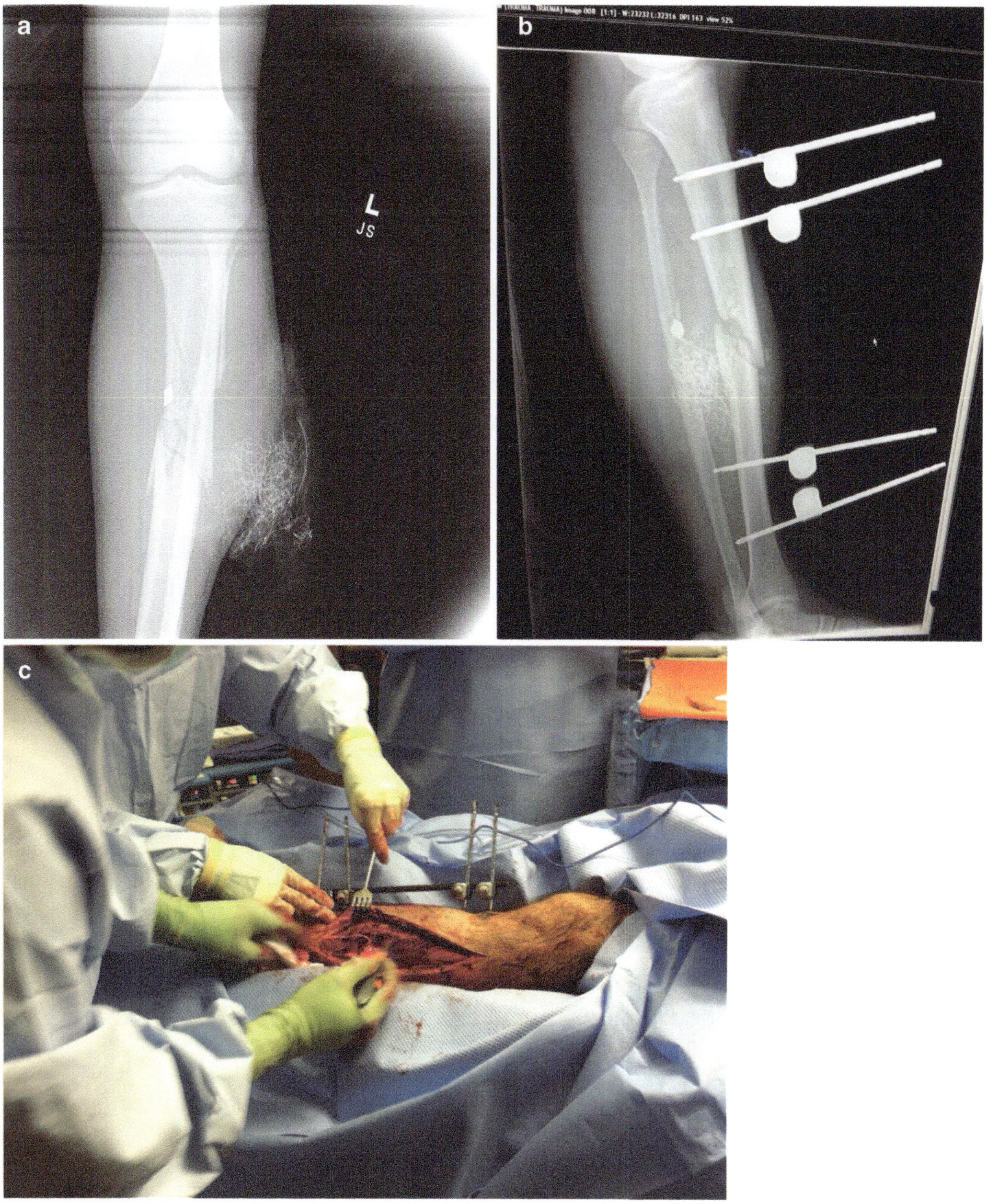

Fig. 6.2 (a) X-ray of gunshot injury to tibia with fracture. (b) Postoperative X-ray with anterior external fixation frame. (c) Tibia with external fixator having fasciotomy

is trained to apply the tourniquet if bleeding is evident. This does not necessarily indicate that arterial bleeding has been identified. Often these tourniquets have been placed under unfavorable combat conditions, sometimes by inexperienced soldiers or medics who are working under considerable stress. It is the surgeon's responsibility to make an accurate assessment of the true nature of the injury. Following initial ATLS protocols with resuscitation and initial evaluation, the tourniquet should be slowly released to see if it is needed for control of major bleeding. This is

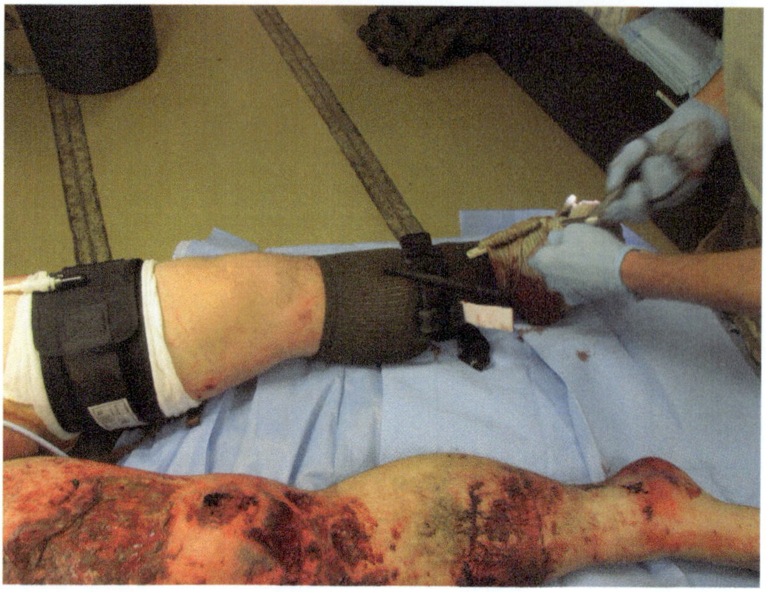

Fig. 6.3 Tourniquet for lower extremity IED injury

especially true if the patient is not going immediately to surgery at which time the tourniquet would be replaced with a pneumatic tourniquet.

It is further critical to establish the timeline of the injury. Remember that after 6 h of warm ischemia, time cell death begins to occur at a variable rate due to prolonged hypoxia. After 8 h, cell death occurs on a massive scale resulting in the likely need for amputation, damage to kidneys, and permanent disability. The key point here is to keep an eye on the clock. In a mass casualty or high-stress situation, or a situation where patients with higher surgical priorities have delayed the care of a patient with a tourniquet in place, time can quickly slip by, potentially resulting in unnecessary complications. Isolated below-the-knee injuries may not be the initial priority for the OR and a tourniquet should not be left on if not needed. If, however, a tourniquet is removed, remember that a patient who is undergoing further resuscitation may yet break loose a clot and begin to bleed significantly. An extremity that has had a tourniquet removed should not be covered or neglected pending surgery for this reason.

Antibiotics should be given as early as possible. Based on the injury to the patient for lower extremity and soft tissue and open fractures, cefazolin 1–2 g. IV Q8H or similar antibiotic should be given initially. Consult the updated clinical practice guidelines for antibiotic administration once you arrive into theater.

6.3 Debridement

Debridement of these high-energy injuries tends to involve much more of the extremity than similar civilian injuries. Extension of the traumatic wounds proximally and distally needs to be conducted in order to determine the extent of muscle and soft tissue damage and contamination throughout the zone of injury, as well as to facilitate proper debridement and irrigation. With land mines and buried-type IED mechanisms of injury, energy is forced in an upward direction and contamination is therefore blown along tissue planes higher into the extremity than would be normally anticipated. Debris will be found far from the obvious zone of injury. Therefore, it is paramount that the entire lower extremity be radiographically checked for contamination and surgically explored, debrided, and irrigated as appropriate.

Whether to amputate or not is a crucial question that the deployed surgeon will likely face during an initial debridement, with significant anxiety on the part of the surgeon, in many situations. Remember that amputation is just the far end of the spectrum of debridement. Maintaining standard debridement principles will lead the surgeon to the correct answer. Remove obviously dead or massively contaminated muscle, fat, or other soft tissues. Remove avascular tissue if flow cannot be returned. Remove non-articular bone that has been stripped of soft tissue attachment. Do try to preserve major cartilage containing bone fragments. Even though an extremity is heading for obvious amputation at some point, try to preserve as much tissue as possible for later reconstruction, especially in the multiply injured patient. Bone and tissue from a late amputated extremity may serve as graft and flap tissue for another extremity. Preserve as many options as possible for the patient's definitive care.

With blast injuries in particular, the amount of raw bleeding surfaces are massive. Blood loss will be encountered and can be difficult to control. Even as orthopaedic surgeons, we must respect the patient's physiology. Remember to replace at least what is lost during the primary and subsequent debridements. Much good information has been developed and published during the current conflicts on the use of blood products in a 1:1:1 ratio of PRBCs, fresh frozen plasma, and platelets. Manage your patients' physiology. Being able to discuss physiological parameters and indicators with your general surgery colleagues will allow you to be a better proponent for your patient and the management of his extremity wounds, which will greatly impact his eventual outcome.

With high-energy gunshot injury, the cavitation effect of the bullet is likewise larger than the injury itself. Therefore, extending the skin incision and exploration of the entire traumatic wound area for devitalized tissue and debris is necessary.

When possible this debridement should be done with the tourniquet deflated to better evaluate the viability of the muscle and soft tissue.

6.4 Vascular Nerve and Tendon Injuries

Vascular injuries to the lower extremity are covered in a separate chapter in this book. It is essential to identify major vascular injuries of the lower extremity when possible prior to debridement and stabilization of the lower extremity fracture. These vascular injuries need to be explored with the help of your general surgical colleague. With an ischemic foot, determination needs to be made if the vascular injuries have the potential to be re-vascularized, and if so then temporary shunting should be performed in this damage control situation. With a viable foot and a single vessel injury, this vessel should be identified, ligated, and tagged.

Nerve injuries found on exploration of the lower extremity should not have attempted primary repair. The proximal and distal ends of the nerve should be identified, tagged, and documented for further evaluation at a level 4 or 5 treatment facility.

Tendon injuries are common with these high-energy blast injuries; it is rare that a tendon is lacerated such that a primary repair can be performed. Debridement of devitalized tendon should therefore be performed, with the expectation that, if possible, a tendon graft can be placed at a later date.

6.5 Stabilization

Stabilization of the tibia following debridement can be performed with either an external fixation frame or with splinting if the injury will allow. Most of these injuries will be best managed with external fixation. Remember that this is damage control and that the fixator will be replaced and or augmented at subsequent medical treatment facilities. The fracture does not have to be perfectly reduced; the fixator is placed as a stabilization device for the extremity both to control movement of the fracture and to stabilize the soft tissue. Anterior tibial frames are generally adequate with crossing the knee or ankle as needed depending on the location of the fracture. Distal superior malleolar fractures are best managed with delta frames across the ankle, and proximal tibia fractures are adequately stabilized with frames spanning the knee (Fig. 6.4a, b).

Splinting of closed lower energy tibia fractures or stable gunshot injuries can be performed.

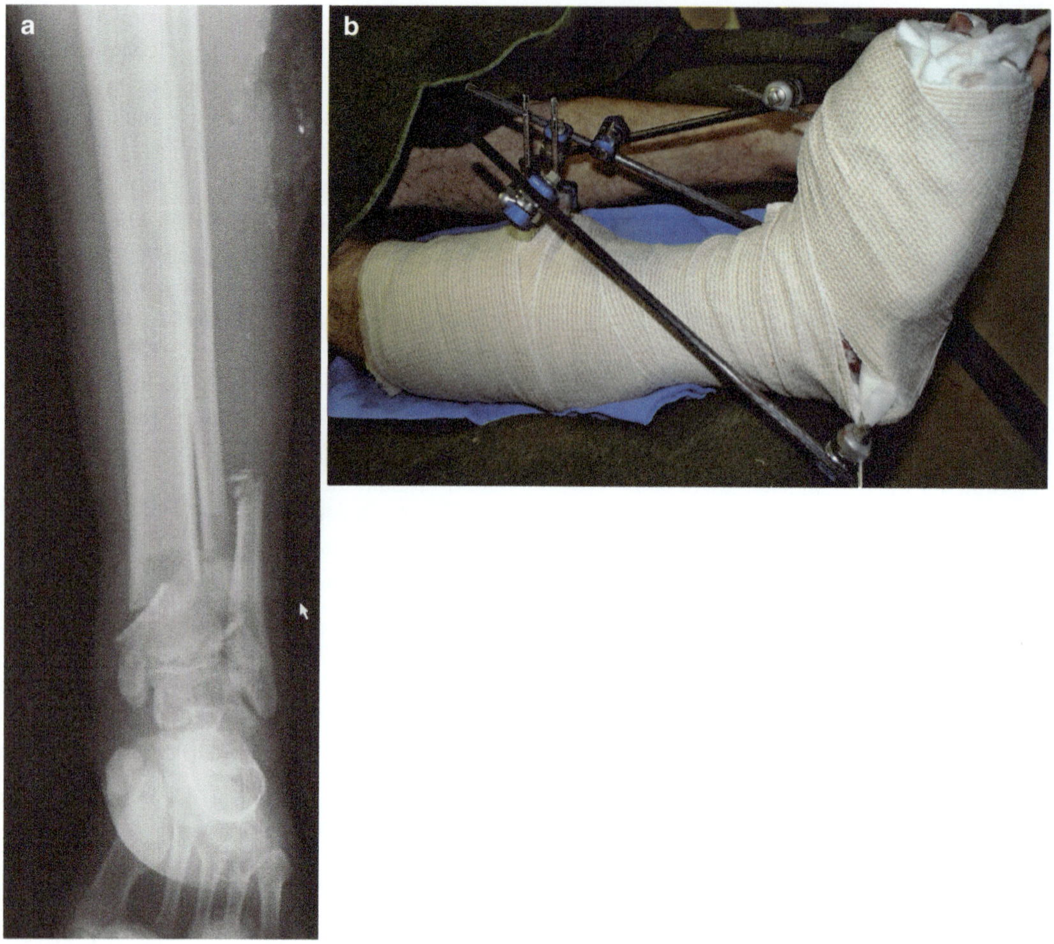

Fig. 6.4 (**a**) Distal tibia fracture from rollover accident. (**b**) External fixation spanning distal tibia fracture across the ankle. Two anterior Schanz pins and a centrally threaded Steinmann pin through the calcaneus

It is best to avoid plaster behind the heel to avoid skin breakdown in this region.

In the lower extremity the most practical insertion position for Schanz pins is straight anterior. At most level 2 medical treatment facilities, image intensifiers are not available so that placement of the Schanz pins needs to be done by feel. Make a stab incision large enough to avoid skin tenting. With the self-tapping and self-drilling pin available in the combat external fixation packets, no predrilling is necessary. When placing the Schanz pin by hand, create a little davit in the bone by tapping the Schanz pin. This is to avoid the pin moving down the crest to the anterior tibia. It may be necessary to start the Schanz pin in a more medial to lateral direction until the first threads catch the bone at which time the pin can be straightened anteriorly. You will feel the pin go through the proximal cortex because of the difficulty with the hand drill. Once it enters the medullary canal, the effort becomes easier until you hit the far cortex at which time you want to count 8–10 complete turns and stop. Place the two pins proximal and distal with the greatest span possible followed by placement of the two near pins using the pin clamps as guides. Following completion of the frame, it is important to get AP and lateral X-rays of the tibia mainly to check that the Schanz pins have been properly placed in the posterior cortex all the way through but not extending too far into the soft tissue to

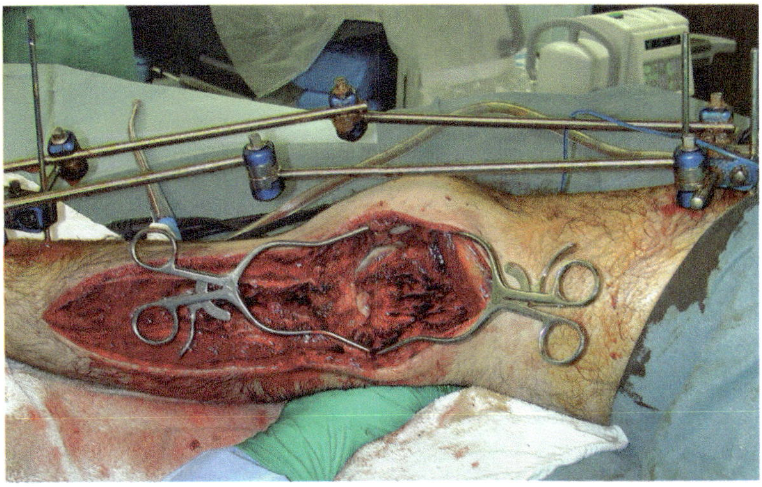

Fig. 6.5 Proximal tibia and distal femur fracture spanned with an external fixator across the knee with fasciotomy incision

thwart potential soft tissue damage. Adjustment can be made as needed. Remember that this is a temporizing stabilization device for bone and soft tissue. While proper alignment is something to strive for, exact reposition of the fracture and excessive length are not necessary. Freely span the knee for proximal tibia fractures. Remember that anteriorly placed thigh pins have a narrow window of safety between the branches of the femoral nerve superiorly and the knee capsule inferiorly (Fig. 6.5). A laterally based thigh construct is safest, but tends to be bumped and to get caught on straps, lines, and clothing during transport. An anterolaterally based thigh construct is perhaps the best compromise for this patient population.

6.6 Compartment Syndrome

The use of fasciotomy is outlined in a separate chapter of this book. These high-energy injuries are much more susceptible to compartment syndrome even with the extensive open nature of the injury. Since these patients will be lost to follow up by you and will be medevac'd either by helicopter or fixed wing to subsequent treatment facilities, liberal use of fasciotomies is recommended when indicated (Fig. 6.2c). Prophylactic fasciotomies should be constrained either to those patients with a high index of suspicion or to those patients who have sustained a vascular injury that has subsequently been repaired or shunted. An unnecessary fasciotomy is highly preferred to missing a compartment syndrome and ending up with its intendant and devastating consequences.

6.7 Final Thoughts

Remember that the initial trip to the operating room is for debridement, skeletal stabilization, and vascular control. You are working in a fairly austere environment where life, limb, and eyesight are the key. Beware of personal projects. Our primary tenet is to "first, do no harm." Though the surgeon may be bored near to death and the need in the community for quality orthopaedic care great – remember that when we leave, the patient must be further managed with the resources at hand. Unless we have passed on the technology and training to the local national community to do this, then the patient may be far better served by limiting the degree of our treatment to what may be successfully managed in the wake of our departure.

Remember that resources are scarce and time is important. Thorough debridement is your goal, but this will be the first of multiple debridements and if a question of viability exists in a somewhat under-resuscitated patient, leaving the tissue for evaluation at a second debridement may be a good choice.

You are the entry level into the echelons of care system. Your decisions can set the patient up for success or for failure throughout the course of his injury management and recovery. Doing too much can be as devastating as doing too little. Talk to and know the surgeons at your left and right limits and those that will be accepting your patients at the next echelon of care. A working relationship and one-on-one communication is the absolute best way to optimize care for the combat-injured patient throughout his transport and care within the deployed military health-care system.

Transtibial Amputation

7

Benjamin K. Potter

Extreme remedies are very appropriate for extreme diseases

–Hippocrates

Contents

BLUF (Bottom Line Up Front) Box

1. In the absence of traumatic amputation, the decision to amputate often does not need to be made at the first debridement. The same is true of the salvage of a compromised knee joint when the ability to salvage a transtibial level is in question. However, do not retain grossly nonviable or unsalvageable parts or extremities.
2. Initial amputations should be *open and length-preserving* – salvage all viable tissues for late reconstructive options.
3. Avoid the temptation to make your initial cuts the final ones, "pick" the definitive amputation length or level at presentation, or craft formal, described flaps at the initial debridement
4. Do not sacrifice residual limb length or amputation level by amputating through proximal fractures; these can often be salvaged through late utilization of conventional (and unconventional) techniques
5. Early management of vessels should include secure ligation regardless of bleeding or thrombosed status.
6. Early management of nerves should leave them long and near the wound edge to permit appropriate late traction neurectomy after the final amputation level is determined.

B.K. Potter, MD
Department of Orthopaedics, Walter Reed National Military Medical Center, Bethesda, MD, USA

Department of Surgery, Uniformed Services University of Health Sciences, Bethesda, MD, USA
e-mail: benjamin.k.potter.mil@health.mil

L.B. Bone, C.N. Mamczak (eds.), *Front Line Extremity and Orthopaedic Surgery*,
DOI 10.1007/978-3-642-45337-3_7,

7. Definitive management of vessels is secure distal ligation; definitive management of nerves is traction neurectomy well proximal to the terminal residual limb.
8. Robust, healthy distal soft tissues, securely stabilized to the bone, maximizes residual limb health and function, is the desired endpoint, and is achievable in virtually all transtibial amputations.

7.1 Introduction

First and foremost, any major amputation should be approached as a reconstructive procedure and not an ablative one, a treatment failure of attempted limb salvage, or simple consequence of severe injury. That said, in the field hospital setting of the recent conflicts where explosive blasts represent the most common mechanism of injury, a majority of the amputations seen or "performed" will be traumatic in nature – the distal limb is already gone or nearly so, and the difficult decisions center more on what to do with regard to what remains of the extremity rather than debate regarding the feasibility of successful limb salvage versus immediate amputation (discussed elsewhere).

Education has been described as what remains after you have forgotten what you have learned – as such, if the reader remembers and internalizes only two things from this chapter, the first should be to begin with an open, length-preserving amputation in any post-traumatic setting. The second should be to pursue a stable, robust distal soft tissue envelope by any means necessary. Doing the former minimizes initial procedure time, prevents immediate infection, and conserves maximal viable tissue; this preserves subsequent reconstructive options for the patient and the next surgeon, whether that surgeon is at a higher echelon of care or – in the case of local national care or humanitarian aid – you. The latter maximizes the definitive quality of "your amputation" and the patient's ultimate residual limb – the soft tissue envelope is at least as important as the osseous platform in these regards.

As discussed elsewhere in this text in greater detail, initial procedures following severe explosive blast or other combat-related multisystem trauma focus on damage control resuscitation and surgery. The initial priorities are therefore aggressive whole blood or 1:1:1 component resuscitation, control of hemorrhage, provisional stabilization of pelvic and long bone fractures and dislocations, and debridement of gross contamination. As the saying does – the first procedure at any emergency is to take your own pulse – if this is your first time treating combat or natural disaster trauma, do not be overwhelmed (Fig. 7.1). Get your bearings, move quickly and decisively, and do what you think is right.

7.2 Initial and Early Management

For limbs at risk, in the absence a patient in extremis requiring a prolonged procedure (i.e., revascularization) for provisional limb salvage, the decision to amputate generally does not need to be immediate. In a controlled setting with a stable patient, one may in fact consider initial limb salvage as the ultimate tissue-sparing amputation – all possible, injury-specific reconstructive options remain (e.g., fillet of foot flap, turnup plasty). Conversely, initial amputation may be considered the most definitive form of debridement possible, and grossly nonviable and unsalvageable terminal extremities should undergo completion of amputation in order to avoid sepsis, reperfusion syndrome, and rhabdomyolysis or risk severe hemorrhage during transport due to failure of a doomed vascular reconstruction.

Initial amputations and debridement of traumatic amputations should be performed in an *open, length-preserving fashion.* Open implies simply that no attempt is made to definitively close the amputation at the time of the initial

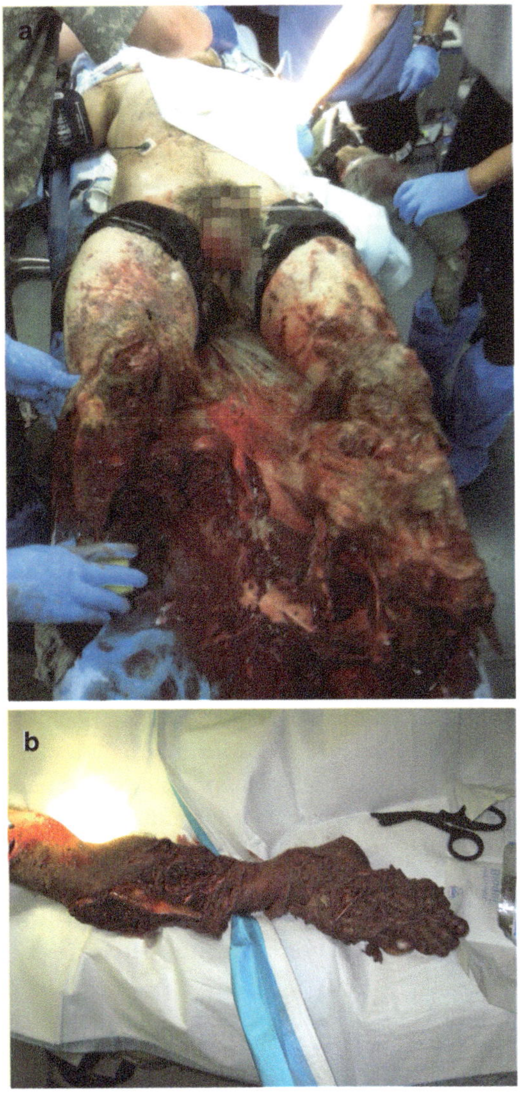

Fig. 7.1 (a) Preoperative photograph of an allied soldier with bilateral lower extremity traumatic amputations and systemic polytrauma following a dismounted complex battle injury from an improvised explosive device blast. Rapid, multidisciplinary resuscitation and surgery was successful at both saving the patient's life and salvaging the mangled left upper extremity. (b) Preoperative photograph of the mangled distal right lower extremity of a local national Afghan civilian following an untoward encounter with a roadside improvised explosive device. Despite the apparent soft tissue compromise and contamination, a transtibial amputation was successfully maintained and healed without complication following serial debridements

procedure. Length-preserving means to spare viable bone and, more importantly, soft tissue for assessment of delayed viability during subsequent procedures, thus maintaining all practicable coverage alternatives ranging from atypical closures, rotational soft tissue flaps, or simply skin graft donor sites. Guillotine and open circular amputations are antiquated techniques held over from bygone eras also known for crude anesthesia, rudimentary asepsis, and limited hemorrhage control. These techniques compromise important residual limb length and sacrifice local coverage options, leaving essentially only further shortening via proximal revision and free tissue transfer as the available alternatives for definitive closure. Even if you are operating by flashlight on a makeshift stretcher in a tent or trailer, you can do better. Moreover, a well-performed open, length-preserving amputation takes minimally more time to complete than a guillotine amputation. Do not, therefore, either perform a guillotine amputation in efforts directed at efficiency or attempt to craft "textbook" definitive soft tissue flaps or guess the final level of amputation during this index procedure. Simply save what is viable and debride the rest (Fig. 7.2).

As implied by this chapter on transtibial amputations, every effort should be afforded to salvage a viable knee joint and preserve a transtibial level. Transtibial amputees have better function, less energy expenditure for ambulation, faster self-selected walking velocity, and easier prosthetic socket fitting than most of the more proximal counterparts. Therefore, if the proximal tibia is present and viable, the knee joint should be preserved even if adequate local soft tissue for definitive coverage appears to be lacking. Local rotational flaps and/or formal free tissue transfer may prove feasible at higher echelons of care (Fig. 7.3a, b). Likewise, do not amputate through proximal fractures or joints as a matter of convenience or simplicity. Proximal fractures can generally be later definitively stabilized through either conventional or unconventional means, union achieved, and a more distal amputation level successfully maintained (Fig. 7.3c).

Vessels should be securely and individually ligated at the index procedure in order to prevent late hemorrhage, regardless of whether they appear thrombosed or in spasm at the initial

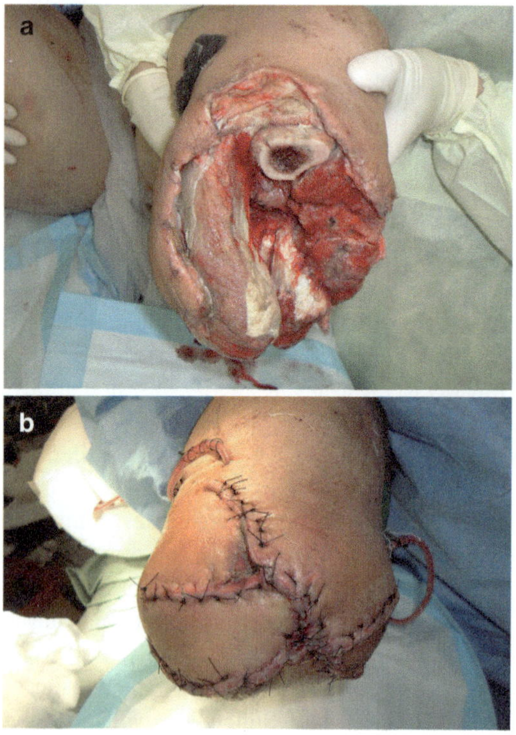

Fig. 7.2 Intraoperative photographs of an open, length-preserving transtibial amputation (**a**) and the subsequent "flaps of opportunity" closure (**b**) that the initial preservation of atypical flaps made possible

debridement. Nerves, however, should be left long at the initial amputation in order to ensure that an appropriate traction neurectomy can be performed at the time of attempted definitive closure once the final amputation level is determined. Early neurectomy makes the nerves more difficult to locate during subsequent procedures and may mislead the definitive surgeon to believe the nerves have already been appropriately dealt with, when in reality he or she is closing at a level well proximal to the initial neurectomies.

Leave the residual limb wound open. There are essentially no indications for closure at the time of initial amputation following severe trauma. Even in the setting of a "clean," "textbook" amputation proximal to the zone of injury, you risk little by packing and returning to the operating suite 24–48 h later for reassessment and closure, whereas premature closure risks much, particularly for patients with limited access to subsequent care. Even in combat and disaster conditions, a second-look procedure is better than risking the likely late infection after the patient is lost to follow-up or transferred to another facility, which may or may not have greater resources and wherewithal than your own.

Rather, pack the wound with antibiotic-impregnated polymethylmethacrylate beads, a negative pressure wound therapy "VAC," or moist gauze soaked in Dakin's solution or sterile saline, and place a compressive dressing. Compressive dressings should always extend well proximal to the knee joint for transtibial amputations to prevent progressive telescoping and a tourniquet effect or increased distal swelling following transfers and knee motion. Depending on your patient's nationality, the weather, and the isolation of your setting, your patient may or may not be "on the ward" in 24–48 h. If they are, return to the operating room in the light of day for a repeat debridement and irrigation. Tissue viability declaration is almost universally delayed following blast injuries, and you may also be able to perform a more thorough and diligent debridement after the patient has been adequately stabilized and resuscitated.

7.3 Definitive Management

If you find yourself in a setting where you, in fact, are both the patient's first and definitive surgeon (e.g., local national allied, insurgent, enemy prisoners of war, and civilian humanitarian care), then definitive closure should be attempted in due course. Generally, this should be attempted when the patient is physiologically stable and the residual limb wound appears healthy following a 2nd or 3rd (or 4th or 5th…) operative debridement. Despite constant emphasis on preserving viable tissue and options, it is naturally permissible to make definitive cuts and closure decisions during this definitive procedure.

First, select the level of bone transection that the local soft tissue envelope can practicably support in a robust fashion. Avoid overly long definitive residual limbs. The general rule of thumb for

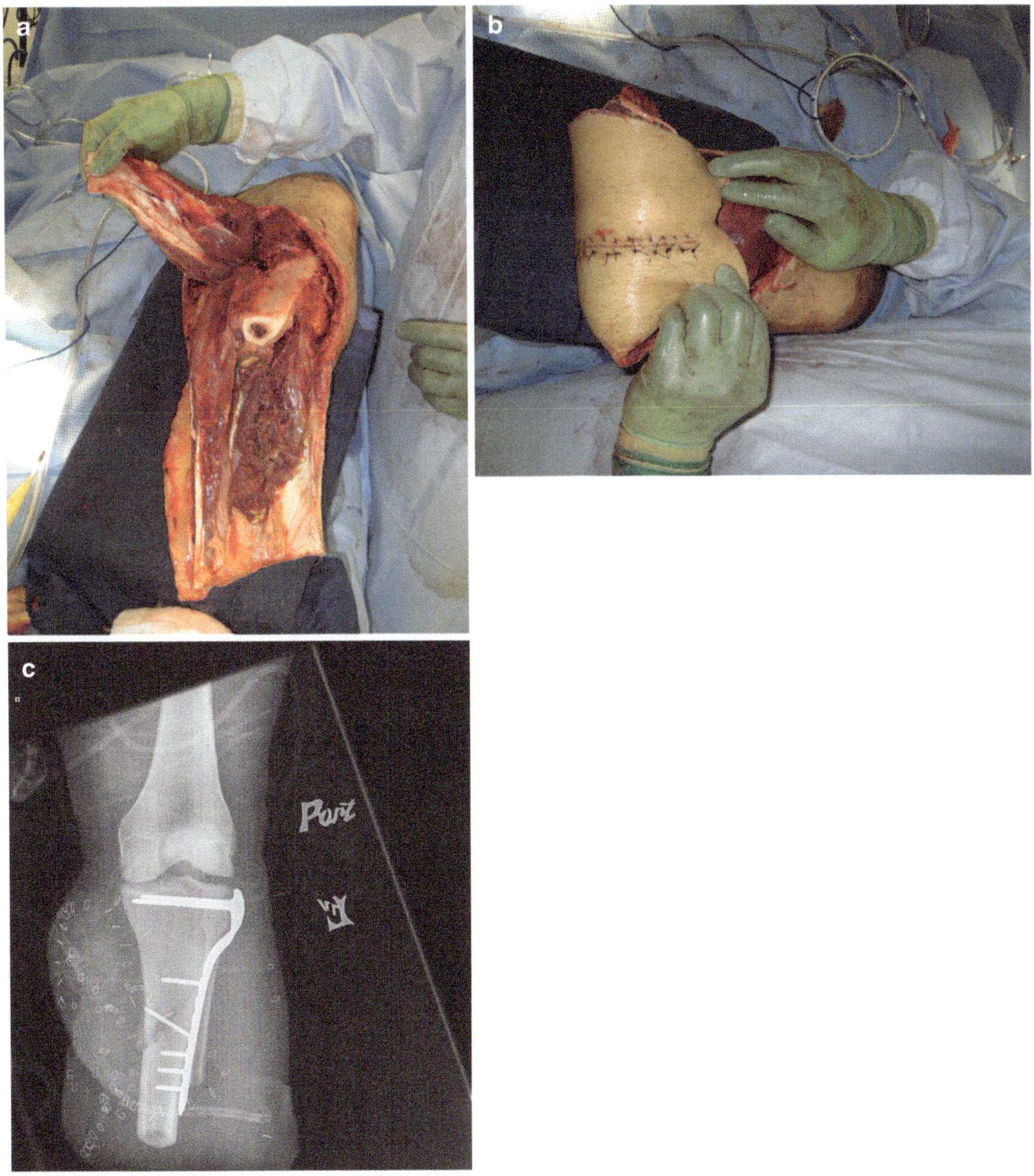

Fig. 7.3 Intraoperative photographs during (**a**) and following (**b**) a medial gastrocnemius flap to augment deficient proximal medial soft tissue coverage of a long transtibial amputation and cover an associated type IIIB proximal tibia fracture. An initial open, length-preserving amputation made this length and level salvage possible, and the lateral gastrocnemius and soleus have been maintained to maximize distal padding after rotation of the flap. An anteroposterior postoperative radiograph (**c**) of the same residual limb demonstrating the results of open reduction and internal fixation of the fracture and rotational flap coverage. Stabilization of the fracture, rather than amputating through or proximal to it, permitted salvage of an optimal (~16 cm) transtibial amputation length. The fracture healed uneventfully despite an early infection of the distal residual limb

optimal transtibial amputation length is 2.5 cm of residual tibial length per 30 cm of patient height, but often you can add 1–1.5 cm to this. This generally falls with 13–16.5 cm regardless of height – leaving both adequate room for a socket and prosthesis and robust distal padding provided

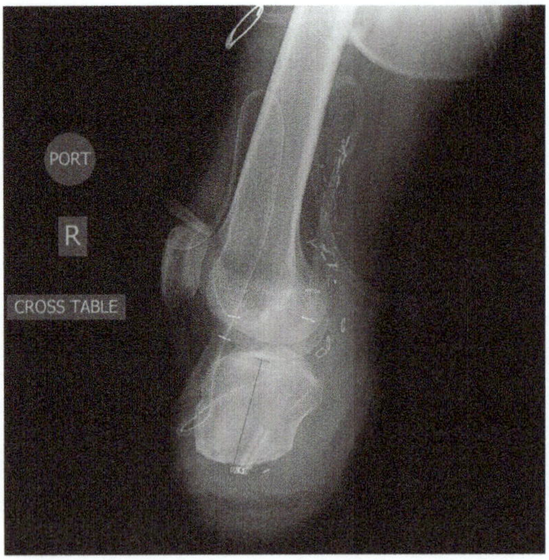

Fig. 7.4 Lateral radiograph of a short transtibial amputation just distal to the tibial tuberosity, thus preserving both the critical patellar tendon and the hamstring insertions. The patient was a functional ambulatory in a conventional prosthesis and a limited runner, despite his short residual limb which required a free tissue transfer to salvage his knee joint and amputation level

that conventional flaps are available. The absolute minimal length for a functional transtibial amputation is around 5 cm of tibia, at or just distal to the tibial tuberosity (Fig. 7.4). For short transtibial amputations with<8 cm of residual tibia, removal of the prominent fibula can be considered with suturing of the biceps/lateral collateral ligament complex to the adjacent proximal tibia or securing them with an intraosseous suture anchor, if available.

Given the largely unproven, theoretical functional benefit and documented higher rate of complications and reoperations in combat-injured patients, there are no good indications for the creation of a distal bridge synostosis (i.e., the Ertl procedure and modifications thereof) in a disaster and developing country scenario, particularly given the likely rudimentary prosthesis options available. However, in cases of overt tibiofibular instability or proximal tibiofibular dislocation, proximal stabilization can and should be performed with a screw, wire, or suture bridge following indirect or direct reduction (Fig. 7.5) in order to avoid problems with symptomatic fibular instability, distal fibula prominence, or knee instability. For longer, standard length transtibial amputations, this technique is preferred to fibulectomy to avoid concerns regarding the biceps and posterolateral corner as well as simplifying prosthetic socket fit by producing a more cylindrical, less conical, distal residual limb.

Smooth sharp bone edges and bevel the anterior tibia to avoid painful erosion of the soft tissue envelope over time. Resect redundant periosteum to prevent late bone spur formation. Leave the residual fibula, when present, 1–1.5 cm shorter than the tibia to reduce prominence, and bevel the terminal fibula slightly in a distal-anteromedial to proximal-posterolateral direction so that the least prominent area of distal fibula sits most proximal in the residual limb.

Redo individual vascular ligations of the posterior tibial, anterior tibial, and peroneal arteries and veins at the time of definitive closure. At a minimum, the initial ligatures are colonized after remaining in a contaminated wound for some period, and often they are far less secure at this point than you or the surgeon before you ostensibly left them.

Perform proximal traction neurectomies during the final procedure, at the time of planned definitive closure. All named nerves – the tibial, superficial peroneal, deep peroneal, saphenous, and sural – should be identified and cut well proximal to the terminal residual limb. If in the proximal one third of the leg, look for both median and lateral/fibular contributing branches of sural nerve. If the residual tibia is shorter than 6–8 cm and no meaningful anterior compartment musculature remains, consider common peroneal neurectomy proximal to fibular neck to guard against a large, superficial symptomatic neuroma in this region.

Local gastrocnemius rotational flaps are simple useful, adjuncts for inadequate regional soft tissue coverage (Fig. 7.3). When practicable (i.e., the soft tissue deficit is anterior or lateral), rotation of the lateral gastrocnemius muscle belly is preferred, as the more robust medial head is

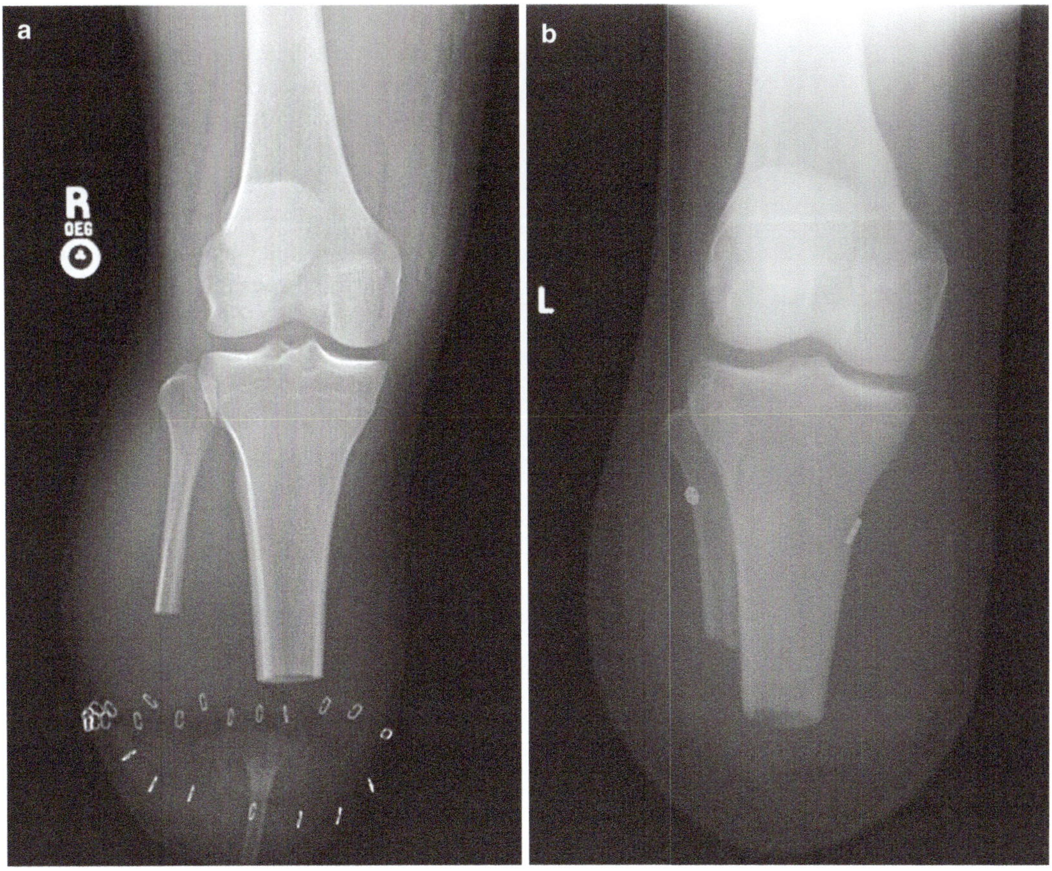

Fig. 7.5 Anteroposterior radiographs demonstrating tibiofibular instability and diastasis due to disruption of the interosseous membrane and proximal tibiofibular joint before (**a**) and after (**b**) reduction and stabilization. A commercial suture bridge device has been utilized, but such stabilization can also be performed utilizing a screw, buried wire, or transosseous suture tied over a post or bone bridge

thus retained for distal terminal padding. Split thickness skin grafts perform reasonably well on residual limbs provided they are placed over healthy, robust muscle tissue. Skin grafts are a poor coverage option over bone or periosteum and will inevitably break down under the best of conditions. As such, if this must be performed and local rotational flaps are not a viable alternative (and free tissue transfer microsurgical expertise is not available), further shortening or revision to a more proximal amputation level should be considered. Despite the benefits of transtibial amputation touted elsewhere and herein, a more proximal amputation with excellent coverage will almost always outperform a more distal amputation with a marginal or chronically ulcerated soft tissue envelope.

Likewise, despite the emphasis on retaining viable soft tissue for atypical closure and coverage options, a posterior myofasciocutaneous flap, when present, remains the preferred alternative for distal transtibial amputation coverage. For thin patients, the soleus muscle is retained; for larger patients with bulky or grossly edematous posterior flaps, the soleus may be resected or beveled. The gastrocnemius tendon and/or fascia are attached just proximal to the tibial bevel through drill holes or, alternatively,

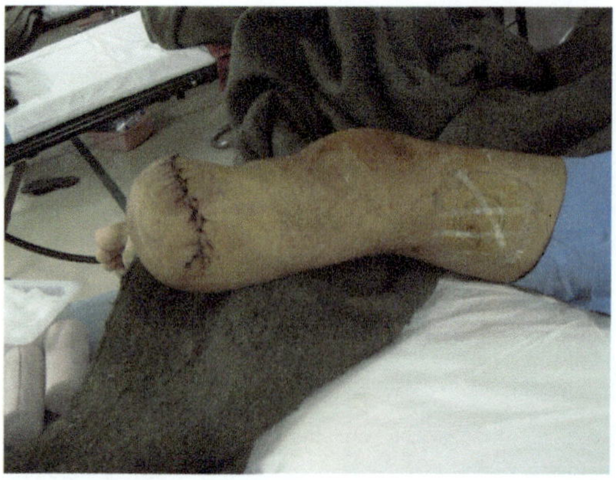

Fig. 7.6 Clinical photograph of the closed transtibial amputation of an Afghan National Army service member who sustained a severe hindfoot blast injury due to an improvised explosive device. A conventional, robust posterior myofasciocutaneous flap was available and utilized for distal residual limb coverage

sewn to the anterior tibial periosteum. This is reinforced with absorbable suture medially and laterally to the soleus bridge/medial tibial periosteum and stout anterior compartment fascia, respectively. Closure should be performed over a deep drain – a Penrose or similar passive device will do if closed suction drainage is unavailable – and skin flap elevation and resulting devascularization are minimized. The skin is closed with an absorbable dermal layer followed by cutaneous monofilament vertical mattress or Allgower-Donati stitches to maximize skin edge eversion and apposition (Fig. 7.6). The addition of topical antibiotic powder to the wound and incisional, low setting negative pressure wound therapy remain useful, if unproven in this setting, adjuncts to ward against deep and superficial infection and early wound dehiscence, respectively. Sutures are removed 2.5–3 weeks postoperatively. If prosthetic support is available through local or nongovernmental organization support, the patient may be fit with their initial prosthesis once the soft tissue envelope is adequately healed, generally at 4–6 weeks after definitive closure.

Vascular Injuries of the Lower Extremity

8

Rodd J. Benfield

Contents

BLUF (Bottom Line Up Front) Box

1. Clinical signs of arterial injury are classified as hard and soft signs. Hard signs go to the operating room. Soft signs require further evaluation.
2. The presence of a peripheral pulse does not exclude significant vascular injury. Investigate objectively with ABIs.
3. Angiograms can be extremely helpful in patients with multiple penetrating injuries to an extremity (i.e., IED, shotgun blast). Know the technique of on-table angiography. A single-shot angiogram may miss arterial injuries. Perform two views when possible.
4. Pneumatic tourniquets are extremely helpful in getting proximal control of arterial injuries.
5. Don't blindly clamp a bleeding wound. Direct pressure or pneumatic tourniquet is preferable.
6. Locally infused heparinized saline is preferable to systemic heparinization in multiply injured patients.
7. Always consider the use of a vascular shunt.
8. Mark the proximal and distal ends of the vein graft before you remove it to ensure the interposition graft is placed in the "reversed" position to accommodate the venous valves.

R.J. Benfield, MD
Department of Surgery, United States Navy, US Naval Hospital Guam, PSL 490, FPO, AP 96538, Guam, USA

Department of Surgery, Uniformed Services University of the Health Sciences - F. Edward Hebert School of Medicine, Bethesda, MD, USA
e-mail: rodd.benfield@med.navy.mil

L.B. Bone, C.N. Mamczak (eds.), *Front Line Extremity and Orthopaedic Surgery*, DOI 10.1007/978-3-642-45337-3_8, © Springer-Verlag Berlin Heidelberg 2014

9. Try to attend a cadaver-based vascular exposure course.
10. An atlas of anatomic exposures in vascular surgery is invaluable.

8.1 Introduction

Injury to the lower extremity encompasses approximately one quarter of all modern combat injuries. These most frequently result from blast or penetrating mechanisms. Oftentimes, these injuries are devastating and involve massive destruction to nerve, vessel, bone, and soft tissue resulting in a nonviable extremity. The ability to definitively control extremity hemorrhage and rapidly restore perfusion can certainly save a life and possibly improve the chance of salvaging a viable extremity.

8.2 Clinical Signs of Vascular Injury

Clinical signs of arterial injury are classified as hard and soft signs. Hard signs include pulsatile external bleeding, expanding or pulsatile hematoma, absent distal pulses, presence of a thrill or bruit, ischemic limb, and shock in the presence of a suspected vascular injury. Patients with hard signs require operative intervention. Soft signs include small, stable hematomas and a history of bleeding, minor bleeding, and proximity injuries. These patients require further evaluation.

8.3 Investigations for Vascular Injury

The presence of a peripheral pulse does not rule out arterial injury. Measurement of the ankle-brachial index (ABI) using Doppler pressures is an excellent initial study to investigate suspected arterial injury. An ABI <0.9 is suspicious for arterial injury and is an indication for further investigation. A patient with penetrating or blunt trauma who has a normal distal pulse exam and ABI ≥ 0.9 does not require further evaluation.

Color flow duplex ultrasonography is an excellent study to investigate for arterial injury but is not commonly available in the combat setting.

CT angiography (CTA) is available at many larger level 3 facilities and can give valuable information regarding missile trajectory as well as possible direct visualization of arterial injury. In facilities with CT capability, multiply injured patients often have CT scans of the head, neck, and torso, and the addition of extremity CTA may be valuable. As always, an unstable patient or a patient with hard signs of vascular injury is better served in the OR than the CT scanner.

Arteriography remains the gold standard for evaluating vascular injury. Common indications for arteriography are multiple penetrating injuries with an abnormal vascular exam (i.e., shotgun or IED injuries) and most blunt vascular injuries. Although formal angiography may be available at select level 3 facilities, the technique of on-table angiography is good to know (Fig. 8.1).

The on-table angiogram is usually performed in the operating room. 25–50 cc of non-diluted contrast is introduced into the proximal artery via a 20G Angiocath. The contrast is injected as quickly as possible and the x-ray is taken just before the syringe is empty. Both AP and lateral views should be obtained to avoid missing significant injuries.

8.4 Techniques for Proximal Control

Control external bleeding immediately (Fig. 8.2). Direct pressure is the best initial move. Avoid blind placement of clamps in a bloody field. As intuitively tempting as it may be, it rarely works and frequently damages surrounding structures. A pneumatic tourniquet may be invaluable provided the injury is distal enough to accommodate its placement. It can then be inflated and deflated at will in the operating room. Field tourniquets are best removed in the operating room and replaced with pneumatic tourniquets if necessary (Fig. 8.3).

Whereas direct pressure and use of tourniquets suffice in a distal injury, vascular injury in

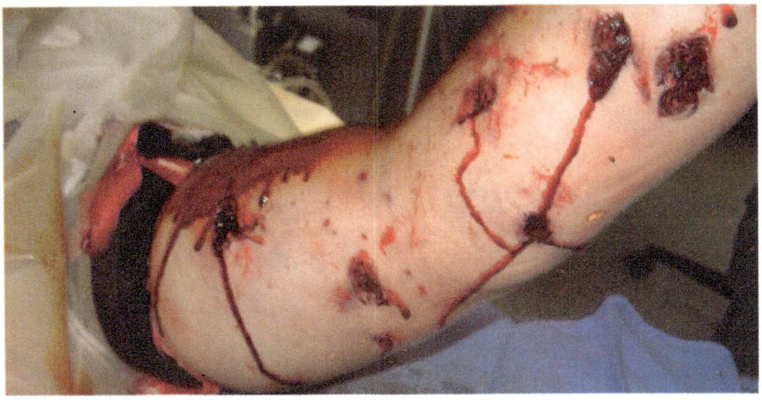

Fig. 8.1 Multiple penetrating injuries to the extremity with abnormal ABI. CT angiography or on-table angiography provides valuable information for these injuries

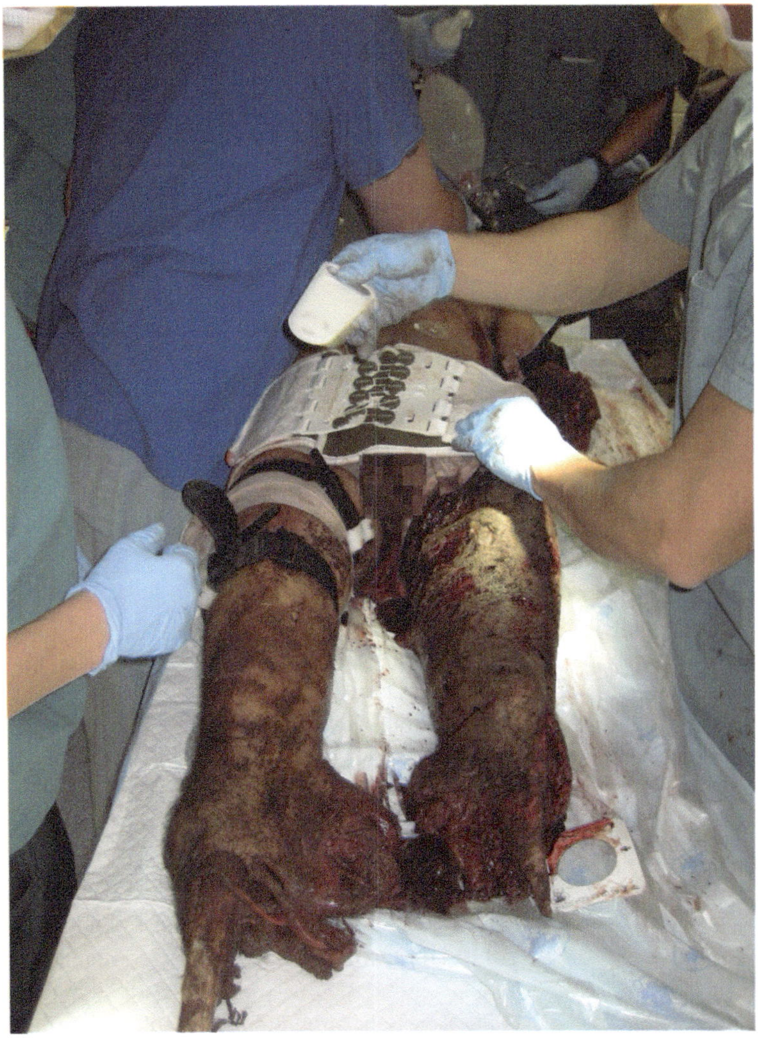

Fig. 8.2 Patient shown with field tourniquets providing proximal control of hemorrhage

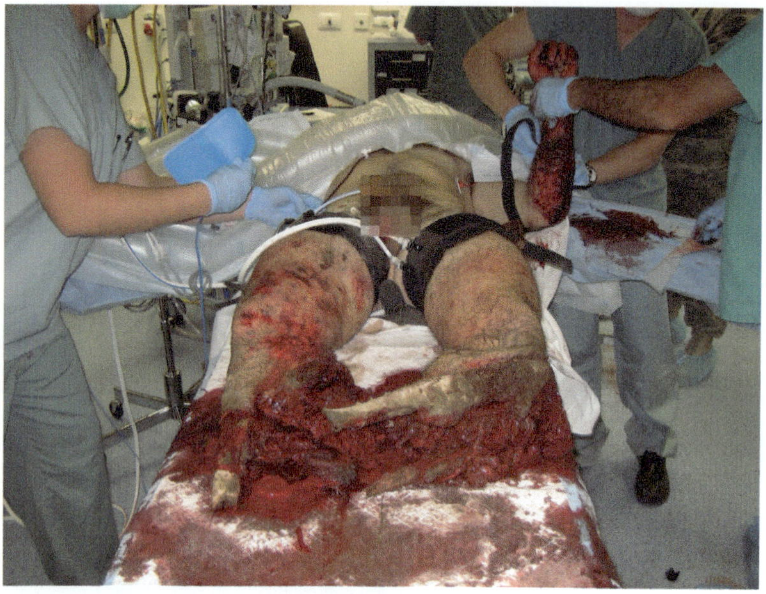

Fig. 8.3 Patient shown after placement of pneumatic tourniquet and removal of field tourniquets in the operating room

the proximal groin poses a significant challenge. Three solutions to this problem exist: laparotomy, retroperitoneal control, and direct exploration.

8.4.1 Laparotomy

If there is an urgent indication for laparotomy, then proceed. Control of the external iliac artery is straightforward from this exposure.

8.4.2 Retroperitoneal Control

Retroperitoneal control can be obtained via an oblique lower abdominal incision placed 2 cm parallel to and above the inguinal ligament ("hernia incision"). The external and internal oblique muscles are divided. The dissection is carried down to the preperitoneal fat, and the peritoneal sac is gently retracted cephalad and medially to expose the psoas muscle and overlying external iliac vessels. This approach can take some time and should not be attempted in an exsanguinating patient.

8.4.3 Direct Control in the Groin

Direct control of the femoral vessels through a vertical groin incision is the fastest and most straightforward approach. A vertical incision is made over the femoral pulse or halfway between the anterior superior iliac spine and the pubic tubercle extending cephalad over the inguinal skin crease. First open the fascia lata and feel for the arterial pulse.

Next open the femoral sheath to expose the artery. Stay anterior in the peri-adventitial plane. Next control the common femoral artery (CFA), superficial femoral artery (SFA), and profunda femoris artery. The CFA and SFA are easily encircled with vessel loops for control. Do not attempt to dissect out the profunda femoris artery as the lateral femoral circumflex vein crosses in front of it and behind the SFA at their confluence and leads to difficult to control bleeding if injured.

There is a marked changed in the diameter of the CFA marking the takeoff of the profunda and SFA. To control the profunda, pass a vessel loop from lateral to medial behind the CFA and above the takeoff of the profunda. Then pass the loop behind the SFA from medial to lateral below the takeoff of the profunda. Then repeat the procedure and you will have successfully encircled the profunda femoris artery.

In a difficult groin with a large hematoma, the vessels may not be identifiable. In this case, you may divide the inguinal ligament to expose the more proximal lying external iliac vessels.

Alternatively, you may divide the inguinal ligament transversely 2 cm above and parallel to its inferior edge to enter the preperitoneal space to identify and control the external iliac vessels.

At this point consider the physiology of the patient, the overall trauma burden, the number of other casualties, and your resources available to determine if damage control with shunt placement is the most reasonable option.

8.5 General Techniques for Repair of Arterial Injuries

After controlling external hemorrhage, prep and drape the bilateral extremities to allow contralateral saphenous vein exposure for conduit. Prep both feet in the neutral position to allow palpation or Doppler evaluation of distal vessels. A longitudinal incision placed directly over the injured vessel allows for proximal and distal extension for vascular control.

Once proximal and distal control is obtained, debride injured vessels to grossly normal appearing tissue. Pass balloon (Fogarty) catheters proximally and distally to remove residual thrombus. Do not pass these catheters more times than absolutely necessary as they injure the endothelium and predispose to thrombus formation. Flush proximally and distally with heparinized saline solution (2,500 units heparin mixed in 250 cc 0.9 %NS or 5,000 units in 500 cc 0.9 %NS).

8.5.1 Shunt Placement

Consider shunt placement which will allow time for wound debridement, irrigation, and damage control resuscitation. Additionally, external fixation of fractures while the artery is shunted will provide a stable platform with the extremity reduced to its normal length upon which to perform a definitive vascular repair.

Shunt placement is performed as follows. Proximal and distal control is obtained with Silastic vessel loops or Rumel tourniquets. The proximal vessel is released to flush clot and the shunt is advanced into the vessel proximally. A distal thrombectomy is performed with a balloon catheter (Fogarty catheter). Heparinized saline is then flushed distally and the shunt advanced distally and secured. Confirm distal perfusion. When using Argyle shunts, I find it useful to tie a silk suture around the middle of the shunt to use as a position reference once the shunt is placed and the distal ends can no longer be visualized.

8.5.2 Vessel Repair

All vascular repairs must be done without tension. Prior to final closure, the vessel should be forward and back bled to clear air and debris. In injuries to both artery and vein, repair the artery first in order to minimize ischemic time followed by venous repair.

Venous injuries are repaired in a similar fashion to arterial injuries. In a stable patient venous repair should be performed as it may enhance the arterial repair. In a tenuous patient, however, venous repair is not mandatory and the vein may be ligated. If this is performed, loose placement of a compression dressing distal to the injury will help control the resultant edema and its long-term sequelae.

Lateral suture repair may be used for minimal, low-velocity wounds that, when repaired, don't compromise the lumen >25 % or result in a thrill. Stab wounds may be amenable to this type of repair, but beware of using this for high-velocity injuries as the injury to the surrounding vessel often requires debridement.

Patch angioplasty may be performed for larger, tangential, low-velocity wounds. Autogenous vein is preferred over synthetic in traumatic injuries.

End-to-end anastomosis is often mentioned but rarely is this technique able to be performed without tension in the young, healthy, spasmed arteries encountered in combat injuries.

8.5.3 Interposition Grafts

Interposition grafts are frequently required to repair combat injuries. Autogenous vein graft is preferable to prosthetic graft for repair of extremity vascular injury due to the high rate of contamination and risk of infection. The contralateral greater saphenous vein is preferred as this preserves ipsilateral venous outflow through the superficial venous system when the deep veins are injured. *Take care to mark the proximal and distal ends of the vein prior to harvesting to ensure the proper "reverse" placement required to accommodate the venous valves.* Marking the anterior surface with a skin marker along the length of the vein prior to harvesting also helps to ensure the graft is not twisted when it is implanted.

Exposed vein grafts will desiccate and lead to blowout, so it is essential that these grafts be covered with soft tissue. The sartorius and gracilis muscles may be mobilized and used to cover grafts. Alternatively, the grafts may be tunneled subcutaneously through uncontaminated tissue.

8.6 Exposure and Repair of Specific Injuries

8.6.1 Superficial Femoral Artery (SFA)

To best expose the SFA, slightly abduct and flex the hip and gently flex the knee. Support this positioning with stacked sterile towels placed under the lateral surface of the knee. Place your incision longitudinally along the superior border of the sartorius muscle taking care to avoid injuring the GSV. Retract the sartorius (anteriorly in the upper and middle thigh and posteriorly in the lower thigh) to expose the fascia between the adductor magnus and vastus medialis muscles which defines the popliteal canal (Hunter's canal). Open this fascia to encounter the neurovascular bundle containing the SFA.

8.6.2 Popliteal Artery

For trauma, the safest and fastest exposure to the popliteal artery is the medial approach. Position the leg as described above for the SFA exposure. Make a longitudinal incision along the anterior border of the sartorius muscle between the sartorius and vastus medialis muscles. Incise the deep fascia just posterior to the femur to enter the popliteal fossa and palpate the popliteal artery against the posterior surface of the femur. Preserve the paired, adherent popliteal veins.

To expose the distal popliteal artery, make a second incision 1 or 2 cm behind the proximal posterior border of the tibia. Incise the deep fascia and retract the gastrocnemius and soleus muscles posteriorly to enter the distal popliteal space, again taking care to avoid injury to the popliteal vein.

At this point, an interposition graft may be placed, tunneled in the intracondylar position, and the remaining popliteal artery excluded with proximal and distal ligation.

If exposure of the entire popliteal artery is required, connect the two incisions and take down the tendinous attachments of the sartorius, gracilis, semimembranosus, semitendinosus, and medial head of the gastrocnemius muscles to expose the entire popliteal neurovascular bundle (Fig. 8.4).

8.6.3 Below the Knee

Since only one of the three arteries to the lower leg is required to maintain perfusion, an angiogram may provide important information to guide the operative plan. With one or two arteries intact, control of bleeding is all that is needed. Tedious exposure and repair of these small vessels is not necessary in this situation. Angiographic embolization, if available, is an excellent modality for hemorrhage control if one or two of the three vessels remain intact.

If exposure and repair is required, start in the distal popliteal fossa as described above and trace the arteries distally. Retract the gastrocnemius muscle posterior to expose the soleus muscle, and detach it from the posterior tibia to trace the distal popliteal to the takeoff of the anterior tibial artery, and then follow the tibial peroneal trunk to the takeoff of the more superficial posterior tibial and deeper peroneal arteries.

Finally, the anterior tibial artery may be found in the mid and distal lower leg through the anterior

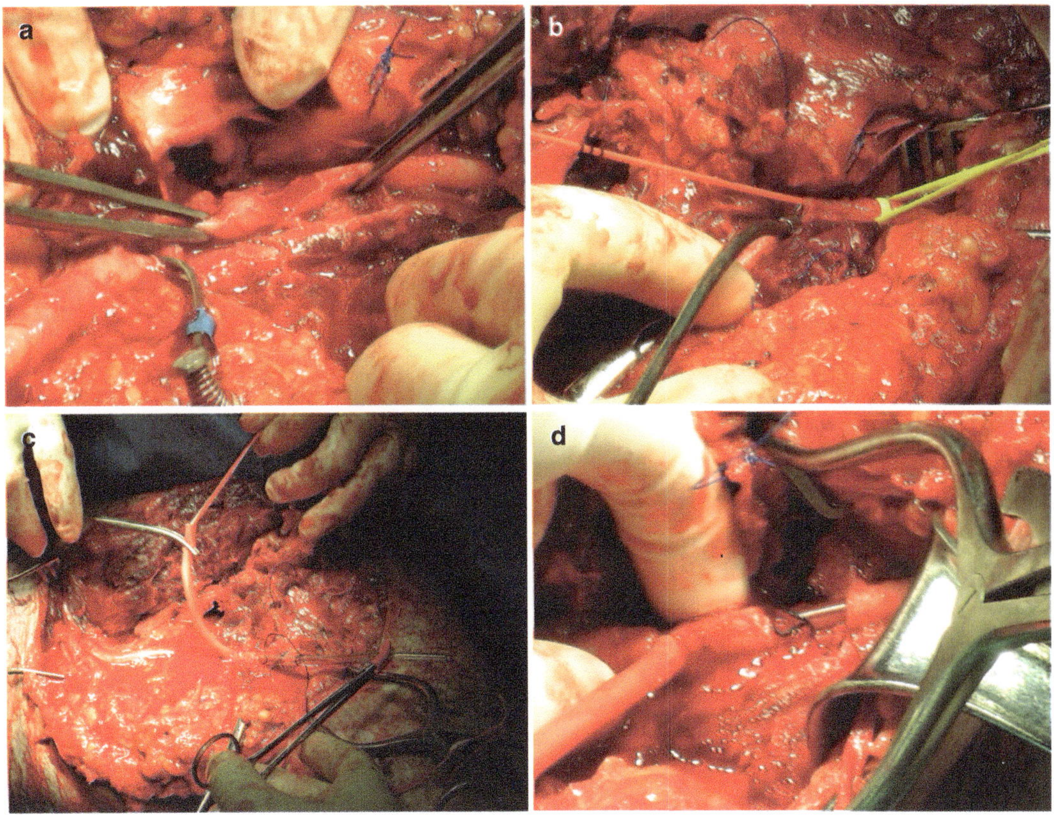

Fig. 8.4 (**a**) Popliteal artery injury shown. (**b**) Fogarty balloon catheter being passed. (**c**) Vascular shunt being placed proximally and secured in place with a Rumel tourniquet. Note the silk suture marking the midportion of the shunt. (**d**) Completed shunt in popliteal artery with silk suture verifying adequate proximal and distal position within vessel

fasciotomy incision where it is found between the tibialis anterior and extensor hallucis longus muscles adjacent to the interosseus membrane.

Vascular exposures and subsequent repair of arterial injuries below the knee are difficult and tedious. If a vascular surgeon is available at the next echelon of care, placing a shunt and shipping the patient may be the best option at this point.

Conclusion

I am a trauma and general surgeon who doesn't perform vascular surgery as part of my routine surgical practice. I found the management of vascular trauma challenging yet extremely rewarding. I hope this chapter will prove useful to others who may find themselves in the position of managing vascular injuries due to combat.

As a concluding word of advice, attending a cadaver-based vascular exposure course such as the Advanced Surgical Skills for Exposure in Trauma (ASSET) offered by the American College of Surgeons is invaluable. Many large Military Treatment Facilities now offer this course to military surgeons. Finally, if I had one book to bring with me on deployment, it would be a vascular exposure textbook such as Anatomic Exposures in Vascular Surgery by Valentine and Wind. I referenced this book on deployment far more than any other.

Use of Fasciotomies of the Lower Extremities

9

Robert Gaines

Contents

R. Gaines, MD
Department of Orthopedic Trauma,
Covenant Medical Center,
Lubbock, TX, USA

Naval Medical Center Portsmouth,
Portsmouth, VA, USA
e-mail: orthogaines@gmail.com

BLUF (Bottom Line Up Front) Box: Critical Pearls of Wisdom to Pass Along

1. Know the bony landmarks for release of the lower extremity compartments.
2. The size of the dermotomy matters; skin incisions should extend the length of the compartment.
3. Be familiar with lower extremity anatomy to avoid neurovascular structures.
4. Visualize that the entire compartment is released.
5. Stabilize underlying long bone fractures with external fixation.
6. Never close the fasciotomy site in the combat environment.

9.1 Principles of Compartment Syndrome

Compartment syndrome simply explained occurs when the pressure within a muscular compartment overcomes the pressure head of the arterial system supplying the vital structures of the compartment. This becomes important as the structures within the compartment begin to decompensate as they are starved of oxygenated blood. This process can occur in any muscular compartment bound by fascia and has been described in virtually every part of the body but is most often an issue of the lower extremity. Due to thoracic body armor and improvised explosive

L.B. Bone, C.N. Mamczak (eds.), *Front Line Extremity and Orthopaedic Surgery*,
DOI 10.1007/978-3-642-45337-3_9, © Springer-Verlag Berlin Heidelberg 2014

devices, the lower extremities are the most common sites of combat injuries. From role 2 to the return to the continental USA, the question of appropriate timing and technique of fasciotomy is a pertinent topic.

Surgeons are familiar with the postoperative sequelae of fasciotomies of the lower extremities in the setting of civilian trauma: venous stasis, nerve injury, scarring, and sensitivity to the affected extremity. Despite these potential pitfalls, fasciotomies of the lower extremities, when performed in the appropriate setting, preserve form and function of the lower extremity. Arguably surgeons are more aggressive about performing fasciotomies in the combat environment. Several differences between civilian trauma and combat operations should be considered. The lower echelons of care in a combat arena have limited resources. Two significant injuries could easily qualify as a mass casualty situation for these smaller units. With limited people and supplies, the surgeon may be more aggressive in releasing compartments because they are unsure of how closely a patient can be monitored after surgery. In the civilian setting, there is the opportunity for serial examinations that allow the surgeon to pick up on an evolving compartment syndrome. In the combat theater, the injured soldier may have a delay in their "second look" due to the unpredictable kinetics of the environment. Secondly, the transfer of the wounded is unpredictable. Transport may be delayed in route or completely unavailable which may extend the time the wounded soldier is without direct access to surgical care. The injuries sustained by the soldier, especially blast injuries, impart much more energy to the limb than blunt civilian trauma. The injury to the soft tissue makes the evolution of compartment syndrome unpredictable. Ultimately the patient is moved from one role to the next via multiple flights or ground transportation. All these add insult to the war fighters' injury, increasing the likelihood of decompensation of the perfusion gradient of the limb.

Compartment syndrome implies a significant injury to the soft tissue envelope. To improve the autocrine, paracrine, and endocrine environment of the injured extremity, it is imperative to provide as much stability as possible to the underlying bony injury. In the combat setting, this is most easily accomplished with an external fixator. The primary goal is stabilization of the bone with a secondary, but just as important, goal of supporting the soft tissue. When placing the external fixator, be mindful of the soldier's future surgeries. If the scenario allows, place pins outside of zones required for definitive fixation. Try not to contaminate key tissue planes that will be necessary for future fixation. If this is not possible, stabilize the patient as best as possible for that particular moment in time.

The tenets of treating compartment syndrome are the same for all regions: (1) long dermotomy to expose the entire compartment, (2) release of the entire compartmental fascia, (3) care not to injure nerves and vessels, and (4) maximize stability of any underlying bone injury as soon as possible.

9.2 Thigh Compartment Syndrome

The compartments of the thigh contain the bulk of the muscle mass of the lower extremity. Compartment syndrome of these large compartments leads to large physiologic shifts that extend beyond the thigh. Myonecrosis of the thigh compartments causes injury to other organ systems, and resultant fluid shifts can affect resuscitation efforts. Because of the large muscle mass and greater volume, impending compartment syndrome of the thigh may not be as apparent as that of the more distal lower extremity. The injuries sustained in the battle field, as previously pointed out, are much different than those seen in most civilian trauma. Blast injuries can send debris and contamination far into the soft tissue envelope. The zone of injury is often much greater than the overt external injury would suggest. The evolution of compartment syndrome in the thigh may progress to critical soft tissue compromise without changes in distal pulses, motor, or sensory findings. The thigh is also more difficult to evaluate as subcutaneous adipose tissue may be more abundant in this region of the lower extremity, masking tense compartments deep to this more pliable superficial layer. When compartment syndrome of the thigh is concomitant with fracture of the femur, stabilization of the fracture becomes an important part of emergent surgical intervention. Stabilization of underlying fractures helps to stop the progression of soft tissue injury.

The thigh is divided into three compartments consisting of medial, anterior, and posterior. The anterior and posterior compartments are the first to be released in the event of thigh compartment syndrome. After their release, the medial compartment is evaluated. Often the release of these two compartments provides relief for the medial compartment. In the event that the medial compartment pressures remain increased, this compartment is then released with care to avoid the femoral nerve and vasculature that resides in this compartment.

Release of the anterior and posterior compartments of the thigh is not as technically demanding as some other anatomical regions. A key to this procedure, as is common with all emergent fasciotomies, is an appropriately placed long dermotomy. The incision should line up with the greater trochanter and extend to the level of the distal lateral femoral condyle. To ensure proper fascial release, the skin incision should match the length of the fasciotomy.

After incision through the skin, the iliotibial band will be encountered. This structure should be divided in line with its fibers to expose the fascia over the anterior compartment of the thigh. Then a scalpel or surgical scissor is used to extend the fasciotomy proximally to the level of the greater trochanter and distally to the level of the lateral femoral condyle. Once the fascia has been incised, the vastus lateralis musculature is encountered. This muscle should be retracted superomedially off of the lateral intermuscular septum. Attention should be paid to perforating vessels in this area. When encountered these vessels should be ligated to avoid significant bleeding complications. With the vastus lateralis swept off of the lateral intermuscular septum, the septum is then incised along its anterior surface throughout the entire length of the skin incision. This releases the posterior compartment of the thigh.

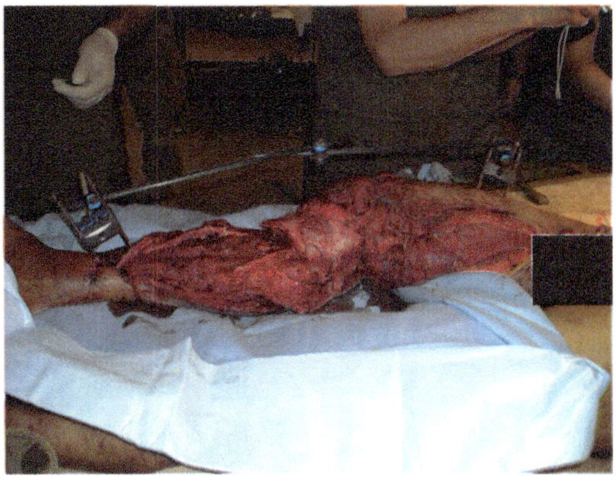

Fig. 9.1 Role 2: This lower extremity demonstrates a large zone of injury with a medial fasciotomy extending from the medial thigh continuing into a medial leg fasciotomy

This is often all that is needed to fully release the compartments of the thigh. After full release of the anterior and posterior compartments, the medial compartment should be reassessed. If after anterior and posterior compartments are released the medial compartment is still in jeopardy, it should be released from a skin incision starting 3 cm distal and 3 cm medial to the femoral pulse. This incision should be medial to the sartorius and over the fibers of the adductor longus. The release of the medial compartment should extend distally. The proximal portion of this incision is close to the femoral artery and vein (Fig. 9.1).

9.3 Leg Compartment Syndrome

Compartment syndrome of the leg is the classic anatomical area associated with this condition. Despite being a well-known process in a very accessible anatomical region, it is often undertreated. The tenets of fasciotomy are the same here as they are in the thigh. The length of the dermotomy matters. There is no room for a small incision for treatment of compartment syndrome due to acute trauma. The two techniques commonly used for the leg are the two-incision and the one-incision technique. The one-incision technique is ill-advised in the combat trauma setting. As not to confuse the issue, only the two-incision technique will be discussed here.

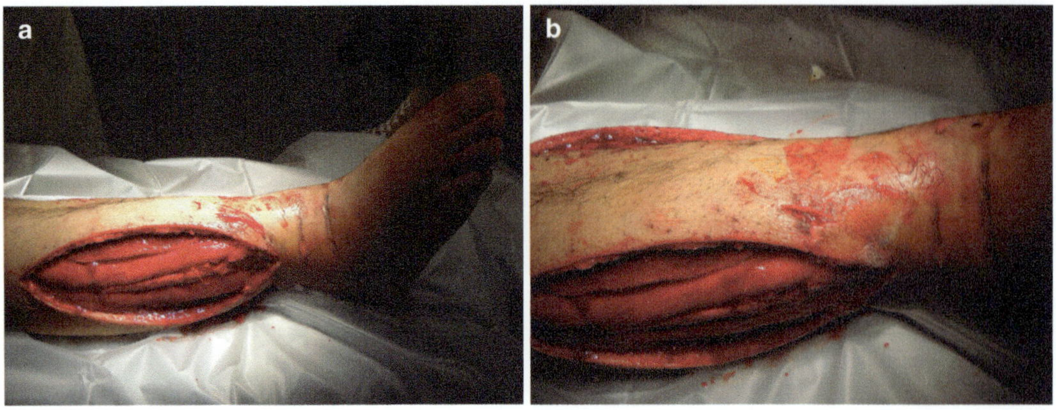

Fig. 9.2 (**a**) Role 2: Lateral fasciotomy to treat a deep contusion from a blast injury causing a leg compartment syndrome without an underlying fracture. Note the blistering of the distal limb. (**b**) Role 2: Anterior view of the leg showing both medial and lateral fasciotomies

The leg is divided into four compartments. Using the two-incision technique, the anterior and lateral compartments are released through a lateral incision, while the superficial and deep posterior compartments are released through a medial incision. The bony landmarks for fasciotomy of the leg are the palpable fibular head, lateral malleolus, and tibial crest. To release the anterior and lateral compartments of the leg, a long incision should be over the anterior compartment, halfway between the fibula and the tibial crest, and run the length of the fibula. After a skin incision is performed, the subcutaneous tissue and skin are bluntly dissected to expose the anterior compartment fascia. A small portal is then created in the fascia with a scalpel. Surgical scissors are then used to extend this portal proximally and distally. Unlike fascial release of the thigh, a scalpel is not recommended to complete the anterior or lateral compartment fasciotomy due to risk of lacerating branches of the superficial peroneal nerve. After the anterior compartment is released, the surgeon should palpate posteriorly from the fasciotomy site to encounter the dense lateral intermuscular septum separating the tibialis anterior from the peroneal musculature (Fig. 9.2a). A common mistake is to release the fascia of the anterior compartment twice and never to encounter the lateral compartment. To ensure that the surgeon is in the lateral compartment, a small transverse incision is often made across the intermuscular septum to further delineate the anterior and lateral compartments. Once the surgeon is confident that they have entered the lateral compartment, scissors are again used to extend the fasciotomy of the lateral compartment proximally and distally. The lateral compartment houses the superficial peroneal nerve. This nerve shows anatomical variation and may have branches in various areas of the lateral and distal anterior compartments. These nervous branches can easily be injured if the fascia is not elevated during fasciotomy. It is recommended to visualize the release along its entire course. It is inappropriate to cut or swipe blindly at the fascia. The surgical scissors should be controlled using the deep blade of the scissor to elevate the fascia while advancing the cutting surface over the compartment musculature.

The medial-sided fasciotomies are used to release the superficial and deep posterior compartments. A skin incision is performed approximately two centimeters posterior to the border of the tibia and stays parallel to the bone. A small amount of blunt subcutaneous dissection allows identification of the superficial posterior fascia. This fascia is then incised along the entire course of the incision. The gastrocnemius and soleus musculature are then retracted posteriorly allowing access to the deep posterior compartment. The fascia overlying the posterior tibialis is then released directly off of the posterior aspect of the tibia (Fig. 9.2b).

9.4 Foot Compartment Syndrome

Compartment syndrome of the foot has been a point of contention in orthopedic surgery for some time. The argument has included the number and structure of the muscular compartments of the foot. Some have argued that due to the small muscle mass, foot compartment syndrome is inconsequential and does not require release. For those who have cared for soldiers with missed or ignored foot compartment syndromes, there is an understanding of the sequelae that result from this process: claw toes, foot deformity, and neuropathic syndromes. Many military surgeons have considered or performed below-the-knee amputations in whole or in part due to the dysfunction caused by untreated compartment syndrome of the foot.

Recently a cadaveric study comprised of careful dissection found that only the hindfoot possessed true compartments. These were described as medial, intermediate, and lateral compartments all with fascial attachments to the plantar surface of the calcaneus. The authors did describe fascia over the dorsal interossei but were unable to find an investing fascia on the plantar aspect of these muscles. Recommendations for incisions for foot fasciotomy vary in their exact location, but most authors agree that a medial incision is required. This medial incision has been described in several different ways including a direct medial incision starting at the sustentaculum and extending distally or a plantar incision off of the weight-bearing line of the medial arch of the foot. Regardless of the exact placement of the incision, the recommendation to release the stout fascia from the plantar surface of the calcaneus remains. There are two stout bands of fascia extending vertically from the undersurface of the calcaneus that must be released to preserve the function of the short digital flexor and quadratus plantae. Through the medial incision, the abductor hallucis musculature is bluntly dissected in line with its fibers until the dense white fascia is encountered on the lateral aspect of this muscle. This fascia is then separated along its entire course from the undersurface of the calcaneus. The final layer of fascia in the hindfoot lies even further laterally and must be released blindly due to the confined space in this part of the foot (Fig. 9.3).

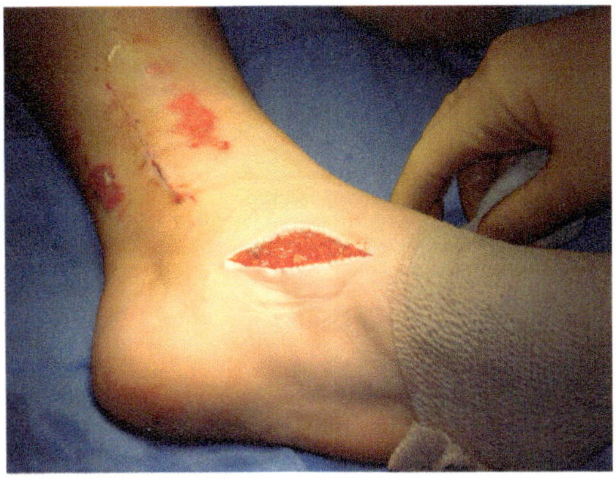

Fig. 9.3 Role 5. Medial incision over the instep of the foot to treat compartment syndrome of the hindfoot resulting after fixation of a distal tibia fracture

For the interossei, two dorsal decisions over the second and fourth metatarsals are described. The fascia overlying the interossei is subcutaneous and easily accessible and released directly from the medial and lateral aspects of the metatarsals. There is no need to continue to the deep aspect of the metatarsal as studies have not found a stout investing fascia in this region. Release of the dorsal fascia is adequate.

9.5 After Care

At the end of the first episode of resuscitative and surgical management, the wounded war fighter should be packaged in preparation for transport or continued resuscitative management. This requires underlying long bone injuries to be stabilized with external fixation or splints and dressings to be placed over open wounds. Wet-to-dry dressings are placed over fasciotomy sites at the lower roles of care. Vessel loops may be used from role 3 facilities and beyond in an effort to keep the skin from retracting (Fig. 9.4). In some situations at higher levels of care, there is opportunity to employ negative-pressure wound therapy. The tenet of care that should not be ignored in any setting in theater is closure of fasciotomy

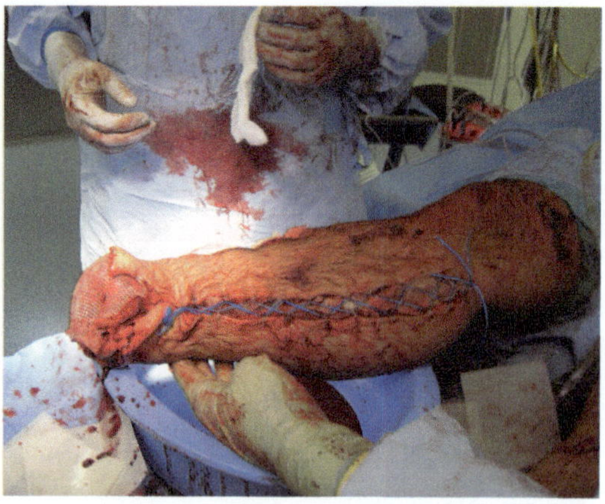

Fig. 9.4 Role 3. Traumatic distal amputation of the leg with two-incision fasciotomy. The medial incision demonstrates a vessel loop bodice to avoid skin retraction

sites in our war fighters. Acute closure of a fasciotomy site in nonsensical and delayed primary closure of fasciotomy sites is reserved for role 4 and 5 institutions. This allows time for injuries to declare themselves and repeat debridements to be performed. Local nationals will occasionally undergo all of their care at the role 3 facility. In this regard delayed primary closure or skin grafting may occur at this level of care.

Transfemoral Amputations 10

Jean-Claude G. D'Alleyrand and Donald Gajewski

Contents

J.-C.G. D'Alleyrand, MD (✉)
Department of Orthopaedic Surgery, Walter Reed National Military Medical Center, Bethesda, MD, USA

Norman M. Rich Department of Surgery, Uniformed Services University of the Health Sciences, Bethesda, MD, USA
e-mail: jean-claude.g.d'alleyrand@health.mil

D. Gajewski, MD
Center for the Intrepid, San Antonio Military Medical Center, San Antonio, TX, USA

Norman M. Rich Department of Surgery, Uniformed Services University of the Health Sciences, Bethesda, MD, USA

BLUF (Bottom Line Up Front) Box

1. Get vascular control, either locally with hemostats or proximally in the thigh, groin, or abdomen. Prep in the entire abdomen for high amputations.
2. *Never* perform a guillotine amputation. These require a fair amount of additional bony resection to allow adequate closure. Leave all viable skin and muscle, regardless of how irregular the tissue flaps.
3. This is debridement surgery. Don't worry about revising the amputation level, aside from removing visibly contaminated bone. Remove as much contamination and frankly necrotic material as possible, finalize your vessel ligation, dress the wound, and evacuate to a higher level of care.
4. Doubly ligate the femoral vessels individually, using a #0 silk suture ligature distally and a #0 silk "tie on a pass" proximally.
5. Bilateral transfemoral amputees are sick patients. They need aggressive resuscitation, with early utilization of blood products. Surgery should be rapid, to minimize blood and insensible fluid losses, as well as hypothermia.
6. Plan on repeating the debridement within 24 h. Do not delay repeat debridement in order to accommodate the air-evac schedule.

L.B. Bone, C.N. Mamczak (eds.), *Front Line Extremity and Orthopaedic Surgery*,
DOI 10.1007/978-3-642-45337-3_10, © Springer-Verlag Berlin Heidelberg 2014

10.1 Introduction

Combat-related transfemoral amputations are associated with major contamination and blood loss. Adequate treatment combines principles of orthopedic trauma surgery and those of critical care. Patients will frequently present in hemodynamic shock. Care for these injuries involves vascular control, resuscitation, and urgent debridement prior to rapid evacuation.

10.2 Principles of Management

Traumatic transfemoral amputees will have sustained substantial hemorrhage prior to arrival to the ED/ATLS tent. The first priority of care will be aggressive resuscitation while simultaneously establishing hemostasis. Patients will typically arrive with one or more tourniquets in place. One tourniquet is frequently not enough to compress the femoral vessels, so it is imperative to check the wounds for active bleeding. If any active bleeding is present, apply additional tourniquets until hemostasis is achieved. If the amputation is very distal through the thigh, the combat tourniquets can be replaced with a pneumatic tourniquet brought from the operating room. This can be prepped in or out of the sterile field as needed. If the wounds extend very proximally, the combat tourniquets will need to be prepped in. If this is the case, the abdomen should be prepped in as well, as control of the aorta or iliac vessels may be required intraoperatively. For very proximal amputations, manual compression of the vessels near the inguinal ligament may be required. Pressure will need to be maintained until intra-abdominal vascular control is established, so the hand and forearm of the assistant will need to be prepped into the field.

After prepping the limb, the first priority is to gain access to the femoral vessels. Search between the vastus medialis, adductor magnus, and sartorius to find the femoral sheath. Individually clamp the superficial femoral artery and vein at the level of the residual femur and release the tourniquet as soon as possible. Transect the vessels below the hemostats and remove the vessel segments distal to this level. The hemostats can be kept in place and revised to formal ligatures after debridement and irrigation. This will avoid the placement of braided, permanent sutures into a grossly contaminated field. If the hemostats are cumbersome around which to work, they can be immediately revised to silk suture as detailed below. High amputations may require additional ligation of the profunda femoris, which should only be done if truly necessary, as this artery is the main blood supply for most of the thigh.

Debridement should be effective yet rapid, to minimize the development of hypothermia and coagulopathy. The traumatic wounds must be extended proximally to allow direct inspection of all degloved portions of the thigh. Attempt to keep the proximal extensions on the medial and lateral aspects of the thigh, but allow the wound pattern to dictate this. Attempt to keep skin bridges as wide as possible, and leave the skin in continuity with the underlying fascia to preserve its blood supply.

It cannot be overemphasized that you should not perform a guillotine amputation. In order to close these wounds and provide a functional limb, there must be adequate skin and soft tissues to pull over the end of the femur to provide power and padding for weight bearing. After a guillotine amputation is performed, the femur will require additional shortening to enable closure, and with the loss of femoral length comes a loss of leverage and power and increased difficulty with prosthetic fitting. Treat this surgery purely as debridement of a contaminated wound, and leave all viable tissue intact, regardless of how bizarre the residual tissue flaps.

Rather than slowly performing a superficial debridement, mobilize each muscle belly and inspect it for a line of demarcation between necrotic and non-necrotic tissue. Perform an *en bloc* resection of the necrotic tissue at this interface. Transection with a scalpel will minimize trauma to remaining tissue. However, Mayo scissors can be used if sharp debridement is too bloody. There will be a zone of transition between necrotic and viable tissue, which will appear contused and ecchymotic. Some of this tissue will eventually undergo necrosis, but some of it will survive and will improve with time and resuscitation. The patient's skeletal length and eventual function will be directly affected by the amount of muscle left for performing myodeses and myoplasties. If the muscle tissue appears structurally intact and not actually necrotic, avoid resecting it and allow it to declare itself at subsequent debridements. In contrast, any unhealthy-appearing fat should be removed. Contaminated or necrotic bone should be excised, but only until bleeding bone is encountered.

With blast mechanisms, debris can be travel along intermuscular planes for great distances. Follow each intermuscular interval proximally until you encounter pristine areolar tissue. Skin that is impregnated with contaminants should be excised. Skin that is nonviable but clean can be retained to provide expendable material for running suture closures. These skin edges will be revised prior to final closure. Minimize inefficient alternating between debridement and irrigation. Perform a thorough debridement by using knife or scissors for blocks of tissue, then rongeurs and curettes for small or loose tissue and debris, then copiously irrigate. One more cycle of debridement may be necessary, and then the procedure should be complete. Use 9–12 l of irrigation per amputation and try to limit surgery to about an hour.

Once debridement is complete, the vessels should be formally ligated, if this has not already been performed. Using a #0 silk on a taper needle, referred to as a suture ligature or "stick tie," pass the needle through the vessel, just proximal to the hemostat. Capture about 30 % of the width of the vessel and tie a secure knot, leaving a tail of several centimeters, thus anchoring the suture to the vessel. Pass both limbs of the suture to the opposite side of the vessel, and tie another secure knot opposite the first one, thereby occluding the lumen. Pass a free #0 silk suture around the vessel, approximately 8–10 mm proximal to the suture ligature, and securely ligate the vessel at this level. Remove the hemostat and repeat this double ligation on the other vessel. Leave cut suture ends about 1 cm long, to help identify the vessels during future debridements. Placing the suture ligatures distally will prevent both sets of sutures from sliding off of the end of the vessel, avoiding catastrophic hemorrhage during transport. This unfortunate event can happen with free tie-only ligation, even with as many as three free ties used. Inspect wounds closely for small bleeding vessels and pack raw, bleeding surfaces for 5–10 min prior to closure, in order to minimize postoperative blood loss.

The wounds should be partially closed with running 2-0 nylon suture in order to prevent retraction of the skin. At the time of definitive amputation closure, it can be difficult to close skin primarily if it has been allowed to retract. If the entire skin envelope can be closed, leave the distal aspect of the wound open to allow drainage. Vacuum dressings can be employed, but this should be done with caution in the setting of the initial debridement. The acutely traumatized tissues may be quite friable and prone to continued bleeding, especially in a negative-pressure environment, so excellent hemostasis should be assured prior to vacuum dressing application.

10.3 Bilateral Transfemoral Amputees

Patients with bilateral transfemoral amputations will have sustained severe hemorrhage and will require aggressive resuscitation with blood products. Combat amputees are almost all young and athletic, so they may be able to temporarily compensate, but they will be approaching the end of their physiologic reserves by the time they present for treatment. A failure to rapidly administer blood products and correct acidosis can have fatal consequences. Patients with very proximal amputations are prone to repeated fecal soilage of their wounds prior to closure, so a prophylactic diverting colostomy may be warranted.

Conclusions

It is not necessary to be facile with amputations in order to provide these patients with the best chance at a good outcome. What is important is to resuscitate the patient, provide hemostasis, and perform a thorough debridement. Wounds should be debrided a second time within 24 h, even if that interferes with evacuation to a higher level of care, as patients may not undergo debridement that day if the transit time is lengthy. If you are diligent with debridement, without removing too much healthy tissue, you will leave the definitive amputation surgeons with all possible options for an optimal reconstruction.

Femoral Fractures

11

Jean-Claude G. D'Alleyrand and Wade T. Gordon

Contents

BLUF (Bottom Line Up Front) Box

1. Debride wounds thoroughly before stabilizing open fractures.
2. Stabilize the fracture however you can. It can always be revised at the next level of care.
3. Stabilization is typically via external fixation. Keep pins out of fracture site and sites for potential future internal fixation.
4. External fixation ideally involves three providers: one for traction, one to reduce the fracture, and one to tighten the fixator clamps.
5. When treating femur fractures proximal to a transfemoral amputation, avoid performing an amputation through the fracture site, if at all possible.

11.1 Introduction

Combat-related fractures of the femur can be caused either by a blunt mechanism or from a penetrating injury, such as a gunshot wound or blast fragmentation. Femoral fractures are frequently associated with high-energy injuries and substantial blood loss. Treatment begins with the ATLS protocol, including hemorrhage control, followed by debridement of traumatic wounds and fracture stabilization, in that order. Stabilization is typically accomplished via

J.-C.G. D'Alleyrand, MD (✉) • W.T. Gordon, MD
Department of Orthopaedic Surgery,
Walter Reed National Military Medical Center,
Bethesda, MD, USA

Norman M. Rich Department of Surgery,
Uniformed Services University of the Health
Sciences, Bethesda, MD, USA
e-mail: jean-claude.g.d'alleyrand@health.mil

L.B. Bone, C.N. Mamczak (eds.), *Front Line Extremity and Orthopaedic Surgery*,
DOI 10.1007/978-3-642-45337-3_11,

external fixation, but must be tailored to the involved region of the femur, associated injuries, and available equipment.

11.2 Principles of Initial Management

Femoral fractures are frequently sustained in the setting of a multisystem trauma. Initial management begins with resuscitation and splinting in the ATLS bay. Once resuscitation is proceeding well, based on a resolving base deficit, treatment should continue with the debridement of open wounds and temporizing stabilization with splint immobilization or external fixation.

Concomitant vascular injury is common, and restoring blood flow to the distal extremity is of utmost priority. The patient may present with tourniquets in place. Tourniquets should be removed in a controlled setting, with the required instruments and equipment necessary for the surgical control of any resulting hemorrhage. It is very important to release the tourniquets slowly, over several minutes, if they have been on for more than an hour or so. After prolonged use, the sudden release of a tourniquet can release vasoactive mediators, which can cause profound hypotension. If pulses are absent below a femoral fracture, a provisional reduction with axial traction will usually restore a pulse. If not, search for additional hard signs of vascular injury and explore the vessels as needed.

11.2.1 Who Goes First: Ortho or Vascular?

The timing of temporizing fixation and vascular repair is often the source of disagreement between orthopedic surgeons and our general/vascular surgery colleagues. Vascular surgeons may insist on revascularization prior to external fixation. However, debridement and fracture reduction following a vascular repair can place that repair at risk of disruption. Moreover, expedient external fixation does not appreciably delay vascular repair. After performing a thorough debridement and stabilizing the fracture, vascular shunt or reconstruction can be performed in a wound bed that is as clean and stable as possible. If distal perfusion has been interrupted for a prolonged period of time, then an intravascular shunt should be placed immediately after prepping the patient. Following debridement and external fixation, the shunt should be closely inspected for signs of dislodgement and revised as needed to a new shunt or to definitive reconstruction.

11.2.2 Debridement and Fasciotomy

Combat-related femoral fractures are commonly open injuries. Standard principles for the debridement of traumatic, open wounds apply. Removal of gross contamination, followed by sharp, aggressive serial debridements of necrotic and devitalized tissue, is performed, followed by wound irrigation.

Fasciotomies of the leg are covered in detail separately in the text and should be performed when indicated. Acute compartment syndrome is difficult to diagnose in the best circumstances and is even more so in an austere environment. Compartment pressure monitoring is not readily available, and pain out of proportion to that expected from an injury is difficult to assess in the polytrauma patient. In these conditions, the surgeon must rely on a high index of suspicion, along with the clinical exam.

Fasciotomies of the thigh are much less commonly indicated than those in the lower leg, and surgeons tend to be less familiar with the technique. There are three fascial compartments of the thigh: the quadriceps, hamstring, and adductor compartments. The quadriceps and hamstring compartments are released through a longitudinal lateral incision, which can also be extended proximally in order to release the hip abductors and gluteus maximus if necessary. Be sure to identify the intermuscular septum in the posterolateral thigh. Release the posterior compartment either behind the septum or through it, to ensure that you haven't made two fascial incisions in the anterior compartment alone. Much less commonly released, the adductor compartment is accessed through a longitudinal medial incision.

The location of this incision, extending into the groin, makes it less desirable with respect to wound complications.

11.2.3 Temporizing Stabilization

External fixation is the method of choice for temporizing fixation of femur fractures. Splinting should be considered only for very distal injuries about the knee, as well as clinical scenarios where the time or resources necessary for external fixation are not available.

11.3 Treatment for Diaphyseal Fractures

External fixation is the mainstay of treatment for these injuries. In general, we place femoral fixator pins anterolaterally. Anterior pin placement offers the advantage of keeping fixators from protruding past the edges of the litter, which potentially may facilitate patient transport. However, there are several branches of the femoral nerve which course through the anterior thigh. This, combined with the anterior nature of the suprapatellar pouch, contributes to an anterior safe zone that averages only 20 cm [1]. Also, anterior pins tether both the rectus femoris and vastus intermedius, which may contribute more to post-fixation stiffness than pins that only transfix the vastus lateralis. For these reasons, we prefer anterolateral pin placement.

Generally speaking, two Schanz pins in each fragment are sufficient to stabilize these injuries. If there is any doubt about the purchase of those pins, use three pins per fragment. The pins can be placed through a 5-hole Hoffmann pin clamp or they can be incorporated into a cluster by connecting the pins in a given fragment with a single bar. These pin clusters, or the pin clamps, are then connected to each other with additional bars that span the fracture (Fig. 11.1). Prior to doing so, an assistant should provide longitudinal traction and rotation while the surgeon manipulates the fragments with the clamps or bars. Once the fragments feel reduced, a third person then tightens the frame. In the case of a segmental fracture, intercalary fragments do not need to be fixed to the frame, unless doing so adds vital stability to the construct.

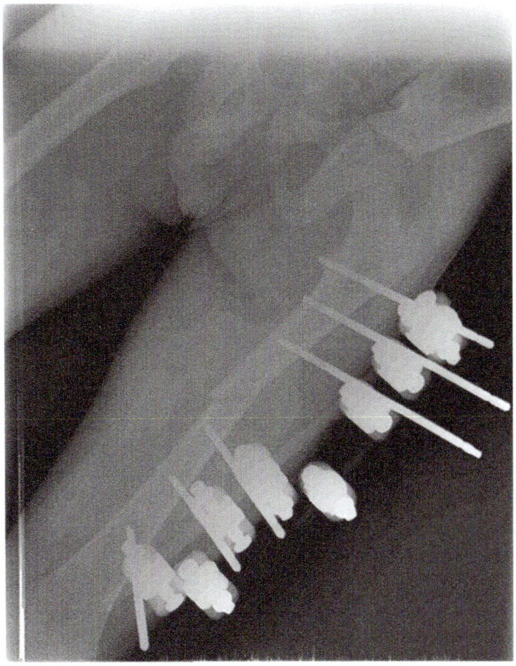

Fig. 11.1 External fixation of a femoral shaft fracture. Due to a shortage of 5-pin clamps, the Schanz pins in each fragment were interconnected with a bar. The fracture was reduced and the bars connected to one another with a third one. Note that the pins in the distal fragment were inadvertently placed more anteriorly than desired

Typically, you can palpate the fracture site and you should try to keep your pins several centimeters away, in order to lower the chance of seeding the fracture hematoma. If external fixation is not a viable option, the legs can be strapped to one another or they both can be strapped to the litter prior to transport.

11.4 Treatment for Proximal and Distal Fractures

11.4.1 Proximal Fractures

If a short proximal segment precludes the placement of two transverse pins, one pin can be placed obliquely from the greater trochanter down to the lesser trochanter. This can be done

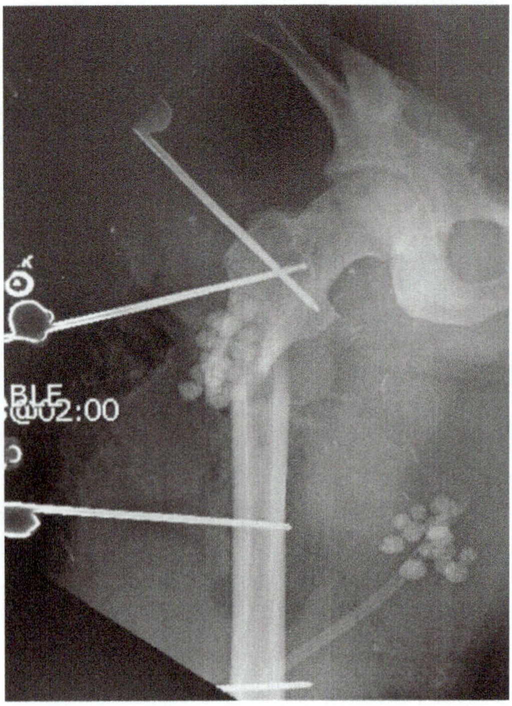

Fig. 11.2 External fixation of a subtrochanteric femur fracture. Due to the short proximal segment, an oblique trochanteric pin was placed to complete the construct

by cutting down over the greater trochanter, feeling over the anterior neck, and using your left index finger as a guide for placement of the pins. A second pin can be placed transversely at the level of the lesser trochanter, completing the construct (Fig. 11.2). Conversely, one or two pins can be placed into the neck and head of the femur; however, this is best done using fluoroscopy. If all else fails, the proximal fragment can be spanned by placing two or more pins into the gluteal pillar of the pelvis. While applying traction, connect the iliac crest pins to those in the distal fragment. This construct should be one of last resort, as the pelvic pins are rather tenuous.

11.4.2 Distal Femoral Fractures

Some distal fractures are length-stable and are thus amenable to splinting. These are limited to AO type B fractures, where one condyle is still connected to the shaft, as well as incomplete or non-displaced fractures. Fractures that are prone to shortening should be stabilized with external fixation. Extra-articular fractures can be usually fixed like diaphyseal ones, taking care to place pins transversely to avoid penetration of the knee joint. For length-unstable intra-articular fractures, spanning fixation should be performed (Fig. 11.3). The femoral pins should be placed proximal to the midpoint of the thigh, to avoid contaminating possible future plate fixation. The tibial pins should be as proximal as possible, starting just below the tibial tubercle and moving distally, to provide maximum rigidity to the construct.

11.5 Femur Fixation with an Ipsilateral Amputation

Femoral fractures proximal to an ipsilateral amputation should be managed in the same manner in which they would be in an intact limb. Femoral fractures in the setting of a transfemoral amputation are usually amenable to standard external fixation techniques. In cases where the distal fracture fragment is very short, splinting or even an amputation dressing may provide adequate initial stability. Rarely, tissue necrosis may mandate amputation through the fracture. If so, care should be taken to preserve all viable tissue, no matter how irregular the tissue flaps, as maintaining length of the residual limb is critical to the patient's ultimate level of function (Fig. 11.4).

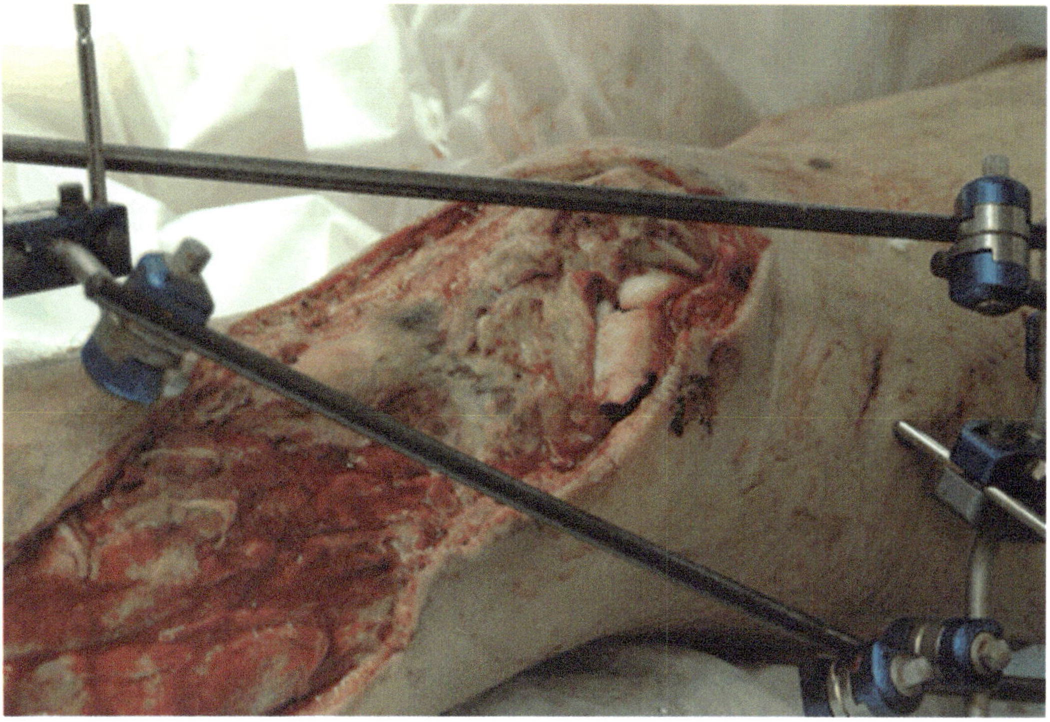

Fig. 11.3 The comminuted, intra-articular nature of this fracture precluded any fixator pin placement in the epiphysis. The knee was spanned and the fracture stabilized with the aid of pins in the proximal tibia

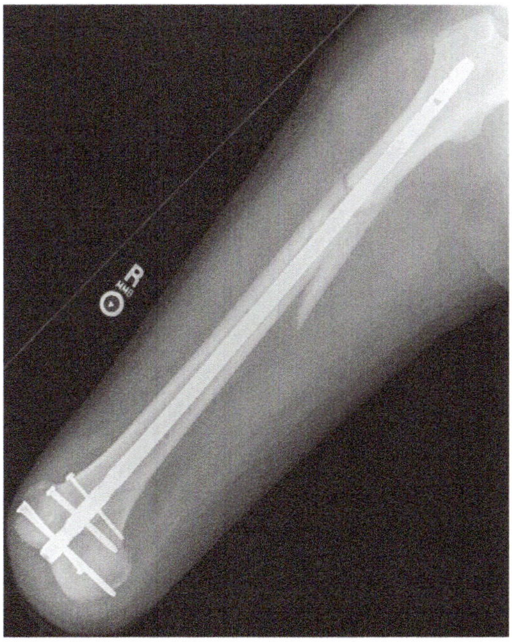

Fig. 11.4 This patient was kept as a knee disarticulation, despite fractures of the shaft and medial condyle. Instead of revising his amputation level through one of the fractures, he was kept at the optimal length allowed by the soft tissues

Conclusion

Patients with combat-related femoral fractures require close monitoring for signs of hypovolemia, and they will frequently require transfusion of blood products prior to evacuation from theater. Unicondylar distal femoral fractures may be amenable to splinting, but the mainstay of initial treatment for femoral fractures is external fixation. Care should be taken to restore skeletal length with the fixator, as this becomes increasingly difficult to do over time. With expedient resuscitation and provisional fixation, these patients can fairly easily be stabilized for evacuation to a higher level of care.

Reference

1. Beltran MJ, Collinge CA, Patzowski JC, Masini BD, Blease RE, Hsu JR. The Skeletal Trauma Research Consortium (STReC). The Safe Zone for External Fixator Pins in the Femur. J Orthop Trauma. 2012;26: 643–7.

Combat Pelvic Injuries and Hip Dislocations

12

Christiaan N. Mamczak and Joseph E. Strauss

Contents

C.N. Mamczak, DO (✉)
Beacon Orthopaedic Trauma Surgery, Memorial Hospital, South Bend, IN, USA

Department of Orthopaedic Surgery, Naval Medical Center Portsmouth, Portsmouth, VA, USA
e-mail: dr_jibwex@yahoo.com

J.E. Strauss, DO
Department of Orthopaedics, Anne Arundel Medical Center, Annapolis, MD, USA

R Adams Cowley Shock Trauma Center, Baltimore, MD, USA

Walter Reed National Medical Center, Bethesda, MD, USA

BLUF (Bottom Line Up Front) Box

1. Combat pelvic ring and acetabular fractures carry significant risks for morbidity and mortality due to the unique mechanisms of injury.
2. Stable and unstable fracture patterns occur along with atypical variations and combined ring-acetabular injuries.
3. Downrange treatment priorities include surgical hemostasis, pelvic ring stabilization, reduction of hip dislocations, and wound decontamination.
4. No definitive fracture fixation downrange.
5. Open pelvic injuries with associated perineal blast wounds and urogenital destruction are unfortunately common and challenging.
6. A multidisciplinary team of general and orthopedic surgeons working together is the best medicine for complex injury patterns requiring proximal pelvic vessel hemostasis and pelvic ring stabilization.
7. Only examine pelvic stability once and then temporize pelvic volume reduction with a sheet or binder centered on the trochanters.
8. Unstable pelvic ring injuries must be ex-fixed with either iliac crest or supra-acetabular frames before turning

L.B. Bone, C.N. Mamczak (eds.), *Front Line Extremity and Orthopaedic Surgery*, DOI 10.1007/978-3-642-45337-3_12, © Springer-Verlag Berlin Heidelberg 2014

patients prone or lateral for posterior wound debridement and prior to transport.
9. Avoid permanent large vessel ligation if possible; this will lead to flap necrosis and revision amputations to a higher level.
10. Partial or complete hemipelvectomy is a last resort lifesaving surgical measure to treat massive intrapelvic bleeding that fails vessel ligation and pelvic packing techniques.

12.1 Introduction

Combat injuries to the pelvic ring and acetabulum have traditionally carried high mortality rates. Improvements in acute casualty care, a more efficient medevac system, damage control resuscitation techniques, and trained orthopedic surgeons downrange can contribute to increasing survival rates for those patients wounded with pelvic injuries. Nonetheless, the combat environment contributes various elements that can delay or limit care and ultimately contribute to critically unstable patients or even mortality. Deployed orthopedic surgeons can expect a variety of stable and unstable pelvic ring and/or acetabular fracture patterns caused by either traditional blunt trauma or blast mechanisms of injury. The downrange orthopedic care of pelvic injuries is limited by the austere operating environment and a lack of surgical resources. The initial treatment priorities focus on acute resuscitation, hemorrhage control, provisional pelvic ring stabilization or femoroacetabular reduction, and the identification and treatment of associated injuries. This damage control algorithm allows for stable patient movement out of the combat theater for later definitive fracture fixation.

12.2 Combat Pelvic and Acetabular Fracture Patterns with Associated Pathophysiology

Approximately 80 % of the combat pelvic ring and acetabular fractures are the result of improvised explosive devices (IEDs). Blunt trauma mechanisms account for nearly 15 % of the injuries usually from tactical vehicle accidents, or crush injuries, and the remaining 5 % of fractures are caused by high-energy gunshot wounds. The

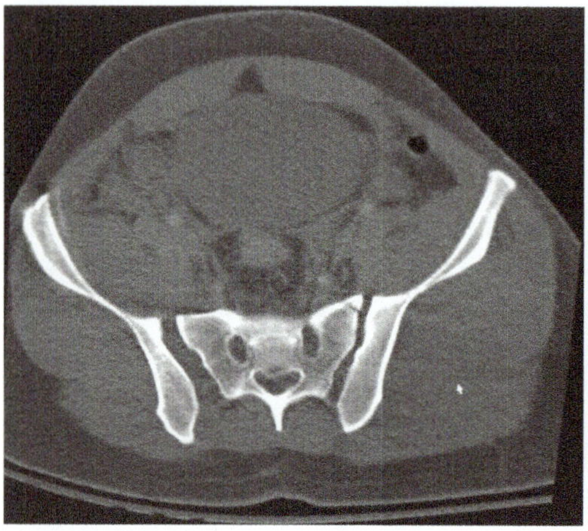

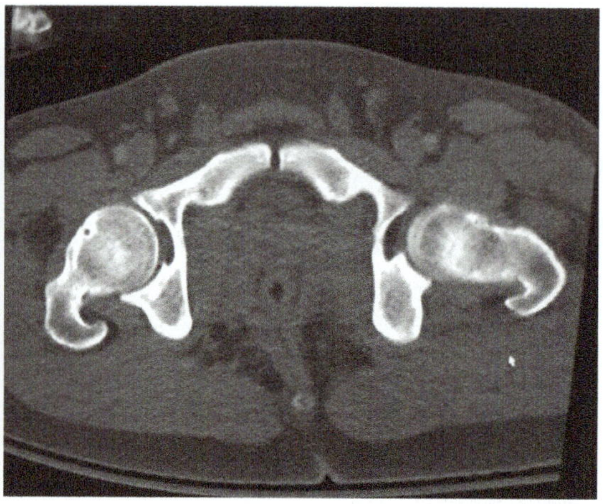

Figs. 12.1 and 12.2 CT images demonstrating an atypical pelvic ring injury with posterior only injuries including widened SI joint and contralateral sacral fracture without anterior ring injury (symphysis or iliac wing). This patient was treated with a pelvic examination under anesthesia and transported with a pelvic binder and serial soft tissue assessments

mechanism of injury can often serve as a guide to understanding the type and pattern of pelvic ring injury. Current classification systems like the Young and Burgess, OTA, and Tile have traditionally helped surgeons understand the pathophysiology of these injuries and guide treatment. However, unlike civilian injuries that tend to follow a more predictable pattern, there is much variability that exists in combat pelvic and acetabular trauma making one classification system less universal (Figs. 12.1 and 12.2). Combined mechanisms and atypical patterns become the norm. Determining pelvic stability is critical to survival. Most cases of IED exposure during dismounted foot patrols result in unstable open-book pelvic fractures, and early pelvic volume reduction is paramount to survival (Fig. 12.3). Blunt mechanisms and troop vehicular injuries are more frequently lateral compression-type fractures. Combat acetabular fractures occur less frequently and are also difficult to classify because of their unusual fracture patterns. Posterior hip dislocations with or without an associated acetabular fracture are more common with tactical vehicle accidents and blunt trauma. Open pelvic fractures have always had a high mortality rate of 50 % or higher due to risks of early exsanguination and subsequent risks of sepsis. More than half of all combat pelvic fractures are open fractures, whereas approximately one-third of acetabular fractures are open.

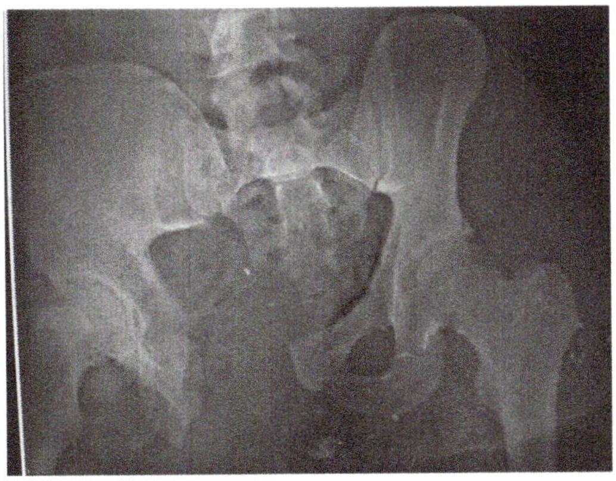

Fig. 12.3 AP pelvic radiograph of an APC-3 open, unstable pelvic ring injury in a DCBI casualty with three extremity amputations. This injury was treated with a team approach with ex-lap and temporary proximal vessel control by the general surgeons and pelvic external fixation and revision amputations with I&D by the orthopedic surgeons

The Dismounted Complex Blast Injury (DCBI) represents a specific polytrauma pattern that carries the highest morbidity and mortality. These high-energy IED casualties present with traumatic bilateral lower extremity amputations, unstable pelvic ring fractures, and perineal blast involvement. The DCBI is a life-threatening injury with a high association of concurrent intra-abdominal, vascular, and/or urogenital injuries (Figs. 12.4 and 12.5). These casualties are by far the most challenging cohort of patients to treat while deployed as most present critically unstable with uncontrolled intrapelvic hemorrhage.

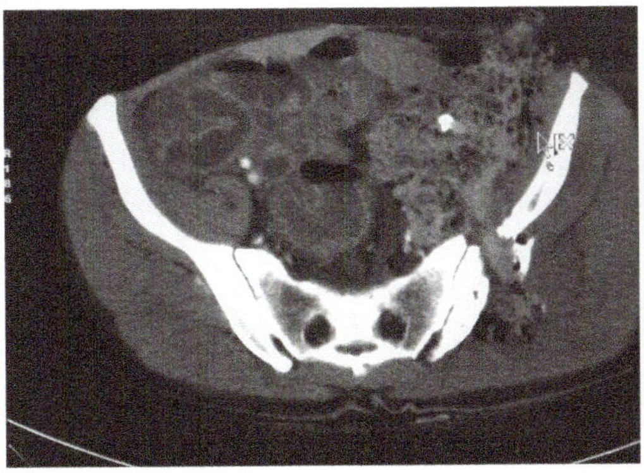

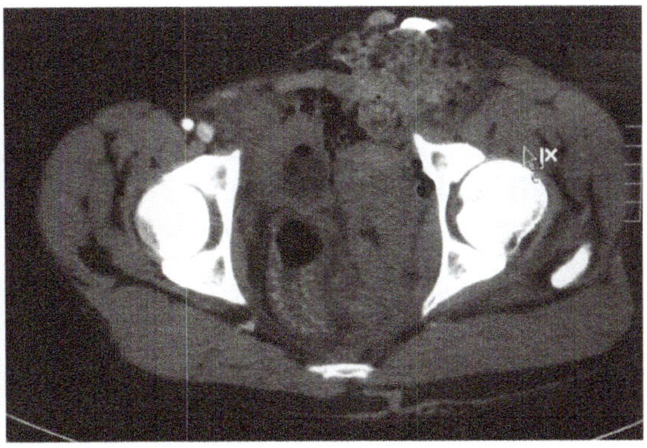

Figs. 12.4 and 12.5 CT images depicting an open iliac wing fracture with complex soft tissue injury and ipsilateral femoral vessel lacerations from a dismounted IED encounter. This patient was treated with exploratory laparotomy with irrigation, debridement, vessel repair, and negative pressure wound therapy

Timing is critical to survival. Damage control resuscitation and emergent surgery are directed at hemorrhage control, decontamination of wounds, pelvic fracture stabilization, and revision amputations.

Hemodynamically unstable patients with pelvic and acetabular fractures present a complex challenge to the combat surgeon and trauma team. A thorough understanding of the injury mechanisms, associated injuries, and treatment protocols can guide management of these complex, life-threatening injuries. Peripelvic arterial and venous plexus bleeding is very common with high-energy IED blast injuries to the pelvis and acetabulum. Hemorrhage control measures from the initial point of injury to eventual damage control surgery for proximal vessel control should remain a priority as this is critical for patient survival. Appropriate evaluation of the abdomen, chest, head, and other potential sites of injury and bleeding cannot be overstressed. Additionally, a thorough examination of the pelvis and perineum is required to rule out open fractures and nonorthopedic injuries to the rectum and GU/GYN systems. On a rare occasion, resuscitative thoracotomies can be performed to augment the resuscitation process when all else fails. Preliminary JTTR data suggest a 4 % overall survival rate after this procedures given the complexity of the injuries, hemorrhagic shock, multisystem organ failure, and sepsis. The routine use of resuscitative thoracotomies is discouraged in nonpenetrating chest injuries and should be reserved only for complex casualties that lose vital signs immediately en route or within the trauma bay or operating room.

12.3 Initial Patient Evaluation and Treatment Algorithm

The initial patient evaluation and treatment phase for patients with pelvic and/or acetabular fractures follows the standard Advanced Trauma Life Support (ATLS) protocol. Index stabilization of the pelvis in the field (Echelon/Role 1 "Buddy Aid") is performed with a sheet or foot, ankle, or knee taping if possible. However, this is often not done as pelvic ring injuries go unrecognized and the uncontrolled pelvic volume contributes to further blood loss and hemodynamic instability. Field tourniquets are applied to minimize further exsanguination from associated lower extremity amputations.

Patients are evacuated to Forward Surgical Teams (FSTs, Echelon/Role 2) or Combat Support Hospitals (CSH or Role 3) where improved surgical capability and equipment become available. Damage control resuscitation protocols continue upon arrival to these higher echelons of care. Patients with pelvic injuries and multiple extremity amputations tend to consume massive amounts of blood products and multiple surgical assets including various operative teams, surgical equipment, and OR time. Institution of a walking blood bank early is imperative at Echelon/Role 2 and Role 3 facilities as resources can be quickly consumed by a single patient. Triage of these life-threatening injuries, especially in the multiple casualty scenario or a DCBI, is vital in order to determine patient survivability and assessment of the available surgical assets and blood products. Remember that timing is everything! All traumatic pelvic wounds should be evaluated in a systematic fashion to determine the extent of associated injuries to the rectum, perineum, and genitourinary systems (Fig. 12.6). Foley catheters are necessary to evaluate GU injuries with either retrograde urethrograms or cystograms. They also allow monitoring of end-organ perfusion and the success of the resuscitative effort through urinary output. When necessary, field tourniquets are replaced with pneumatic ones, particularly in cases where continued hemorrhage occurs. Total limb tourniquet time must be documented with a goal of expedited surgical hemostasis and removal of the tourniquet as soon as possible.

Physical examination of the pelvis should be conducted by a skilled provider and performed only once. Repeated examinations can cause clots to be dislodged and exacerbate bleeding. In situations where fracture stability is unclear, stabilization of the pelvis with a compression sheet or binder is recommended until further guidance is available from an orthopedic surgeon. Pelvic or

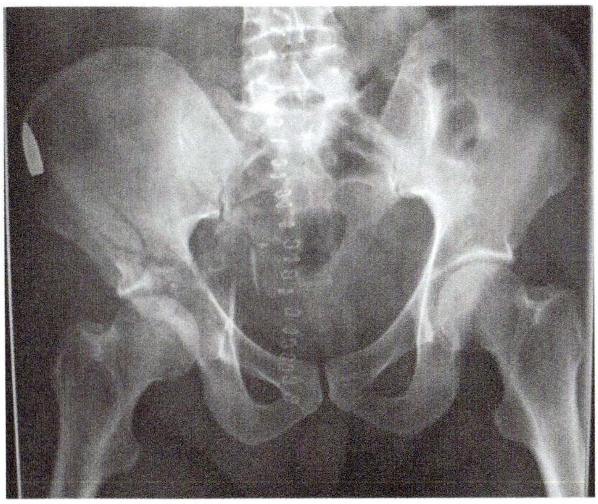

Fig. 12.6 AP pelvic radiograph with penetrating high-velocity GSW and complex, comminuted acetabular fracture and traumatic rectal laceration treated with exploratory laparotomy with irrigation, debridement, rectal repair, and diverting colostomy. Associated visceral and neurovascular injuries are common in penetrating and blast mechanisms

acetabular fracture patterns not associated with cardiovascular or pelvic instability do not require temporizing stabilization and can be admitted to the ward with serial exams to assess vital signs and urine output. The majority of the hemorrhage associated with pelvic trauma is venous in nature and may be successfully controlled in the trauma bay with simple maneuvers that reduce and stabilize intrapelvic volume. Pelvic binders are effectively applied by centering the binder over the femoral trochanters and the symphysis pubis. Assistants should apply pressure on the trochanters to assist in ring reduction while another provider securely fastens the pelvic binder or clamps the pelvic sheet.

Hip dislocations must be urgently reduced under conscious sedation in the trauma bay or the operating room. Unfortunately, there are no means for skeletal traction during medevac transport. Closed fractures with intra-articular fragments are not treated until they arrive in Role 4 or 5 hospitals out of the combat theater. Hip stabilization with abduction sheets or pillows and a knee immobilizer are the only available conservative means in theater. Persistently unstable acetabular fracture-dislocations that fail these treatment measures require hip-spanning external

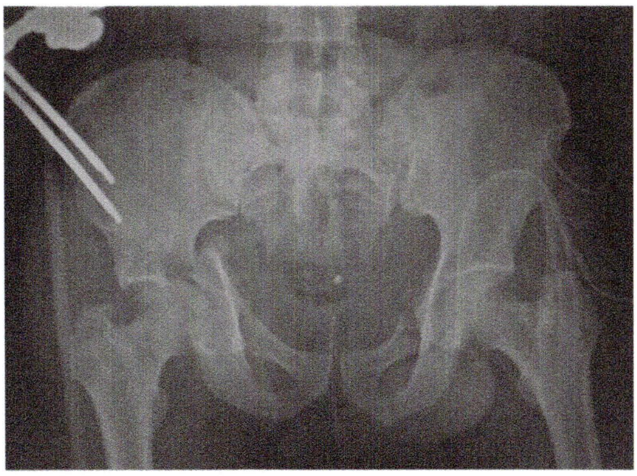

Fig. 12.7 AP pelvic radiograph of a comminuted transverse-posterior wall acetabular fracture and combined contralateral ring injury. The lack of skeletal traction in transport and a long working distance demonstrate the relative instability and poor control of hip-spanning external fixation

fixation to prevent further injury to the articular cartilage and surrounding neurovascular structures (Figs. 12.7 and 12.8).

Adjunctive studies should be limited to trauma bay radiographs of the chest and pelvis in the hemodynamically unstable and stable patients with pelvic or acetabular fractures. In these cases, CT scanning is generally avoided and used only when objective measures of head injury suggest the possible need for neurosurgical intervention. Otherwise, unstable patients are taken emergently to the OR for surgical intervention. Selected extremity radiographs and additional views of the pelvis with inlet, outlet, and judets are obtained only if patient stability permits. Once these steps are completed, the patient is transported directly to the operating room for initial damage control surgery. Intraoperative use of fluoroscopy at Role 3 facilities is a valuable tool to further assess pelvic stability through a dynamic exam.

Since the majority of unstable pelvic injuries are due to high-energy IED injuries, the initial surgical care of the DCBI patient is best achieved using a team of surgeons including general and orthopedic working concurrently. The initial goals of damage control surgery involve hemorrhage control, pelvic ring external fixation, and wound decontamination. For example, the general sur-

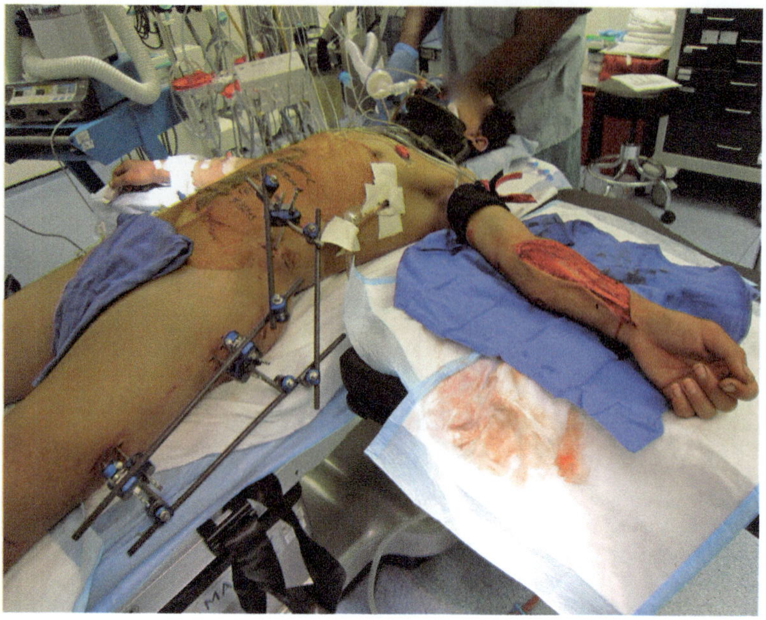

Fig. 12.8 Example of hip-spanning external fixation with a multiplanar construct and a distributed working distance that does not violate potential future surgical incision sites

geons can achieve proximal intrapelvic vessel control and address intra-abdominal injuries while an orthopedic team focuses on the lower extremity amputations. A third team can address upper extremity injuries if necessary. These coordinated efforts maximize OR efficiency and limit prolonged physiologic insult to a severely injured patient. Prior to surgery, the most critical procedures should be listed keeping in mind reasonable parameters to terminate surgery if the patient becomes too unstable. Assurance of hemostasis and removal of all nonviable tissue, including skin, fat, fascia, muscle, and bone, are essential to reduce the load of contamination and necrotic tissue in the wounds. These patients will require repeat surgeries and reevaluation on a regular basis. Their traumatic wounds typically progress; meaning tissue that may have appeared viable at one setting may require debridement at the next operative intervention.

12.4 Pelvic External Fixation

Unstable pelvic ring fractures are provisionally stabilized with lower extremity internal rotation and taping or pelvic sheets and binders until formal operative external fixation is applied. Avoid prolonged use of pelvic binders for greater than 24 h to minimize soft tissue pressure ulcers. It is best to replace binders with pelvic external fixation when the patient is stable or resources are available. External fixation provides the best downrange stability and allows access to complex soft tissue injuries of the abdomen and perineum. This construct permits safe patient transport to higher echelons of care without losing control of the pelvic volume and disrupting clot formation (Figs. 12.9 and 12.10).

Downrange pelvic external fixation is performed using either iliac crest or supra-acetabular pins constructs. Patient stability, operative resources such as fluoroscopy, and surgeon experience help dictate which frame option is optimal at the index treatment. In the hemodynamically unstable patient or DCBI pattern, a resuscitative frame using iliac crest pins is preferred because it is not as fluoroscopic or time intensive as supra-acetabular pins. In the austere environments where resources are limited by equipment, fluoroscopy, and surgeon comfort level, iliac crest pins are also the recommended method. Supra-acetabular pins are often reserved for the hemodynamically stable patient where fluoroscopy is available (Echelon/Role 3 or higher). Surgeons unfamiliar with this technique

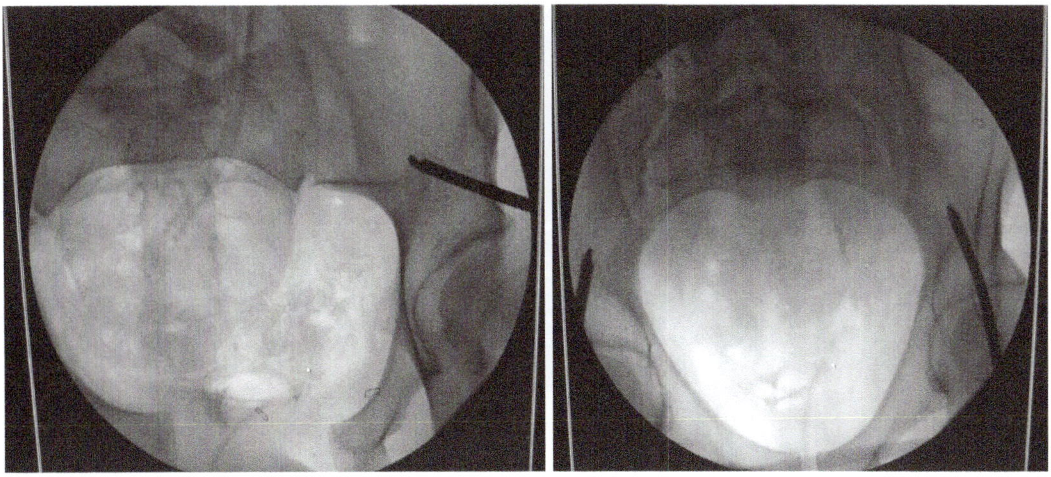

Figs. 12.9 and 12.10 Intraoperatively, fluoro images depict the value of pelvic ring stabilization with external fixation (supra-acetabular pins in this case). Reduction of pelvic ring volume decreases intrapelvic potential bleeding space, enhances hemostasis and clot formation, and provides pain control and access to soft tissue injuries during transport out of theater where definitive fixation occurs

should proceed with the more standard iliac pin constructs.

12.4.1 Technique for Iliac Crest Pins (Resuscitative Frame)

A 3–4 cm incision is made 2 cm posterior to anterior superior iliac spine (ASIS) in line over the iliac crest. Sharp dissection continues directly down to iliac crest bone by incising between the external oblique abdominal fascia and the tensor fascia lata. Next, palpate the inner and outer tables of iliac wing and place a 2.0 mm Kirschner wire or hemostat inside the iliac wing along the inner table as a trajectory guide for the intended half pins. This will help direct pins to remain within the inner and outer iliac tables. A common fault is placing the pins too vertical where they penetrate the outer table without substantial bony purchase. Insert at least three 5 mm half pins into each iliac wing with a centimeter of spread between pins. Pins should optimally engage the inner and outer tables for at least 5 cm; hence, multiple pins assure better stability in case one pin is poorly directed. The incision can be loosely approximated around the pins with a few sutures. Pin-to-bar clamps are placed two fingerbreadths above the skin. Reduction bars are orientated anteriorly and centered over the pubic symphysis where bar-to-bar clamps secure and hold the closed or open reduction. Stacking the pin-to-bar clamp constructs will increase stability. A third transverse bar may be added for additional multiplanar stability. All clamps are retightened and the adequacy of reduction is assessed with fluoroscopy when available. When applicable, take advantage of open celiotomy wounds to reduce and clamp the pubic symphysis or assess the posterior ring reduction through direct palpation (Fig. 12.11).

12.4.2 Technique for Supra-acetabular Pins (Sport Frame)

These pins are centered on the anterior inferior iliac spine (AIIS) and directed toward the dense cortical bone just superior to the greater sciatic notch. Inexperienced surgeons should not attempt this technique, as there are risks of acetabular penetration and hip sepsis with incorrect placement. The starting point and trajectory of the pins are confirmed over the AIIS with fluoroscopy using obturator outlet ("AIIS teepee") and iliac views. A 1–2 cm incision is made with blunt

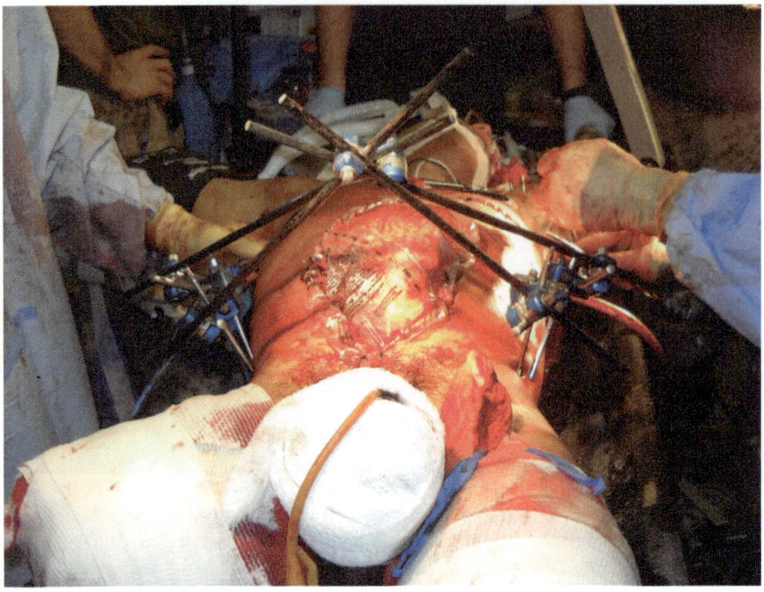

Fig. 12.11 Post-op DCBI casualty treated at a Role 2 FST with iliac crest pelvic external fixation with proper multi-pin placement and multiple bar stabilization after symphyseal reduction was achieved through the open ex-lap wound. This is the recommended frame for orthopedic surgeons operating without fluoroscopy

instrument dissection made down onto the AIIS. Ensure that the pin is greater than 1 cm above the acetabular dome and out of the hip capsule (iliac view). A single 5–6 × 225–250 mm half pin is advanced into each hemipelvis. The obturator inlet view confirms pin placement within the inner and outer tables and the iliac view confirms final position above the sciatic notch. Since a solid tube of bone runs from the AIIS to the PSIS near the midline of the pelvis, these pins offer the greatest control for pelvic reduction and stabilization. Pin-to-bar clamps are placed two fingerbreadths above the skin. In thin patients without open wounds, a single transverse bar can be attached across the anterior pelvis between pins to maintain the reduction. In cases of large abdomens or open abdominal wounds, a two-bar construct should be used with bars orientated anteriorly and medially from each AIIS pin. Stacking additional bars increases frame rigidity. These sport frames are low profile and facilitate patient mobilization but tend to limit hip and waist flexion to about 70° (Fig. 12.12).

12.4.3 Stabilize the Pelvis Before Turning Prone

Patients with complex perineal blast wounds to the buttocks require external fixation for unstable pelvic injuries prior to turning them in a lateral recumbent or prone positions. Sometimes, these wounds can be addressed from the supine position with elevation of the legs. When in doubt, err on the conservative side, and take the patient to the ICU for monitoring, correction of coagulopathy, and further resuscitation. Return back to the OR in 4–6 h for repeat irrigation and debridement and a more thorough evaluation of all wounds, especially posterior wounds that may require special positioning. An aggressive, efficient debridement is essential to debulk highly contaminated open pelvic blast wounds. Do not get lost in the complexity of these wounds and set time limits of 2–3 h for index surgeries and debridements. It is understood that all contamination will not be removed at the initial operative debridements. Patient survival is the goal.

12.4.4 External Fixation for Acetabular Fractures

In unstable acetabular fractures in which the femoral head remains displaced and impacted into the acetabular socket or in cases with large fracture fragments, hip-spanning external fixation may be used to decrease joint reactive forces against the articular surfaces. The success of these hip-spanning ex-fix frames is limited due to

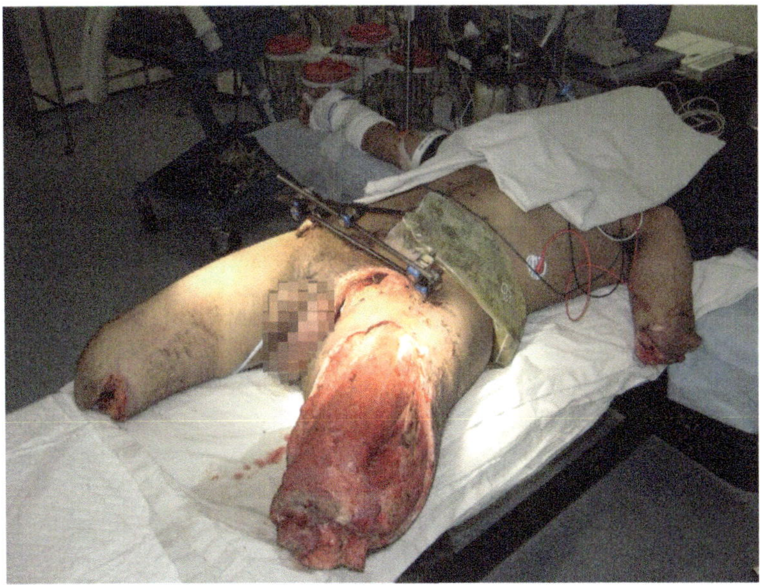

Fig. 12.12 Post-op DCBI casualty treated at a Role 3 MTF with supra-acetabular pelvic external fixation with proper pin placement guided by fluoroscopy and multiple bar stabilization after symphyseal reduction was achieved through the open ex-lap wound. Note the diverting colostomy utilized in this case of open pelvic fracture where wound sepsis is a major complication

the long working distance between iliac crest and femoral shaft pins. Supra-acetabular pins should be avoided. Multiplanar frames increase the stability across a long working distance and can help combat the deforming forces across the joint (Fig. 12.8). Poorly constructed uniplanar frames are usually insufficient to maintain a reduction (Fig. 12.7). Often, the simple use of a knee immobilizer and makeshift abduction pillows will suffice for maintaining joint reduction for transport. Skeletal traction is challenging, cumbersome, and no longer recommended for patient evacuation out of theater.

12.5 Peripelvic Vascular Injuries

The morbidity and mortality associated with pelvic fractures can be directly linked with injuries to the peripelvic vascular tree. The arterial and venous network around the pelvis is extensive and unfortunately prone to laceration with greater degrees of pelvic ring instability and fracture displacement.

Vascular injuries, especially within the iliac system or iliofemoral junctional region, are common and sometimes difficult to repair or shunt (Figs. 12.4 and 12.5). Proximal vascular control of the iliac vessels is imperative for the unstable patient with the DCBI pattern. This is performed through a laparotomy (intra-abdominal) or retroperitoneal approach. Assisting the general surgeons with these approaches is a great way to understand the anatomy of the iliac vasculature and the techniques utilized to effectively control hemorrhage. Temporary iliac vessel ligation with Rummel tourniquets may be necessary until the injured vessel is shunted, repaired, or ligated. Every effort should be made to prevent permanent common or internal iliac vessel ligation. Retroperitoneal pelvic packing with combat gauze or saline-soaked Kerlix may be required for additional hemostasis. Certain Role 3 hospitals have an interventional radiologist who can assist with selective angioembolization for adequate hemostasis in these critically injured polytrauma patients.

In those rare cases of massive intrapelvic bleeding with associated high proximal amputations, the decision to ligate the iliac vessels as a lifesaving measure is a balance between hemorrhage control and tissue viability that maximizes the length of amputations. Every effort should be made to advance temporary vascular control to the most distal and viable level.

Partial or complete hemipelvectomies are accepted damage control measures to handle the most severe cases of massive retroperitoneal bleeding and open pelvic ring injury. These retroperitoneal venous plexus injuries are extremely challenging and patients can quickly expire on the operating table. Timing is critical to survival: some injuries despite heroic measures are non-survivable.

12.6 Open Pelvic Fracture Care

Open pelvic fractures generally carry significant risks for morbidity and mortality. The complexity greatly increases when these injuries occur from higher energy combat wounding patterns where soft tissue defects are more extensive and blast bioburden heightens the risk for infection. Associated injuries to the urogenital and the colorectal systems should be expected and require a multidisciplinary team approach for surgical care. Historically, most open combat pelvic injuries have been non-survivable. However, recent advances in protective body armor and acute combat casualty care have led to a recent trend of survivors (i.e., DCBIs). An array of open fracture patterns occurs depending on the mechanism of injury.

Index care focuses on lifesaving resuscitation, pelvic ring stabilization, femoroacetabular reduction (if applicable), and wound decontamination as previously mentioned. The treatment for these injury patterns is surgical. Exploratory laparotomy allows visual access to treat associated vascular and visceral injuries (i.e., bladder or colon). A quick pre-op plan with general surgeons will reinforce orthopedic damage control principles and emphasize the definitive treatment techniques for open pelvic and acetabular fractures. Taking a few moments to do this can prevent burning bridges for future care.

Diversion of the fecal and urinary streams is important in preventing unnecessary continued contamination to complex open wounds. Sigmoid colon interruption with diverting colostomy must be performed away from potential future surgical incisions and implants (Fig. 12.12). The same is true for suprapubic catheters. If temporary vessel ligation is necessary for hemostasis, every effort must be made to avoid permanent ligation of large named peripelvic vessels in order to avoid ischemic necrosis of soft tissue flaps. On a rare occasion, partial or total hemipelvectomy can be a lifesaving procedure for complex open fractures with massive intrapelvic bleeding.

Open combat wounds are never closed downrange. Depending on the complexity of the wound, open pelvic injuries can be cumbersome to dress. Adequate surgical debridement and irrigation are the primary means to prevent necrosis and sepsis. Yet, infection is a constant concern. Bactericidal dressings such as the antibiotic bead pouch or Dakin's wet-to-dry coverage offer temporary infection control during patient transport and between surgical debridements. Negative pressure wound therapy (NPWT) can be a useful alternative for temporary wound coverage as it also decreases the bioburden. However, NPWT is not without challenges in the combat zone. First, complex soft tissue wounds around the pelvis are not always "VAC-able" as it is difficult to maintain a seal and there are detriments to a wound stewing in its own drainage. Second, NPWT can be highly dangerous in vascularized wounds and hypocoagulable patients with persistent oozing. Lastly, NPWT equipment is limited downrange and patient transport personnel may not monitor machines to assure there is an adequate seal and proper suction. Traditional wet-to-dry dressings overwrapped with a compressive Kerlix or Ace wrap are a reliable method for dressing these difficult wounds.

12.7 Critical Factors for Patient Monitoring and Transport

Due to the high morbidity and mortality associated with combat-related pelvic fractures, it is imperative that patients are transported with the necessary means to monitor their potentially volatile hemodynamic status. This includes adequate central and peripheral IV access for continued resuscitation and a Foley or suprapubic catheter to assess end-organ perfusion. Pelvic ring reduction along with external fixation frames and hip relocations should have one last check for stability prior to transport. Open wounds require adequate dressings and NPWT machines necessitate adequate battery life for the duration of transport either in or out of the combat zone. If the patient remains critically unstable, then continued hemostatic resuscitation and/or surgical hemostasis is necessary before transport. If there is a delay in transport, open wounds require repeat irrigation and debridement every 24–48 h. Extensive repeat surgical cases that can lead to substantial blood loss and hemodynamic instability due to surgical intervention should not occur within 6–8 h of transport.

Conclusion

Combat pelvic and acetabular fractures can vary from simple, stable, and closed injuries to extremely complex, open, and life threatening (i.e., dismounted complex blast injury). The unique combination of blast, penetrating, and blunt mechanisms of injury contributes to the intricacy. Despite high historic rates of battlefield mortality, modern combat casualty care innovations have led to an increasing number of survivors with pelvic and acetabular fractures. The priorities of initial downrange orthopedic care involve assessment of pelvic stability, surgical hemostasis of the complex peripelvic vasculature, pelvic ring stabilization with external fixation, reduction of hip dislocations, and wound decontamination before transport uprange. Polytrauma is the norm and a team of general and orthopedic surgeons working concurrently is the most efficient system for achieving numerous, critical goals during the index surgery while decreasing the risks of prolonged surgery and a second physiologic insult. Know when to quit in the operating theater; further hemostatic resuscitation in the ICU goes a long way in preventing unnecessary morbidity and mortality. When in doubt, seek peer advice with other orthopedic surgeons downrange as you are never alone.

Frontline Orthopedic Care for Hand Injuries

13

Eric P. Hofmeister and Donald E. Bittner

Contents

BLUF (Bottom Line Up Front) Box

1. Study and know the anatomy of the hand.
2. In the setting of mass trauma, do not neglect an examination or an assessment of the injured hand.
3. Attempt all measures to save the length and vascularity of the thumb.
4. Employ liberal use of fasciotomies to include the thenar and hypothenar eminence and intrinsics and include an acute carpal tunnel release.
5. Splint or surgically stabilize all structures out to normal length to maintain the tension relationship on the soft tissues.
6. Understand and incorporate functional splinting to ensure that the metacarpophalangeal joints are held in flexion, the wrist in slight extension, and the interphalangeal joints in extension to slight flexion during transportation ("Intrinsic Plus" Position).
7. When making incisions across a flexor crease, be sure to use Z- or curved-type incisions to avoid postinjury stiffness.
8. Save any viable tissue, even if you're unsure if it could be used at a later date (spare parts surgery).
9. Identify, tag with colored suture, and document all cut structures (i.e., tendons, nerves, and blood vessels).

The views expressed in this article are those of the authors and do not reflect the official policy of the Department of the Navy, Department of Defense, or the US Government. No benefits in any form have been received or will be received from a commercial party related directly or indirectly to the subject of this article.

E.P. Hofmeister, MD (✉) • D.E. Bittner, MD
Department of Orthopedic Surgery,
Naval Medical Center San Diego,
San Diego, CA, USA
e-mail: eric.hofmeister@med.navy.mil

L.B. Bone, C.N. Mamczak (eds.), *Front Line Extremity and Orthopaedic Surgery*,
DOI 10.1007/978-3-642-45337-3_13, © Springer-Verlag Berlin Heidelberg 2014

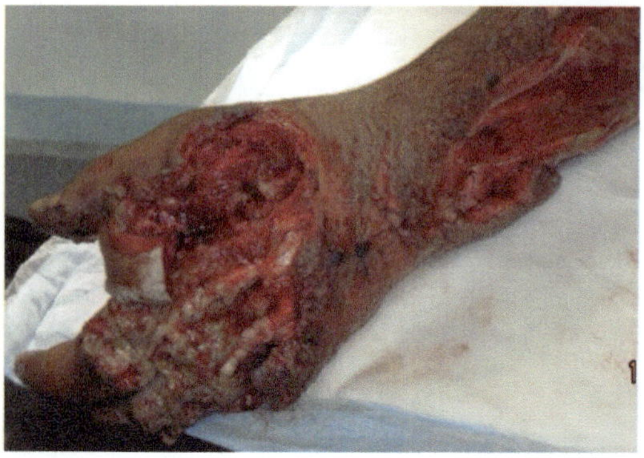

Fig. 13.1 Examples of typical severely injured hand encounter on the battlefield (Courtesy of Donald E. Bittner, CAPT, MC, USN, Naval Medical Center San Diego)

Injuries to the hand in the combat environment can range from trivial, small lacerations to extensive-, explosive-type injuries, leaving the hand and upper extremity mangled. With the improved personal protective equipment and advances in vehicles, morbidity and mortality on the battlefield have been greatly improved. However, the extremities remain vulnerable to injury. Although many of these injuries can appear quite daunting on first inspection, it is important to keep a very systematic approach to examining the hand. The goal of initial treatment is to:

1. Debride nonviable tissue, especially muscle
2. To remove the gross contamination from the wound
3. To identify structures that are injured
4. To splint and stabilize the hand in a functional position to allow for further debridement and reconstruction in the future

Hand injuries can be a combination of blunt, blast, and burn trauma, sometimes all in the same casualty (Fig. 13.1). One must think of all these entities at the same time while treating these patients, as no one entity can be addressed separately with a good outcome.

13.1 Anatomy

The hand has incredibly complex anatomy. The hand is made up of eight carpal bones, five metacarpal bones, and three phalanges in the index, middle, ring, and small fingers, while the thumb has two. Additionally, there are variable appearing bony sesamoids within the hand to include possibly two at the volar aspect of the thumb, index, and small metacarpophalangeal joints. The bones of the hand are all held in place by an intricate network of ligaments. Each digit has flexor tendons and extensor tendons along with small but very important intrinsic musculature to include the thenar, hypothenar, lumbrical, and interossei muscles. The main blood flow to the hand is volarly through both the radial and ulnar arteries with variance on which is the more dominant contributor. In addition to collateral flow, the hand may also receive vascular input from a persistent median artery located within the carpal canal.

Innervation of the radial 3-1/2 digits is predominantly the median nerve while the ulnar nerve supplies sensation to the ulnar 1-1/2 digits. The dorsoradial aspect of the hand and digits also receives sensory innervation from the radial nerve; however, only the deep motor branch of the ulnar nerve and the deep branch of the median nerve supply muscular innervation to the hand intrinsic muscles. Additionally, there is a rich anastomosis of venous network and lymphatics located predominantly in the dorsal aspect of the hand. The skin on the hand is quite different with a thicker, more durable glabrous skin volarly and thinner skin with hair dorsally.

Despite this very complex anatomy, it is important when addressing these injuries to keep the treatment as simple as possible as overtreatment or attempted definitive treatment of the severely injured hand can lead to a disastrous outcome. Debridement is the key with stabilization of the bony anatomy. Tissue sparing and tagging neurovascular structures are important. Never close these wounds but attempt to obtain soft tissue coverage over neurovascular structures and tendinous structures whenever possible.

13.2 Mechanism of Injury

The mechanism of injury to the hand in the battlefield can range remarkably in severity from everything as simple as a fingertip crush injury or laceration to a completely complex explosive injury to the hand involving all neurovascular structures, bony anatomy, and soft tissue. These injuries can stem from one of several types of battlefield components. One of the most common causes of battlefield hand injury results from exposure to blasting munitions, which are a unique combination of blast, burn, and blunt trauma. When addressing these injuries, one must think of each of these components separately in order to obtain the proper treatment. Occasionally, gunshot wounds are encountered.

13.3 Initial Evaluation

Upon first encountering a patient with a hand injury, it is important to understand in what environment and situation the injury occurred. For example, open fractures sustained in a swamp or burn pit are much different from an open laceration over a metacarpal fracture resulting from a closed fist striking a wall. Furthermore, it is easy for the provider to get distracted by a horrific hand injury and forget the basics to include ABC (airway, breathing, and circulation), cervical spine protection, ATLS (advanced trauma life support) protocol, and standard resuscitative measures. However, once this is accomplished and prior to the patient being transported, it is very important if time permits to get a good evaluation and properly treat hand injuries. The best way to evaluate the injured hand is by a systematic approach. Before any dressings are removed, it is often easy to get a good sensory exam, including a 2-point discrimination on each fingertip along with a vascular exam of the digits. Doing this exam prior to taking down dressings not only prepares the examiner for what they may encounter but is also easier before the patient becomes less cooperative from the dressing removal or administration of pain narcotics or an arm block. During the systematic exam, each joint should be put through a passive (and active if possible) range of motion with each bone palpated.

In the severely injured patient, it is still important to get as much of an exam as possible. It is essential to make an immediate decision as to what can possibly be saved and what must be debrided and excised. The hand can endure extensive trauma and still remain reconstructible. If the injury is quite extensive, the decision to amputate may need to be decided immediately. In patients with multiple areas of trauma undergoing lifesaving surgery, time can be of essence. If the clinical situation allows, saving as much viable soft tissue and digit or extremity length as possible is recommend to later allow for complex reconstructions and "spare part surgery." Creative downrange thinking can lead to reconstructive salvage options, for example, imminent thumb amputations were successfully treated with pollicization after a great toe was revascularized within the forearm prior to lower extremity amputation.

If time and situation allow, standard radiographs to include AP, lateral, and obliques of the hand in its entirety along with the wrist are warranted. However, transfer of the patient should never be delayed to obtain these studies.

13.4 Fractures

As mentioned, all bones and joints within the hand should be palpated and fractures stabilized if time and situation dictate. Not only does this allow for decrease in pain and narcotic requirements but also decreases fluid production at the fracture site, potentially decreases the infection rates, and keeps the soft tissue on proper tension. Closed fractures can be managed either with splinting or, if markedly malaligned or dislocated, reduced and splinted, or occasionally stabilized, with temporary K-wire fixation or external fixation applied (Fig. 13.2a–d). Open fractures require exploration, debridement, reduction, and stabilization if time and safety to the patient are not jeopardized. Generally, all open fractures in the combat environment should not be closed nor should definitive fixation such as plates and screws be placed downrange. Open fractures can be loosely closed, but they must have the ability to allow for drainage of the wound and all spaces to be open so no deep space

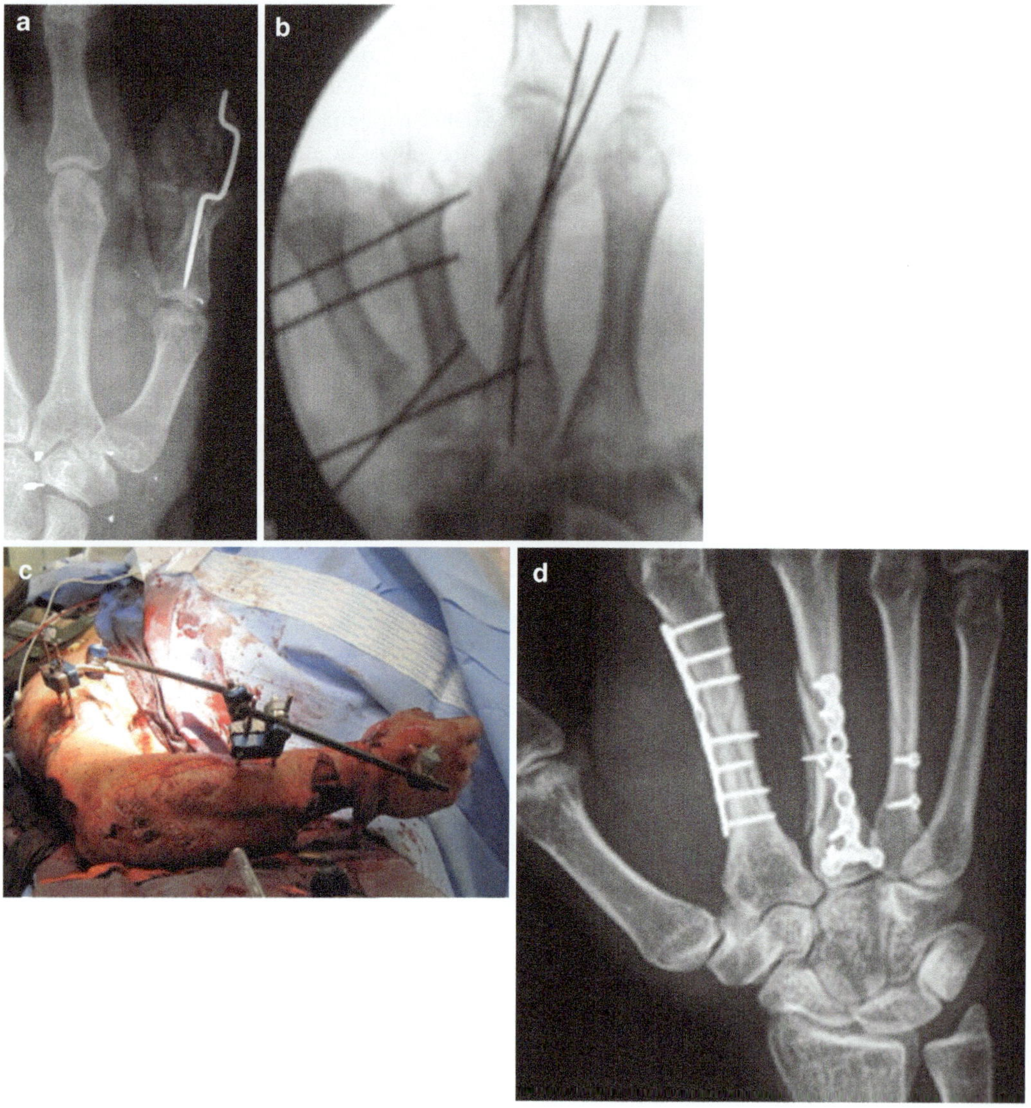

Fig. 13.2 Methods of fixation for fracture stabilization, including spacing metacarpal fixation (**a**), multiple K-wires in a two-finger amputation (**b**), and incorporation into an external fixator of the upper extremity (**c**). Multiple internal rigid fixation as shown in (**d**) is not an appropriate treatment in the battlefield setting (Courtesy of Eric P. Hofmeister, CAPT, MC, USN, Naval Medical Center San Diego)

abscess can form. Fracture stabilization should be kept as simple as possible utilizing minimal hardware. Pinning of fingers can consist of constructs such as cross K-wires, K-wires perpendicular to the fracture, or using an adjacent digit or an adjacent phalanx or metacarpal to help stabilize. These can often be done without the aid of fluoroscopy and again serve to keep the digit or extremity grossly aligned. External fixation can be used to span open fractures and can go from the digit to a metacarpal or even to the distal forearm. When required, they can easily be incorporated into an upper extremity external fixation.

13.5 Vascular Injuries

Although the hand has dual arterial blood supply, occasionally it can remain vascularized despite disruption of both the radial and ulnar arteries. In

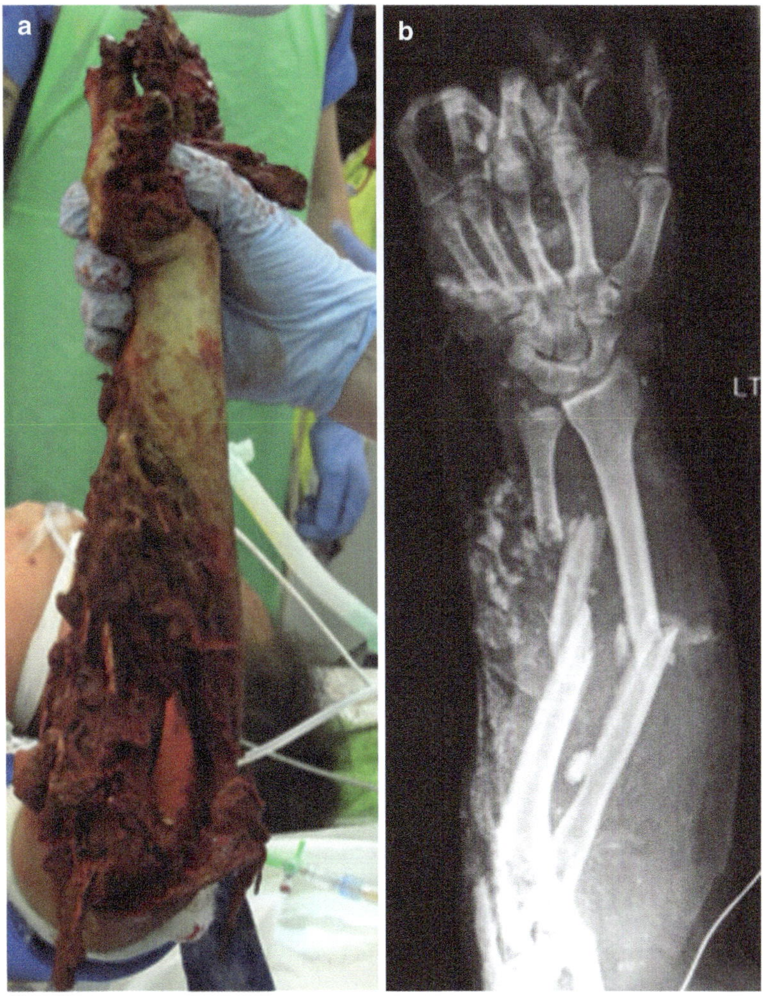

Fig. 13.3 (**a**, **b**) Despite disruption of both the radial and ulnar arteries, a portion of this hand remained perfused and was able to undergo reconstruction and regain some functional use of the hand (Courtesy of Donald E. Bittner, CAPT, MC, USN, Naval Medical Center San Diego)

a battlefield environment with more proximal vascular injuries, these can be repaired or shunted, but injuries distal to the wrist rarely are reanastomosed, grafted, or repaired due to lack of time, experience, and microscopic equipment available to provide a reanastomosis. It should be noted, however, if blood flow is questionable despite disruption of both the radial and ulnar arteries and the patient is healthy and in stable condition, this tissue should *not* be amputated (Fig. 13.3a, b).

13.6 Compartment Syndrome

Although less talked about than in other areas of the body, compartment syndromes of the hand can occur and this is particularly true in blast injuries or massive trauma to the hand. Although the amount of muscle is not great and often the injured patient can tolerate dead muscle from the hand, it can ultimately lead to devastating functional results if not treated properly. There is controversy over the exact number of compartments within the hand, but generally, compartment releases of the hand include decompressing the thenar eminence and the hypothenar eminence, two dorsal incisions to release the dorsal and volar interossei, and a carpal tunnel release. The carpal tunnel incision can be easily incorporated into a forearm fasciotomy taking care to come across the wrist flexor crease at an angle rather than a straight incision (Fig. 13.4). Preventing compartment syndrome of the hand prevents severe posturing and stiffness, and release of the

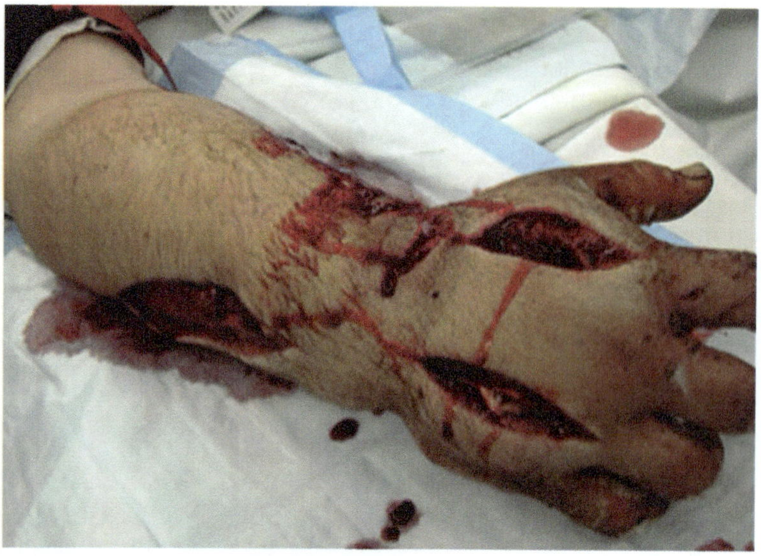

Fig. 13.4 Incisions on the dorsal hand and forearm required for release of all dorsal compartments of the hand (Courtesy of Eric P. Hofmeister, CAPT, MC, USN, Naval Medical Center San Diego)

carpal canal can greatly improve and restore function to the median nerve.

Often, blast injuries to the forearm can "jump joints" and extend into the hand. If there is any question, these injuries should be treated aggressively and compartment releases should be completed. Tissue that appears only slightly abnormal can quickly evolve to extremely abnormal over a 6- to 8-h period as these patients undergo aggressive resuscitation and potentially long and noisy medical evacuations and often cannot respond subjectively due to being intubated, heavy narcotic use, or arm blocks. Despite doing extensive compartment releases, once the swelling in the hand has subsided, often skin grafting is only required at one incision site or not required at all.

13.7 Nerves and Tendons

During the evaluation of the traumatized hand, severed nerves, flexor and extensor tendons, and muscles may be identified. Although these are generally not repaired in the theater, occasionally nerve repairs can be done if the wound is not contaminated, the patient is otherwise stable, and the equipment and expertise are available. Situations that may allow for consideration of a repair in the battlefield include sharp nerve lacerations of either the median, ulnar, common digital, or proper digital nerve of the hand. Isolated lacerated intrinsic muscles or extensor tendons may also be repaired; however, flexor tendons or tendons and nerves that are injured with gaps such as that which would occur in a blast injury should not undergo reconstruction while in the battlefield environment and are best suited for a plethora of reconstructive methods at larger specialty treatment facilities.

If a structure is repaired, postoperative splinting is required. Even with an isolated hand injury, the patient will not be able to stay in theater if proper facilities and rehabilitation are not available. It is very important to identify any lacerated structures, tag with colored sutures on each end for easier identification at definitive reconstruction, and incorporate skin and/or muscle to maintain or create a soft tissue envelope over these structures to prevent desiccation and destruction.

13.8 Muscle

Any small muscular structures in the hand must also be evaluated for debridement, as these can hold a plethora of fine partial debris and bacteria. Muscle viability can be judged by the amount of pullback of the muscle as well as the color while debriding. Electrocautery can aid in the amount of muscle pullback when debriding in the hand;

however, one must be very careful when debriding these areas that they have an idea of where the neurovascular structures are to not cause further damage.

13.9 Skin

Debridement of all soft tissues, especially the skin, is essential in these patients. If thorough debridement is not completed, the infected area could extend past the area of injury and ultimately cause more soft tissue loss and disability. There is a learning curve on deciding the extent of debridement and one must use logic when looking at these wounds. Any area of skin that appears to be macerated, contused, or has an extensive amount of debris must be debrided.

Negative pressure wound therapy assisted closures can be quite beneficial and helpful to injuries of the hand; however, it must be noted that these are often difficult to maintain a secure seal, especially when these injuries involve the digits. Creative methods may need to be incorporated to get a good seal (Fig. 13.5). Nonetheless, negative pressure wound therapy is crucial in a battlefield and is used quite extensively along with Dakin solution packing and wound splinting.

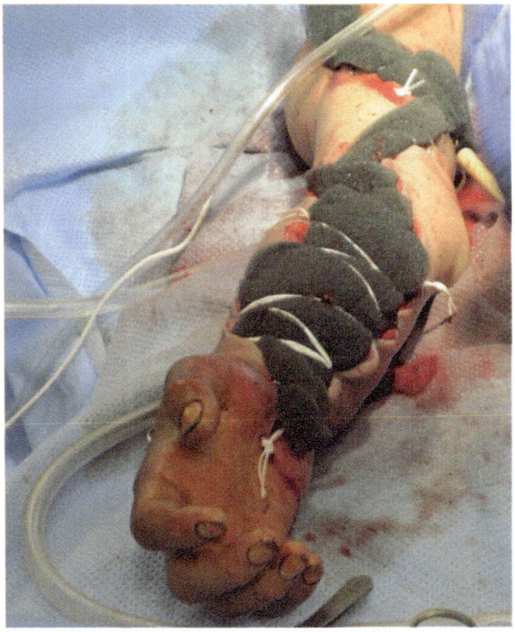

Fig. 13.5 Arm and forearm fasciotomies with acute carpal tunnel release and the use of a wound vacuum-assisted closure (*VAC*) (Courtesy of Eric P. Hofmeister, CAPT, MC, USN, Naval Medical Center San Diego)

13.10 Burns

Burn injuries to the hand can be in isolation such as a thermal burn from an explosive incendiary or an open fire, or it can be in combination with a blast or gunshot wound. Burns to the hand often ultimately require specialized care to ensure optimal results, and the negative long-term consequences with even initially appearing inconsequential burns to the hand must be appreciated.

When evaluating the hand, one must decide whether it is a first-degree, second-degree, or third-degree burn. With second- or third-degree burns, escharotomies of the hand are essential, along with extension into the forearm area to prevent further loss of vascular status from the constricting wounds. Hydrating dressings and burn ointments are critical for tissue preservation, infection prevention, and pain control (Fig. 13.6a, b). Additionally, burns share many of the same types of problems as blast injuries, and therefore in addition to escharotomies, thorough debridement of necrotic and infected tissue, proper wound coverage, and splinting are essential in optimizing treatment.

13.11 Amputation/Combined Injuries to the Hand

Although every effort should be made to preserve the digits of the hand, especially the thumb, one should never do this at the risk of life to the patient. Oftentimes, the hand is the last area evaluated in the extremely critically ill patient and a very quick assessment and treatment must be accomplished. If the injuries to the hand or upper extremity are threatening the life of the patient, then amputation may be warranted. Also, if there is incredible damage with severe soft tissue stripping and/or skeletonization of bones, amputation

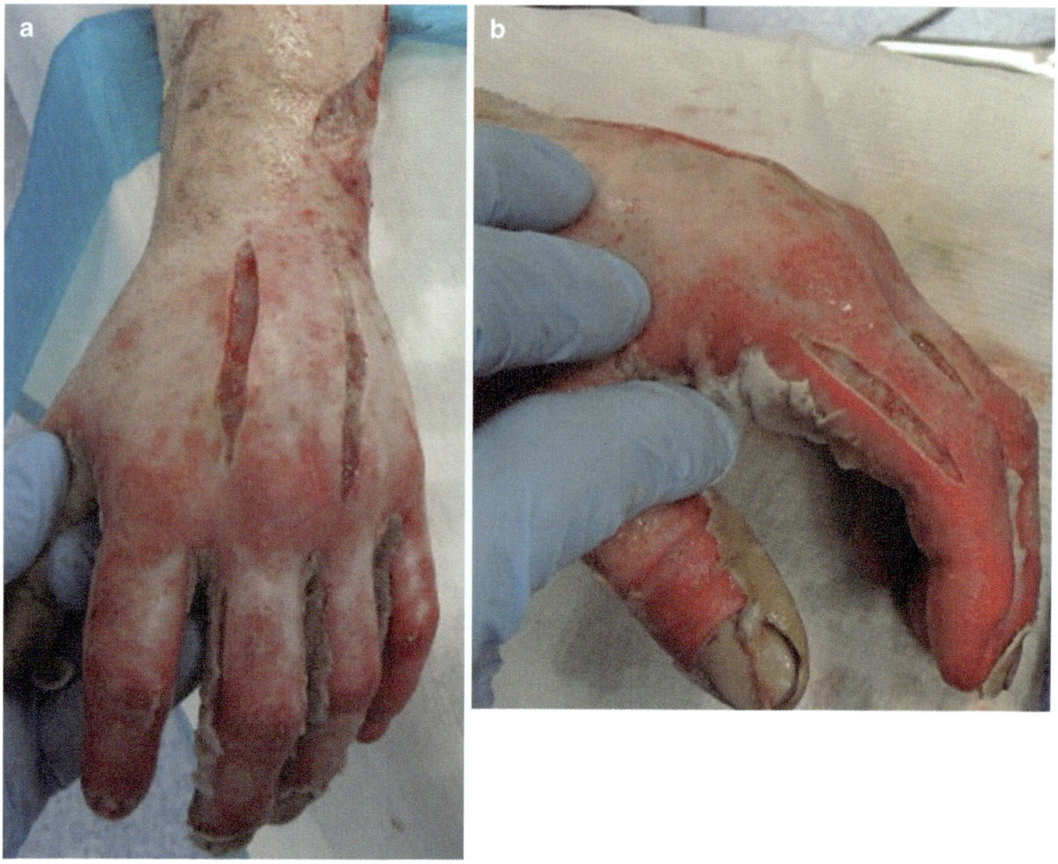

Fig. 13.6 Escharotomies of a third-degree burn of the dorsal hand (**a**) and digits (**b**) (Courtesy of Donald E. Bittner, CAPT, MC, USN, Naval Medical Center San Diego)

may be warranted. Finally, amputation may be warranted in settings where removing a portion of the hand provides improved soft tissue coverage over other vital structures, thereby giving a better outcome (Fig. 13.7a, b). Combined injuries have a component of blast and burn and are often devastating. However, with modern-day microsurgical treatment, soft tissue transfers, and free flaps, optimal function can be restored to the severely mangled hand.

When amputating digits, every attempt should be made to save any vascularized, noninfected soft tissue for wound coverage. A "soft tissue glove" can be accomplished by dissecting directly on the bone as "shelling out" the destructed bony digits, leaving the neurovascular glove intact. Minor debridement of this tissue will allow for a soft tissue glove to pull back over any open areas. Although a very light tacking of the skin and a drain are desirable, no attempt should be made at completely closing these flaps. Attempts to preserve all viable length should be employed with the increasing awareness of free digit transfers or even vascular composite allografts that are available as future reconstructions.

13.12 Splinting

Splinting of the injured hand should always be done and should be an easily mastered skill of those taking care of hand injuries. Fingers can be immobilized in AlumaFoam or prefabricated splints, while more proximal injuries or combined injuries require splinting the entire hand and wrist. Plaster splinting is generally placed volarly;

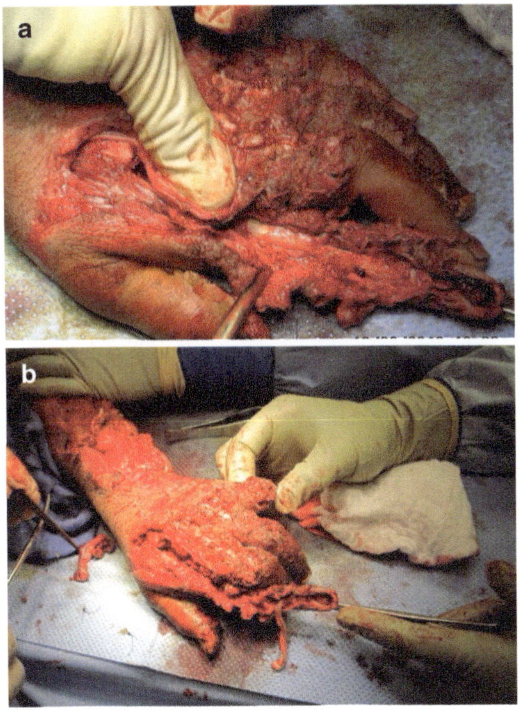

Fig. 13.7 (**a**, **b**) Two cases requiring amputation of a portion of the hand and utilizing the viable soft tissue to improve the soft tissue coverage over other vital structures (Courtesy of Donald E. Bittner, CAPT, MC, USN, Naval Medical Center San Diego)

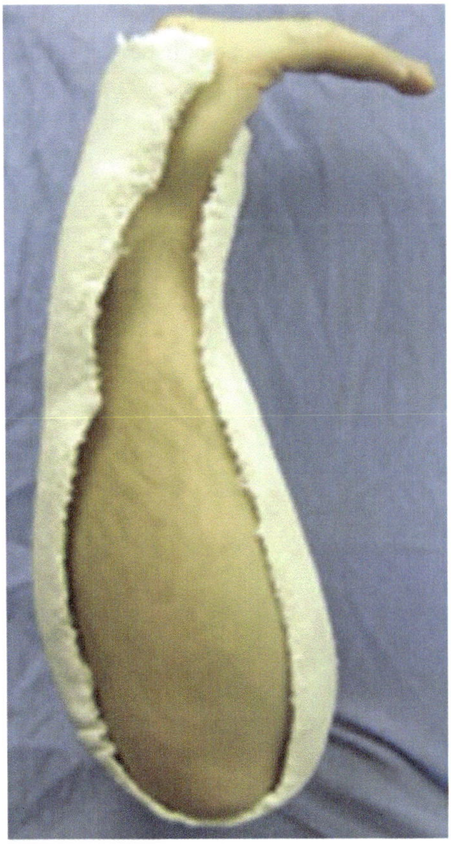

Fig. 13.8 Proper splint application. The wrist should be splinted in slight extension, the metacarpophalangeal (*MP*) joints are held in flexion, and the interphalangeal (*IP*) joints are splinted in extension to slight flexion (Courtesy of Eric P. Hofmeister, CAPT, MC, USN, Naval Medical Center San Diego)

however, if repair of certain tissues has been done, a dorsal extension block splint may actually be more appropriate. In addition to placing nonadherent dressings and bulky dressings to allow for swelling, particularly during long transports with rapid changes in elevation, it is important to keep the hand in a position of function. The wrist should be splinted in slight extension while the metacarpophalangeal (MP) joints are held in flexion to keep the collateral ligaments out to length, preventing MP joint stiffness. The interphalangeal (IP) joints should generally be splinted in extension to slight flexion (Fig. 13.8). If injured, the first webspace between the thumb and the index finger should also be incorporated into the splint and held out to ensure that a webspace contracture does not evolve over the ensuing transportation and serial treatments. If external fixation has been utilized, this often will serve as the splint, and only the addition of soft dressings will be required. This also aids in quick repeat evaluation of the wounds. If the humerus or the forearm has significant fracture or soft tissue instability, these must be splinted to prevent further damage of the neurovascular structures of the hand as "what is upstream" provides neurovascular input to the hand "downstream."

Conclusion

The hand is a very complex and highly specialized area of the body, which can quickly overwhelm the provider or be completely neglected. A thorough, systematic review while keeping the anatomy and mechanism of injury in mind along with prompt treatment can often lead to optimal results. Optimal treatment can be accomplished by adhering to the following principles:

1. Complete and document a thorough hand evaluation and examination preoperatively
2. Thorough debridement
3. Simple fracture stabilization
4. Tagging injured neurovascular structures and tendons
5. Proper wound care
6. Appropriate splinting.

Forearm Injuries

14

Leo T. Kroonen

Contents

L.T. Kroonen, MD
Division of Hand and Upper Extremity Surgery, Department of Orthopaedic Surgery, Naval Medical Center San Diego, 34800 Bob Wilson Drive, San Diego, CA 92130, USA
e-mail: leo.kroonen@med.navy.mil

BLUF (Bottom Line Up Front) Box

1. Remember life over limb. If you have to amputate a limb to save a life, it's worth it.
2. Get an early look at what you're dealing as soon as possible in the trauma bay. You can start preparing the OR while the patient is still being worked up.
3. Check all tourniquets in the trauma bay. If you don't need them, get rid of them. You don't need any more dead muscle than you already have.
4. Know your anatomy. When placing an external fixation, make an incision rather than placing pins blindly in the upper extremity.
5. When performing fasciotomies of the forearm, avoid making an incision that will leave the median nerve uncovered. A radially based flap can help avoid this problem.
6. Get a good vascular exam early, and be prepared to shunt or repair vessels if it will make a difference in saving the hand.
7. Leave nerves long if possible. A long nerve won't make your patient sick acutely and might give more options for reconstruction later.
8. Debride only what you need to debridement. Think about atypical coverage with fillet flaps, skin graft, or free flaps to preserve length.

L.B. Bone, C.N. Mamczak (eds.), *Front Line Extremity and Orthopaedic Surgery*,
DOI 10.1007/978-3-642-45337-3_14, © Springer-Verlag Berlin Heidelberg 2014

14.1 Introduction

Injuries to the forearm in a combat environment can result from a diverse array of mechanisms including blast wounds, gunshot wounds, crush injuries, burns, and blunt trauma. The principles of managing these injuries are similar to other regions of the musculoskeletal system. However, given the difference in function of the upper extremity compared to the lower extremity, and because upper extremity prostheses in their current state are unable to come as close to recreating the function of the native arm, greater attempts should be made to preserve length and function when possible.

14.2 Patterns of Injury

While there are countless patterns of injuries that can be produced from the varied mechanisms mentioned of injury, the blast wounds to the forearm associated with improvised explosive devices will often take on a typical pattern associated with the position in which the arms are held in the "low-ready" position. In this position, with the blast coming from the ground, the ulnar side of the non-dominant forearm and hand receives the majority of the damage, often with some preservation of the more radial structures (see Fig. 14.1). Meanwhile, the dominant arm with the trigger finger is typically held closer to the body in a more protected position. Most often, fortunately, the dominant arm is injured less severely. In penetrating trauma from gunshot wounds, RPGs, or other projectiles, any injury pattern can be seen.

14.3 In the Trauma Bay

Initial management should include due attention to the ATLS protocol, with careful evaluation of vital signs, circulatory function, and ventilatory function. Once these vital functions are addressed, attention can then be given to the extremities. Most often, the trauma team (consisting of a trauma team leader who is usually an ER physician, nurses, and corpsmen) will be the first people evaluating the patient, and as an orthopedic or general surgeon, you are asked to stay back until called for.

Once given the okay by the trauma team leader, the forearm can be examined to evaluate the extent of the injury. Oftentimes, the patient will arrive from the battlefield with field tourniquets in place. As part of the initial assessment of the forearm, and when it is clinically feasible, taking these field tourniquets down to assess circulatory function of the arm is appropriate. In the field environment, these tourniquets are often placed at any sign of bleeding, and often, there is not a significant arterial injury that would require tourniquet control. If the tourniquet is removed and there is only minimal bleeding that can be controlled with gauze and an Ace wrap, then removing the tourniquet will save additional ischemic injury to the distal arm and hand. This also will allow the opportunity to assess perfusion of the hand. If pulsatile bleeding is encountered, a tourniquet can be reapplied, switching to a pneumatic tourniquet if clinically feasible. The broader distribution of pressure to the skin with a pneumatic tourniquet compared to a field tourniquet might prevent additional ischemic injury to the soft tissues below the tourniquet.

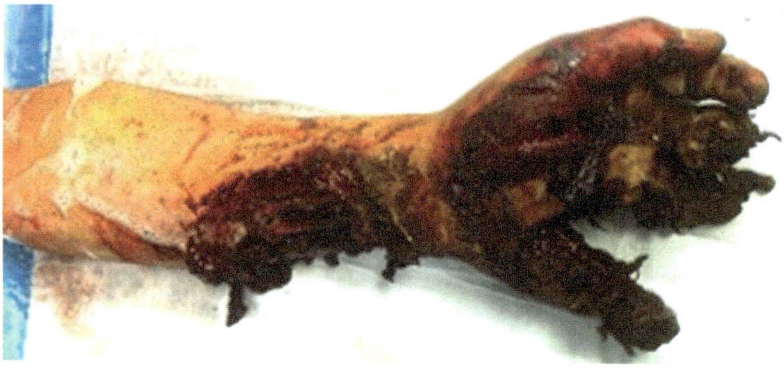

Fig. 14.1 This is a classic wounding pattern from an IED. The most damage is seen on the ulnar side of the hand, with relative sparing of the radial structures

If the patient is awake and cooperative, a neurologic examination should also be performed to assess function of the median, radial, and ulnar nerves. Careful documentation of any neurologic deficits should be communicated to whomever is documenting the note.

All field dressing should be taken down for at least a cursory evaluation of the wounds, and the forearm can be checked for evidence of gross instability and deformity, as well as for evidence of compartment syndrome. Compartment syndrome of the forearm is not uncommon with any of the high-energy mechanisms mentioned previously. While a Stryker or arterial line can be used to formally assess the pressures, this is most commonly a clinical diagnosis based on assessment of the tenseness of the compartments and pain associated with passive stretching of the fingers. It is rarely a diagnostic dilemma. If the compartments feel overly tight, then they should be released.

Once the wounds are assessed, if the patient is not going to be headed straight for the operating room, then plaster or fiberglass splints can be placed as indicated to offer some stability to protect the remaining soft tissues. The information that was just collected in the brief survey of the extremity can then be used to formulate a tentative surgical plan. Then, while the patient undergoes further stabilization and evaluation, the surgeon can begin communicating with the operating room staff to collect necessary equipment, which might include cystoscopy tubing, irrigation, external fixators, shunts, K-wires, or other equipment.

14.4 A Review of the Anatomy

When dealing with a traumatic amputation, it is easy to become disoriented as to which direction is volar, dorsal, radial, or ulnar. A helpful tool through the forearm level is to flex and the forearm stump through the elbow, and then rotate through the forearm until they are oriented so that the two bones line up in a row collinear with the humerus. In this orientation, the radius is always on top, dorsal is to the lateral side of the arm, and volar is to the medial side.

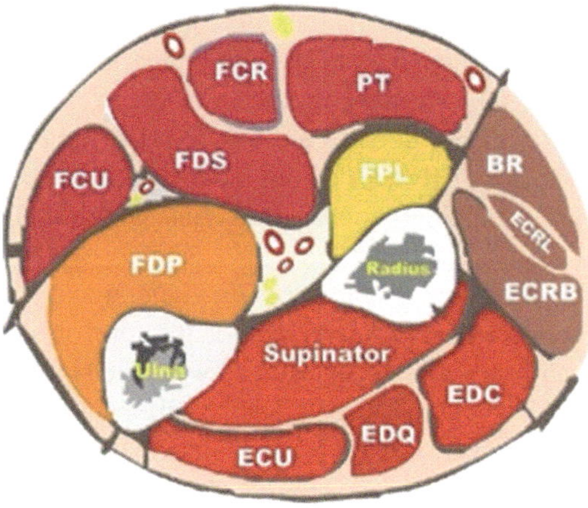

Fig. 14.2 Cross-sectional anatomy through the proximal forearm. *FCR* flexor carpi radialis, *PT* pronator teres, *FDS* flexor digitorum superficialis, *FPL* flexor pollicis longus, *FCU* flexor carpi ulnaris, *FDP* flexor digitorum profundus, *BR* brachioradialis, *ECRL* extensor carpi radialis longus, *ECRB* extensor carpi radialis brevis, *EDC* extensor digitorum comunis, *EDQ* extensor digiti quinti, *ECU* extensor carpi ulnaris (Taken from Chandraprakasam T, Kumar RA. Acute compartment syndrome of forearm and hand. Indian J Plast Surg. 2011;44:212–8)

Figure 14.2 is a cross section through the proximal forearm. The muscles are arranged in layers at the volar forearm, with the wrist flexors (FCR/FCU/PL) on the most superficial layer. The flexor superificialis is just deep to the wrist flexors, and then the flexor profundus is the deepest layer, often invested in its own fascia. The pronator quadratus is the deepest layer at the distal forearm and sends transverse fibers across the volar side of the radius and ulna. In the proximal forearm, the pronator teres extends from the medial epicondyle, across the forearm, and has a long, broad insertion at the midportion of the radial shaft.

On the extensor side, the most superficial muscles are the outcroppers that lead to the 1st dorsal extensor compartment (APL, EPB). These muscles cross over the extensor radialis longus and brevis tendons at the junction of the middle and distal thirds of the forearm. The extensor digitorum, extensor indices, extensor digiti quinti, and ECU tendons all travel in parallel. On the radial most side of the forearm, the brachioradialis runs and has a broad insertion along the radial styloid.

The *ulnar nerve* runs its course behind the medial epicondyle at the elbow and then dives deep in between the two heads of the FCU muscle. It then follows a course deep under the FCU and eventually ends up just radial and deep to the FCU tendon. The ulnar artery runs with it along this course.

In the proximal forearm, *the radial nerve* runs across from the lateral side of the forearm and can be found in the interval between the brachioradialis and the ECRL. The posterior interosseous branch then dives deep into the supinator muscle, which surrounds the proximal 1/3 of the radial shaft just distal to the bicipital tuberosity. The superficial branch of the radial nerve travels with the radial artery deep to the brachioradialis through the midportion of the forearm. Then, the artery continues volar and radial to the FCR tendon. The superficial radial nerve emerges volarly to travel along superficial to the brachioradialis at the distal forearm.

The *median nerve* travels across the antecubital fossa with the brachial artery, and then dives deep under the proximal arcade of the FDS, but superficial to the FDP and emerges with the FDS tendons proximal to the carpal tunnel. The anterior interosseous branch dives deeper and runs along the interosseous membrane. The palmar cutaneous branch comes off the median nerve proper about 5 cm proximal to the level of the wrist crease.

The interosseous membrane is a dense fibrous structure with thickenings that travels between the radius and the ulna along the entire course of the forearm. Just dorsal to this membrane, the posterior interosseous artery and nerve travel. On the volar side, the anterior interosseous artery and nerve travel. These vessels must be ligated when performing a transradial amputation.

14.5 Fasciotomies

In the combat environment, there should be a low threshold for performing fasciotomy. Given the potentially long transit times, and the tendency for the zones of injury to progress over the course of several hours, prophylactic fasciotomies should be performed if there is any question in the surgeon's mind.

While several different incisions have been described for a forearm fasciotomy, consideration should be given to future coverage issues. A carpal tunnel release should be a routine part of the forearm fasciotomy. However, continuing the standard carpal tunnel incision across the midline of the volar wrist can result in significant coverage problems for the median nerve. For this reason, it is my preference to carry the standard carpal tunnel incision transversely across the wrist at the level of the wrist crease and toward the ulnar side. This creates a radially based flap that can be used to easily cover the median nerve even in cases where the skin cannot be primarily closed (see Fig. 14.3). The skin flaps should be kept as full thickness as possible, and the fascia can then be opened in a plane between the FCU and FDS. Through the more distal forearm, the fascia should be completely opened. The incision is then curved back radially across the volar forearm to reach the mobile wad, which can be decompressed through the same incision. Then, the incision is curved back ulnarly and can be extended in an oblique fashion across the elbow crease and carried up the medial brachium to release the anterior and posterior compartments of the arm if necessary.

In most cases, the release of the volar forearm is sufficient. However, if after the volar fasciotomy is performed, there is still concern for tightness of the dorsal forearm, then a separate longitudinal incision can be made over the dorsal forearm to decompress the dorsal compartment, though I rarely found this necessary.

14.6 Vascular Injuries

The radial and ulnar arteries provide redundant vascular supply to the forearm through the deep and superficial palmar arches in the hand. This affords a tremendous benefit in forearm trauma. Because of the dual blood supply, in many cases, an injury to one of these two major arteries can be simply ligated, and the forearm and hand will remain well perfused due to the collateral flow of the other. A Doppler is usually available and should be used to rigorously assess the flow to the remaining distal limb (Fig. 14.4). The Doppler

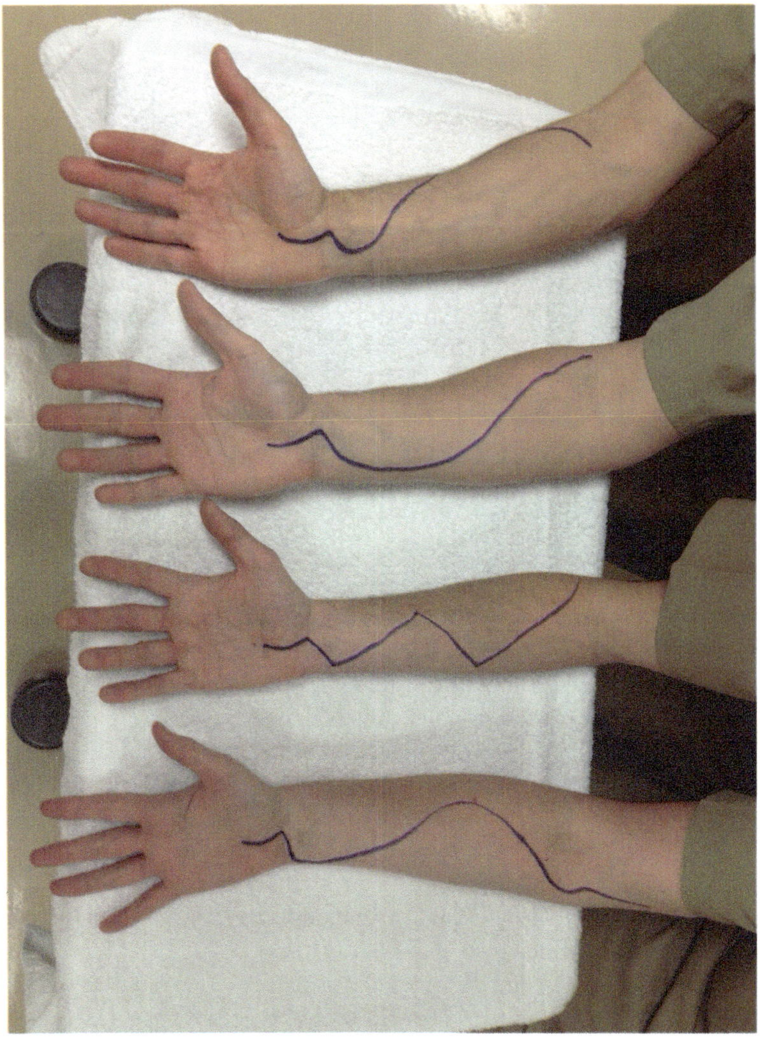

Fig. 14.3 Several different incisions have been described for forearm fasciotomies. My preference is for the bottom incision, as it leaves a large flap that will easily keep the median nerve covered even in the face of significant swelling (Taken from Ronel DN, Mtui E, Nolan WB III. Forearm compartment syndrome: anatomical analysis of surgical approaches to the deep space. Plast Reconstr Surg. 2004;114(3):697–705)

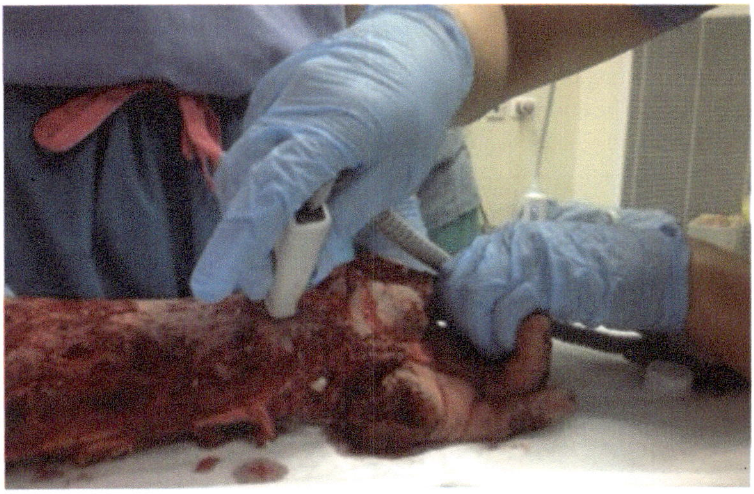

Fig. 14.4 A Doppler is invaluable for assessing vascular flow when patients are coming in hypovolemic with significantly traumatized limbs

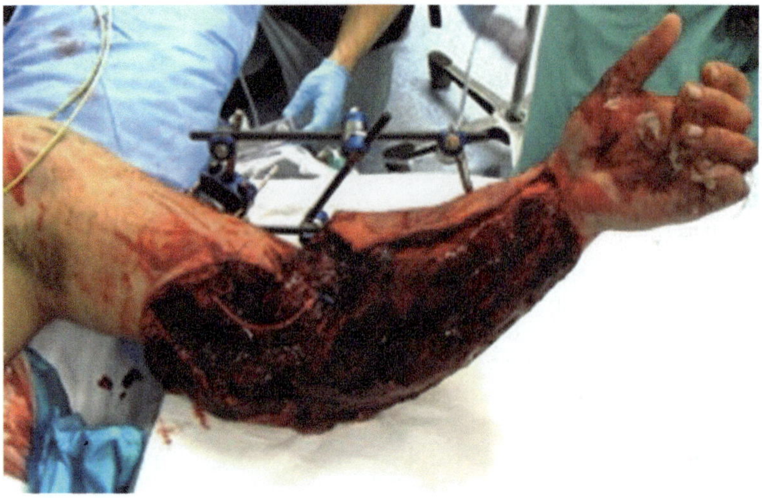

Fig. 14.5 After an IED blast, an initial attempt was made to salvage this patient's arm through the use of a vascular shunt, which can be seen at the level of the elbow. Ultimately, this arm was amputated, as it was felt that the arm was leading to his rhabdomyolysis and the success of a graft through a large hostile bed such as this was likely to fail

can be used to assure patent palmar arterial arches and can also be used all the way out to the fingertips of each digit to ensure that each level is perfused. If the contralateral arm is uninjured, a brachial-brachial index can be taken in a similar manner to an ankle-brachial index to assess whether or not there is any significant compromise in perfusion.

For cases in which there is questionable collateral flow, consideration should also be given to possible arterial repair, grafting, or shunting. In the combat environment, the decision to attempt salvage of the limb must be carefully weighed against the overall clinical condition of the patient. This might be a reasonable thing to do if the zone of injury is small and the distal portion of the limb has not sustained significant trauma. However, if there is a large zone of injury, which would require a long shunt or vascularized graft through a large, hostile host bed, then such a salvage should be undertaken with extreme caution. Oftentimes, the patients are in critical condition, and the additional stress of trying to maintain a significantly traumatized limb might lead to rhabdomyolysis, with subsequent kidney failure and possibly death.

For critically injured patients in whom it is felt safe to attempt to salvage a limb with vascular compromise, a shunt should be used, as this is quickly placed and held in place with simple, circumferential sutures (see Fig. 14.5). The patient can then be stabilized in an ICU setting and even transported to a higher echelon of care prior to undergoing definitive grafting. Definitive grafting procedures can also be performed using vein grafts that can be harvested from the dorsal veins of the forearm or hand or from the lower extremity.

14.7 Debridement Principles

The fundamental principles of debridement of the upper extremity are similar to that for the lower extremities with a few exceptions. First, it must be realized that significant amounts of devitalized muscle are a threat to the patient's life. Rhabdomyolysis as a result of prolonged ischemic time or large loads of devitalized muscle, combined with hypovolemic shock, can lead to multiorgan system failure quickly. Thus, aggressive debridement is a lifesaving procedure. If the limb has to be amputated to limit the hit on the kidneys, then it should be done.

At the same time, every attempt should be made to preserve structures that could serve future purposes once the patient has been stabilized. Because the technical demands of the upper extremity are different than that of the lower extremity, and because the current upper

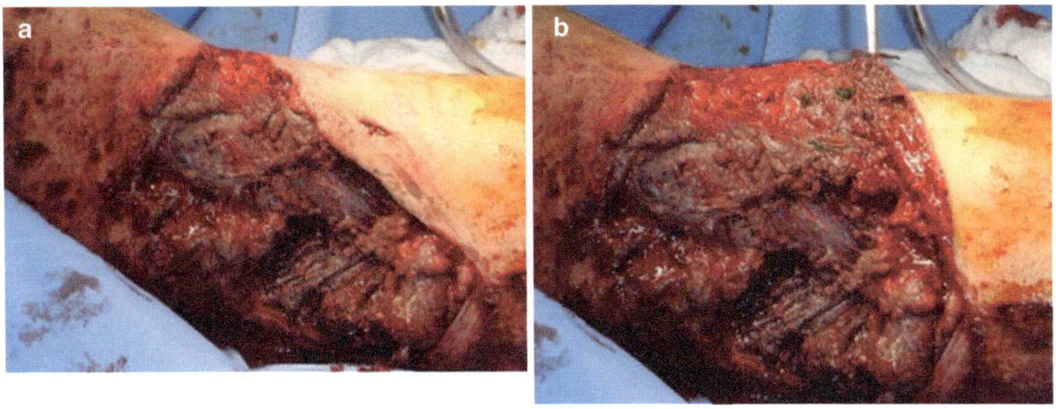

Fig. 14.6 (**a**) Initial inspection of this elbow wound looks like it is fairly clean. (**b**) Upon lifting up the skin flap, gross contamination is still seen. It is essential to leave no stone unturned when debriding combat wounds

extremity prostheses are not as capable of recreating normal function when compared to lower extremity prostheses, attempts should be made to preserve nerve tissue, tendons, and muscle tissue when possible. Extra length of nerves can prove useful for later nerve grafting or for the evolving targeted muscle reinnervation procedures (more on this later). Lengths of tendon can be incorporated into later tendon transfers. Neither nerve nor tendon tissue will contribute to rhabdomyolysis, so if they can be adequately debrided, then they should be preserved. While it might seem counterintuitive to leave these structures long relative to the rest of the limb, their use in future reconstruction cannot be understated. Just tuck the excess length of these tendons and/or nerves under the soft tissues to prevent desiccation, and they can always be cut down later if they are not used.

No stone should be left unturned in debridement of the forearm. The gross contamination that can occur in the combat environment should not be underestimated (Fig. 14.6a, b). The safe method is to assume that any skin abrasion, no matter how small, is likely the result of a projectile that penetrated and is now deep to the skin. Because these projectiles are often traveling at high velocity, the underlying tract of soft tissue injury is often much larger than can be readily appreciated by looking at the superficial wound. We used a small curette in every small wound we could find, and if it penetrated deeper with a little pressure, we would extend an incision large enough to further explore the wound, removing the retained foreign body if it was encountered.

For dressings, our group became big fans of a dilute Dakin's solution rather than Betadine or wound VAC's. We found them much more reliable in keeping the wounds clean. Rolls of Kerlix soaked in this solution were the most efficient technique, followed by dry Kerlix, fluffs, ABD pads, and finally compressive Ace wraps.

Another important consideration in debridement is the use of "fillet flaps." This is the essence of "spare parts" surgery. These flaps are classically described in the hand, but even in the forearm or other areas, they can be useful. The general concept is that any viable tissue can be used for coverage. Thus, always look for opportunities to use good quality, well-perfused tissue distally to cover more proximally. For instance, if the hand is not viable, but some of its skin is still viable, this is a good way to get the end of the limb covered. In Fig. 14.7a, b, the skin on the radial side, all the way up including the thumb, was preserved with its nerve supply and brought back to cover a transradial amputation, while preserving length. This is just one example of how thinking outside the traditional amputation incisions can help to preserve length of the limb.

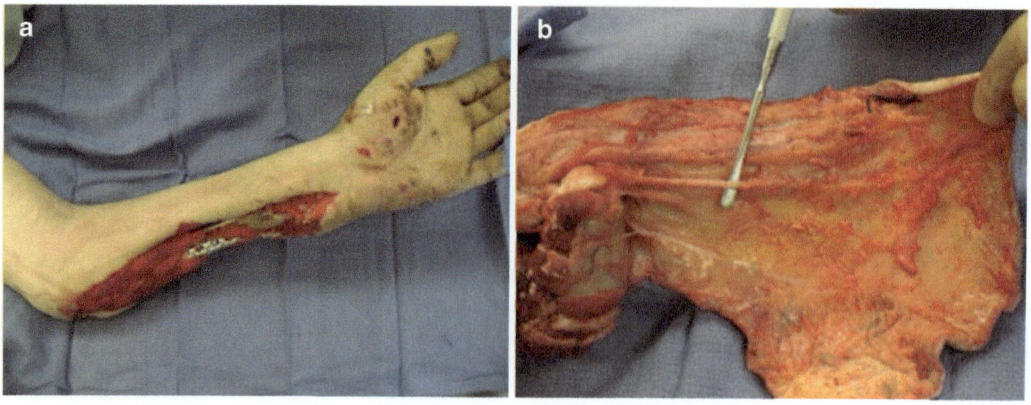

Fig. 14.7 (**a**) In this insensate forearm with ulnar and median nerves out, the patient elected for transradial amputation. (**b**) A fillet flap was developed based on the radial artery (seen behind the Freer) and the superficial branch of the radial nerve was preserved (at tip of Freer) to provide sensibility of the skin flap

14.8 Levels of Amputation

Amputations through the upper extremity can be at any level, really. Starting most distally in the forearm is the wrist disarticulation. While previously it was thought that this is not a good level due to the fact that a prosthesis could not be fit easily, that is no longer the case. With improved prosthetic designs, they are able to fit a myoelectric prosthesis over a wrist disarticulation, and even without a prosthesis, the stump at this level alone is very functional. The retained distal radioulnar joint can provide pronosupination to the patient, which is very beneficial.

Through the transradial level, as long as about 10–12 cm of stump is remaining, a prosthetic can be fit and still take advantage of a working elbow joint. In order to achieve this, it is worth maintaining a fractured proximal radius or ulna if the soft tissue envelope with support is healing.

If 10–12 cm cannot be maintained, then an elbow disarticulation should be performed. The limited bleeding associated with a joint disarticulation is a benefit to this level. However, if an elbow disarticulation is undertaken, every effort should be made to keep nerve lengths as long as possible to allow for later targeted muscle reinnervation.

14.9 Stabilization

On the front lines, stabilization of the forearm is usually straightforward. In many cases, a plaster splint can be used, once an adequate debridement is performed. However, if there is significant comminution, if multiple washouts are anticipated, or if there have been any soft tissue repairs performed, an external fixator is appropriate.

The safest method of placing the pins of an external fixation is to make an incision and do a formal approach to the bone. There are simply too many nerves that can be damaged if you don't have direct visualization of the bone. Common places to place pins are the lateral humerus, spanning the elbow joint (beware of the radial nerve passing from posterior to anterior about 8–10 cm proximal to the lateral epicondyle). If the fracture being stabilized is distal in the forearm, then pins can be placed in the proximal radius by making a dorsal approach in the forearm between brachioradialis and the extensor carpi radialis longus or between the extensor carpi radialis longus and brevis tendons. The radial nerve is close in all of these approaches, so direct visualization of the bone is critical. Alternatively, the ulna is subcutaneous along its entire border, and this can serve as a very safe place for pin insertion.

For the distal pins, the classic external fixator would have two pins in the second metacarpal, but any metacarpal can be used. Again, formal surgical approaches are necessary to avoid damage to the tendons and superficial nerves. If the hand is not remaining, then pins can be placed in the distal radius in the interval between the first and second dorsal extensor compartments (avoiding the superficial branch of the radial nerve), in the distal ulna (avoiding the dorsal ulnar sensory nerve crossing at about the level of the ulnar head), or any place else you can find, as long as you have dissected down to the bone.

14.10 Future Reconstructive Options for the Upper Extremity

Our collective experience throughout the decade of war in Iraq and Afghanistan has led to the blossoming of advanced reconstructive options in the upper extremity. However, as mentioned previously, the level to which the upper extremity prosthesis recreates normal function has not yet reached the level of lower extremity prosthesis. However, prosthetic options are still continuing to evolve.

First of all, the use of free microvascular coverage to provide coverage or preserve length has been instrumental in limiting the number of limbs that has required amputation. Close consultation with plastic surgeons allows for educated decisions on the best ways to achieve coverage for the limbs in which the hand might still be well perfused, but the midportion of the forearm has been significantly traumatize. If the limb can be salvage, and at least some of the nerves are working, then the use of tendon transfers or nerve transfers can achieve some level of function through the hand. When this is not possible and amputations must be undertaken, two other major advances that could be entertained are targeted muscle reinnervation and hand transplantation.

Targeted muscle reinnervation makes use of the nerves that were previously innervating the hand and forearm and reinnervates redundant muscles in the upper arm. Most commonly, the median nerve is taken to the medial biceps, the distal portion of the radial nerve is taken to the lateral triceps, and the ulnar nerve is taken to the brachialis. This effectively takes the number of inputs for a future myoelectric prosthesis from 2 (biceps and triceps) to 5 (lateral biceps, medial biceps, brachialis, long head of triceps, and lateral head of triceps) (Fig. 14.8). The retraining after undergoing one of these procedures is much easier for the patient, since cocontraction maneuvers are not required. For cases in which the upper extremity is amputated much higher, the same technique has been performed by reinnervating either the different portions of the pectoralis or the different heads of the serratus anterior.

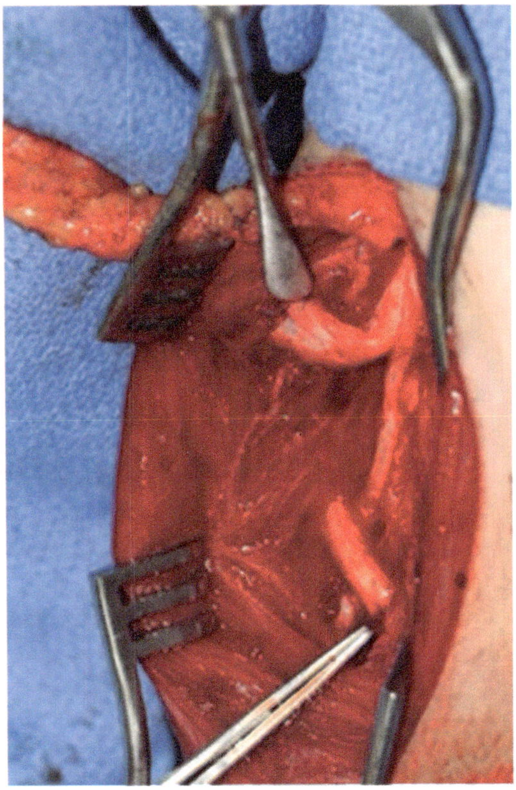

Fig. 14.8 In this patient with a non-dominant arm elbow disarticulation, a targeted muscle reinnervation was done. The tip of the Freer elevator is pointing out the median nerve proximally, which has been coapted to the neuromuscular junction of the medial head of the biceps. The forceps distally are showing the ulnar nerve, which has been coapted to the neuromuscular junction of the brachialis

Finally, hand transplantation has become more readily available at several centers across the country. There is currently a DoD level advisory board in place to help facilitate the option of hand transplantation in appropriate active duty military candidates. The best candidates for a hand transplant are those who are bilateral upper extremity amputees below the elbow or possibly unilateral amputees with the dominant arm missing (note: this is very rare, since in the low-ready position, it is usually the non-dominant arm that is exposed while the dominant arm is held close to the body). The other important consideration in choosing a hand transplant candidate is the heavy burden of requiring lifelong immunosuppresion. A failed hand transplant is most common because the patient was not compliant with taking the immunosuppressive medication. This requires a special patient with a strong social support structure to be successful in this lifelong endeavor. This procedure is best performed at centers that have set up formal multidisciplinary programs to undertake hand transplants.

14.11 Final Thoughts

The fundamental principles of combat surgery in the forearm are much like elsewhere in the body, and it is critical to remember the patient as a whole. Understand that an amputation might actually save their life. Beyond that, when it is feasible, go to the greatest lengths possible to preserve as much as possible, knowing that the prosthetic options for the arm are not nearly as good as those for the legs. The implications of saving a functional upper extremity for a triple amputee cannot be overstated.

Combat Injuries of the Elbow

15

Derek F. Ipsen

Contents

D.F. Ipsen, DO
Hand Surgery Service, Walter Reed National Military Medical Center, Bethesda, MD, USA
e-mail: derek.f.ipsen.mil@health.mil

BLUF (Bottom Line Up Front) Box

1. Know the surgical anatomy of the elbow. Familiarity with the anatomy will aid in rapid assessment and treatment with less probability of iatrogenic injury.
2. Initial evaluation and treatment of the injury should include:
   (a) Advanced Trauma Life Support (ATLS) principles (life before limb).
   (b) Prompt resuscitation and administration of antibiotics.
   (c) Determine viability of the extremity distal to the injury. Limb salvage vs amputation.
   (d) Vascular compromise. If possible, restore perfusion through manipulation, vascular repair, reconstruction, or shunt placement.
   (e) Bony and articular stability. Stabilization of fractures and soft tissue injuries by external fixation or splinting will protect repairs, reduce pain, decrease tissue sheer, and aid those transporting the patient.
   (f) Gross contamination should be removed systematically with care to preserve vital structures.
   (g) Neurologic and soft tissue injuries need proper exploration and accurate documentation.

L.B. Bone, C.N. Mamczak (eds.), *Front Line Extremity and Orthopaedic Surgery*,
DOI 10.1007/978-3-642-45337-3_15, © Springer-Verlag Berlin Heidelberg 2014

(h) Proper dressings for further evacuation include negative pressure wound therapy and traditional wet to dry bandages. Both can be used with splinting or external fixation.

3. Future procedures should be considered at the time of the initial evaluation and treatment.

15.1 Introduction

Improvements in the design of combat body armor have made injuries to the chest, abdomen, and head much less common than in any other conflict in history. Unfortunately, the extremities remain largely exposed due to weight and mobility considerations. As a combat surgeon, you will see more extremity injuries than any other type of injury. For this reason, surgeons who are involved with acute combat casualty care should have a working knowledge of extremity war injury management. Specifically, this chapter will focus on elbow injuries.

15.2 Anatomy

The elbow joint proper is comprised of three principal joint articulations. The ulnohumeral and radiocapitellar joints are responsible for the flexion and extension arc of motion. The proximal radioulnar joint allows for forearm rotation. Injury to any joint component or the surrounding soft tissues can result in loss of normal range of motion and function. The medial and lateral collateral ligaments provide stability in the coronal plane, whereas the bony architecture and capsule provide stability in the sagittal plane. The annular ligament provides stability of the radial head as it articulates with the ulna. Extrinsic muscle tendon units also help provide additional dynamic stability to the elbow joint.

The radial nerve crosses posterior to the humerus in the mid-brachium and then pierces the lateral intermuscular septum anteriorly approximately 11 cm proximal to the elbow joint. It then travels distally and anteriorly to the lateral epicondyle between the brachialis and the brachioradialis muscles before it branches into the posterior interosseous nerve and the superficial branch of the radial nerve (SBRN).

The median nerve courses anterior and toward the midline with the brachial artery but remains medial to it. As it crosses the elbow joint, it descends under the bicipital aponeurosis and between the two heads of the pronator teres muscle. Just past the elbow joint, it divides into the median nerve proper and the anterior interosseous nerve in the same region as the brachial artery bifurcation.

The ulnar nerve pierces the medial intramuscular septum in the mid-brachium from anterior to posterior and then travels posterior to the medial epicondyle before it passes between the two heads of the flexor carpi ulnaris in the forearm.

The musculocutaneous nerve descends anteriorly, between the biceps and brachialis muscles, terminating as the lateral antebrachial cutaneous nerve as it emerges lateral to the biceps tendon in the cubital fossa.

The brachial artery arises from the axillary artery and travels distally in the medial brachium. As it approaches the elbow, it courses laterally under the bicipital aponeurosis, descending under the flexor pronator muscles and dividing into its two principal terminal branches, the radial and ulnar arteries. A rich collateral blood supply exists between the brachium and the forearm. While a rare circumstance, those with complete injuries to the brachial artery in this area may still present with a perfused hand.

15.3 Initial Evaluation

When a casualty sustains an injury on the battlefield (Fig. 15.1), the first responder is usually another member of their unit or their medic. They perform lifesaving procedures in place, such as applying tourniquets and pressure dressing as well as makeshift splints. As soon as evacuation

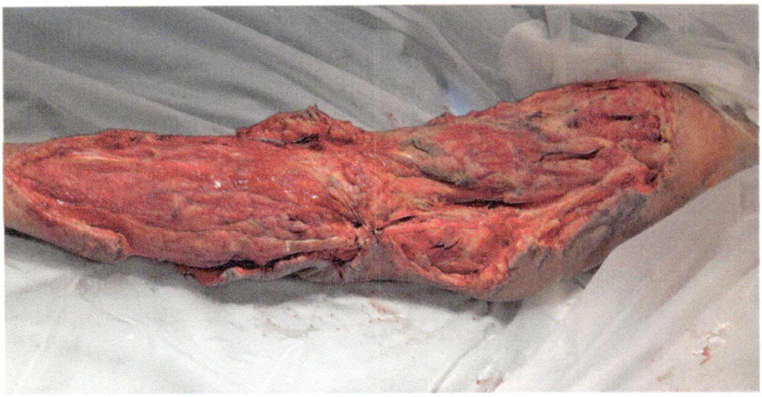

Fig. 15.1 Example of a combat blast injury involving the upper extremity

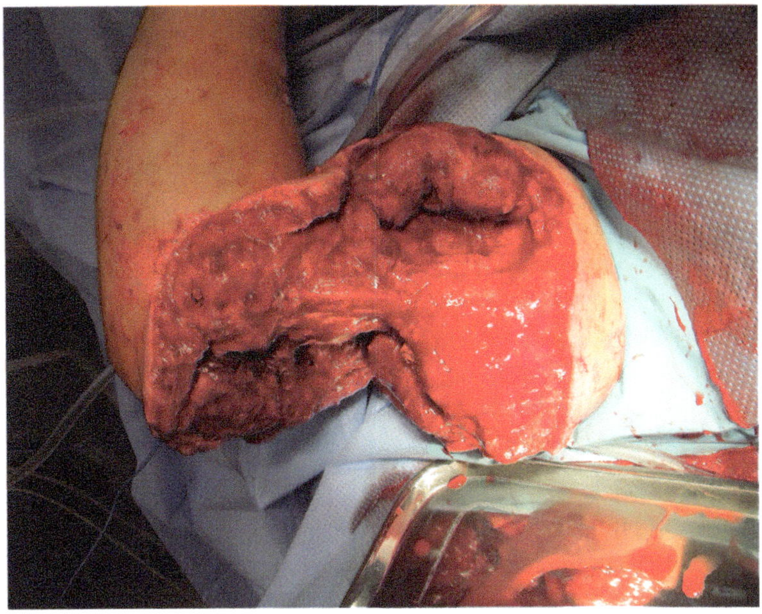

Fig. 15.2 Despite severe soft tissue injury to the brachium and elbow, the distal extremity remained viable

can be arranged, they will arrive at your facility. At this point, a well-rehearsed sequence of events will take place. The A, B, C, D, and E components of the Advanced Trauma Life Support protocol are initiated. Unless the casualty is actively hemorrhaging from an extremity wound or an unstable pelvis, the orthopedic surgeon will be delayed in their initial evaluation while resuscitation is performed. The extremities should be evaluated as soon as possible since ischemia time from a tourniquet may be prolonged due to the evacuation and resuscitation. This can result in unnecessary tissue death if not addressed in a timely manner.

15.4 Viability

The first determination made is the viability of the extremity distal to the injury (Fig. 15.2). This is a decision that all combat surgeons will struggle with at some point. If the amount of damage distally is so severe that the limb cannot be saved, an amputation is in order. When possible, get a second and third opinion. This will help you make the tough decision that ultimately may save the person's life by reducing the chances of infection and toxicity from nonviable tissue breakdown products. Regardless of the decision, proper antibiotics should be administered early.

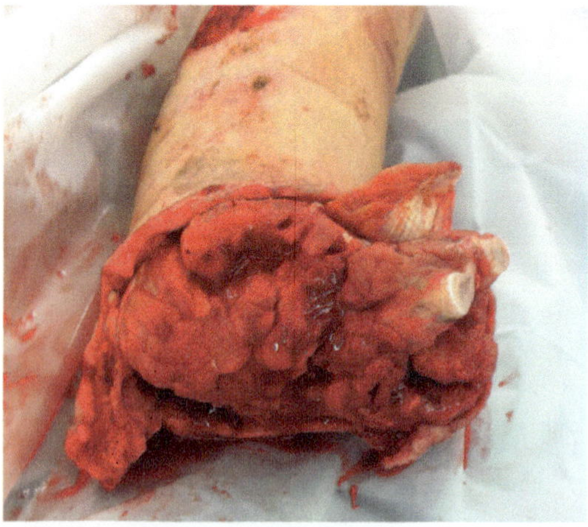

Fig. 15.3 This transradial amputation with limited soft tissue coverage was salvaged with a free tissue flap allowing for native elbow motion and better prosthetic function

When the decision to amputate an upper extremity is made, length preservation is paramount (Fig. 15.3). The initial amputation should be performed through the zone of injury with subsequent revisions as the injury evolves. Advanced reconstruction techniques are very successful at preserving limb length. If the native elbow joint can be preserved, the prosthesis will be much more useful as it eliminates two more degrees of freedom (elbow flexion and extension) that have to be powered from an ectopic source. Even very short proximal forearm segments are helpful for prosthetic wear. It allows for better suspension and less slipping at the skin socket interface. It also provides additional muscle segments to help initiate movement of a myoelectric terminal device. Aggressive traction neurectomies should be avoided so that procedures such as composite tissue allotransplantation (CTA) and targeted muscle reinnervation (TMR) are possible. When an upper extremity is amputated, nerves are transected and no longer have distal targets. Those nerves can be connected to preserved proximal muscles that have more than one site of innervation. This is TMR. Muscles that previously had one innervation and one function now have several sites of voluntary control. Multiple myoelectric receptors can be placed on the same muscle to allow more degrees of freedom for the prosthetic. If CTA is to be considered, nerve length is crucial. Shorter residual nerves mean a longer distance of regeneration after a transplant. As motor end plates remain unstimulated, they begin to degenerate. The closer the anastomosis is between the native nerve and the muscle target on the CTA, the better. This may be the difference between some intrinsic hand muscle function and no functional recovery.

15.5 Perfusion

Once you have made the decision that the limb is salvageable, proceed with the next step and access perfusion. This can be performed by palpating pulses, checking capillary refill, or listening for a Doppler signal if available. In the combat setting, you cannot rely on a warm, pink extremity for perfusion confirmation as the casualty may arrive with severe burns or covered in petroleum products if a vehicle was involved. If the person has a tourniquet in place, it should be removed in a controlled setting. When life-threatening hemorrhage is encountered, the tourniquet is reapplied and the person taken to the operating theater where proximal control can be obtained and maintained. At that time, you can determine if the vessel is amenable to repair and reconstruction or if temporary shunting is the best option. Shunting is the standard of care at Role 2 treatment facilities unless the vessel is easily repaired in a timely manner. More complex repairs and reconstructions should be reserved for Role 3 facilities and above. Any of these procedures can be performed after a thorough debridement in the operating theater. This is also the proper place to access the bony and soft tissue injuries. If you encounter a pulseless extremity with a deformity but no obvious vascular injury, attempt gentle manipulation of the extremity into a more anatomic position then reaccess perfusion. A vessel draped over a fracture can be compressed or may spasm temporarily. Careful manipulation and splinting can hasten the return of a pulse and help avoid unnecessary operative exploration. The compartments of the

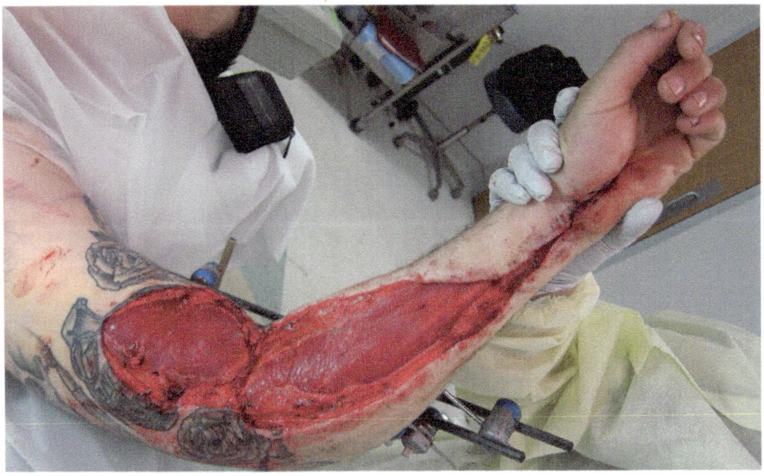

Fig. 15.4 Example of a complete fasciotomy extending from the carpal tunnel to the mid-brachium

forearm and brachium should also be assessed for signs of compartment syndrome. If there is any question about a compartment syndrome being present, then a fasciotomy should be performed (Fig. 15.4). Continue working until the limb is perfused or the rest of the procedures will have no bearing on the end result.

15.6 Stability

Skeletal stability is important for several reasons. As mentioned earlier, it can help maintain a position for maximum perfusion. Stability can also protect a vascular repair or reconstruction. It decreases pain by immobilizing the fracture fragments and allows for comfort and convenience during transport. It also decreases soft tissue sheer that aids the healing process. The two mainstays of skeletal stability in theater are external fixation and splinting. Both work well for injuries about the elbow and both should be used in specific situations. Splinting works well in closed injuries or injuries with a decreased risk of severe soft tissue swelling. It can also be used when external fixation is not possible. A posterior splint made from 10 to 12 layers of plaster should be used. Room temperature water helps prevent thermal injury from the curing plaster. It should be well padded and can be reinforced with a side slab of plaster in effect creating a right triangle at the elbow. The hand or fingers are left free to access neurovascular changes.

If the patient is going to the operating theater for any reason, an external fixator should be considered (Fig. 15.5). Application of an external fixator is quick and safe if you adhere to some basic but very important principles. First, the pin sites need to span the fracture and be placed outside the zone of injury if possible. This allows the pins to be placed in a relatively uninjured location with skin coverage avoiding the placement of foreign objects into a contaminated wound. For fractures involving the elbow, the proximal pins are placed on the distal lateral humerus. The anatomy section should remind you that the radial nerve is in close proximity to these pins. At least two pins are placed and a formal incision exposing the bone should be performed to visualize the radial nerve and protect it. The two distal pins are less technical if the ulna is suitable for placement. The subcutaneous border of the ulna is relatively safe and free of major neurovascular structures. Make a small incision and bluntly spread to bone. If the radius is used, then a formal open approach similar to the humerus should be used. An incision on the radial border just proximal to the thumb outcropper muscles will allow visualization and protection of the SBRN. Bicortical pin placement will ensure good purchase. If an image intensifier is available, check the depth. If not, then the pins need to be placed by feel. The near cortex is hard to penetrate. Irrigation will help keep the pins cool and reduce thermal necrosis. Once the

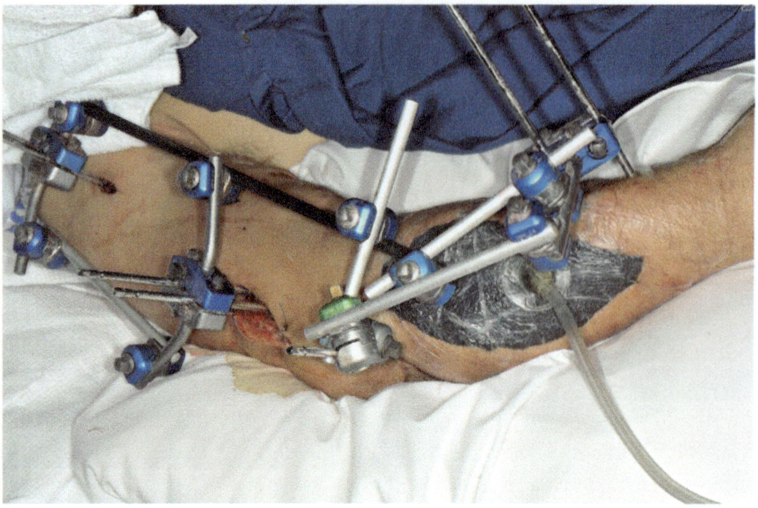

Fig. 15.5 A severe elbow and forearm injury stabilized with external fixation. Notice the complete open incision on the distal humerus

near cortex is breached, the pin will travel easily until it reaches the far cortex. If the pins are being driven under power, the operator will feel the pin penetrate the far cortex as well as hear the pitch change in the drill. Avoid plunging as important neurovascular structures reside on the other side. If the pins are driven by hand, then you have to feel the amount of pressure necessary to breach the far cortex. When the pressure required for advancement suddenly decreases, the pin is through. Next, the pin clusters are connected. Many studies have been done to determine the most stable configurations of external fixation. Those principles should be followed as the wounds allow but the bare minimum should consist of two pins proximal and two pins distal to the fracture with a spanning rod between the two pin clusters. Place the spanning rods close to the skin for stability but not so close that wound care is difficult.

During the initial exploration in the operating room, the fracture fragments are assessed. The fragments should be manually debrided of all foreign material and irrigated until clean. This is in conjunction with a thorough soft tissue debridement. Every attempt should be made to protect soft tissue attachments of the fragments. Gross anatomic alignment is the best position and the elbow should be spanned with an external fixator. Avoid using implants in the acute setting, as the gross contamination present at that time will compound the rate of infection. It is also important not to discard viable or potentially viable fragments if possible, as they will act as fracture keys for later fixation and reconstruction. If the person will not be leaving the area of operation, permanent implants can be considered but only after the wound is clean and stable. For everyone who will be evacuated out of the combat theater, permanent implants should not be used.

Serial visits to the operating room every 24–48 h are necessary until the wounds are clean or until the patient is evacuated to the next level of care.

15.7 Contamination

Injuries incurred while in the combat theater are usually high energy and are accompanied by open wounds with severe contamination. Soil, improvised explosive device (IED) material, clothing, petroleum products, and anything from the surrounding environment can be found in the wound. Many wounds are also accompanied by burns of varying depth and size. All of these factors need to be considered when the initial and subsequent debridements are performed.

The first priority is to remove all grossly contaminated and devitalized tissue. The exceptions to this rule are injured nerves and large fragments of bone that may be useful for later fixation or reconstruction. The evolution of the wound will dictate how often it needs to be irrigated and debrided, but as a rule in the acute phase, every 24–48 h is sufficient. Debridements should be performed in a stepwise manner to ensure all tissue planes are addressed. Continue debridements until the tissue remains viable and gross contamination is gone. At this point, definitive fixation and reconstruction can begin.

15.8 Neurologic and Soft Tissue Injuries

One of the most difficult procedures about the elbow in the late reconstructive phase is nerve reconstruction. This is due to the severity of the injury, the formation of scar tissue, and lack of knowledge about the initial injury. If detailed records do not accompany the patient throughout the evacuation chain, the accepting surgeon will not know the extent of the neurologic injury. As the initial surgeon, there are steps you can take to help ensure the patient will get the best outcome with the least morbidity. First is an accurate exam. When the patient arrives and is conscious, a thorough neurologic exam should be performed, documented, and sent with the patient. If they are not conscious and need to be taken to the operating theater, a detailed exam should be performed. In the damage control setting, this may be delayed but should be performed as soon as possible. Intact nerves should be protected during evacuation (Fig. 15.6). Transected nerves should be left as long as possible, tagged with a dyed, monofilament nonabsorbable suture or a vascular clip in the perineurium, measured from a known anatomic landmark, and protected. The final accepting surgeon will be greatly aided by these steps and good documentation.

Other soft tissue injuries should be treated in a similar fashion. Debridement of all contaminated,

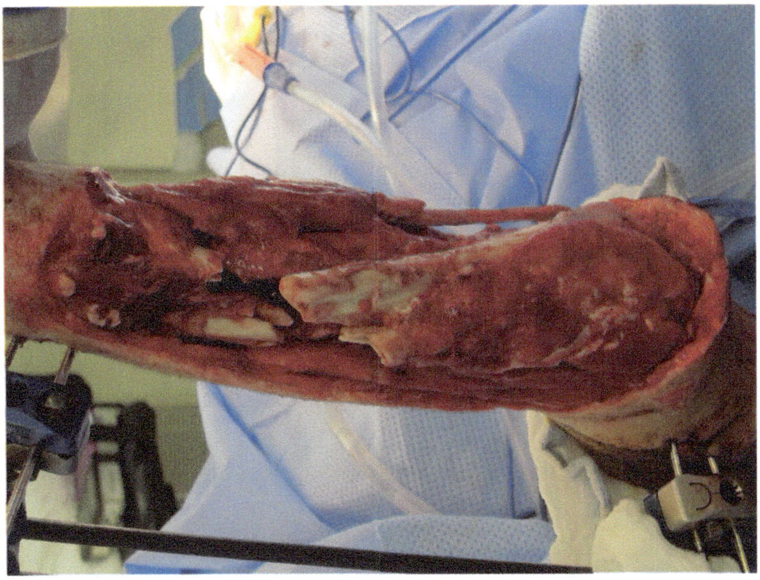

Fig. 15.6 Forearm and elbow injury with an intact ulnar nerve

nonviable tissue is performed in a stepwise fashion. Start with the skin and subcutaneous tissue and work on each layer until the wound is clean. Certain tissues, such as tendons, can look dead at the initial examination; however, after irrigation and a moist dressing, they may be salvageable. Any tendon that crosses the elbow joint should be saved if possible. This can help decrease long-term morbidity as native anatomy is preserved. Only the operating surgeon at the time can make the decision if tissue should be preserved, but thinking ahead can help the patient as well as the next surgeon in the evacuation chain.

15.9 Packaging for Evacuation

When a patient is ready for evacuation to the next level of care, several considerations have to be made. Mode of transportation, length of time to destination, and capabilities of those transporting the patient are just a few. In recent years, the invention and improvement of negative pressure wound therapy have made packaging for evacuation much less complicated. It is a sealed environment with drainage control and can be used with any type of bony stabilization. It can be changed every 48–72 h, thus eliminating the need for daily or twice daily changes of traditional dressings. It does require knowledge of application and support from the transport team. The negative pressure unit requires a power supply when the battery is exhausted so evacuation time is an issue. It does have some limitations. It should never be applied directly to a vascular structure, especially a repaired vascular structure. This can result in exsanguination if the structure ruptures. The standard porous sponge should not be applied directly over nerves or tendons as it can become adherent to them and cause damage (Fig. 15.7). Many surgeons will use antibiotic impregnated methyl methacrylate beads to help sterilize the wound. If they are used under a negative pressure device, care must be taken to ensure no vital structures are compressed between the beads and bone. At the elbow, this requires vigilance since the nerves are in close proximity to the underlying bony structures.

When negative pressure dressings are not available or contraindicated, a traditional bulky wet to dry dressing is used. All active bleeding is controlled in the operating room at the time of debridement and then a bulky dressing is applied. Moist, sterile gauze is placed next to open structures followed by more bulky products to absorb moisture. If an external fixator is not available, then a splint is applied as directed earlier. The

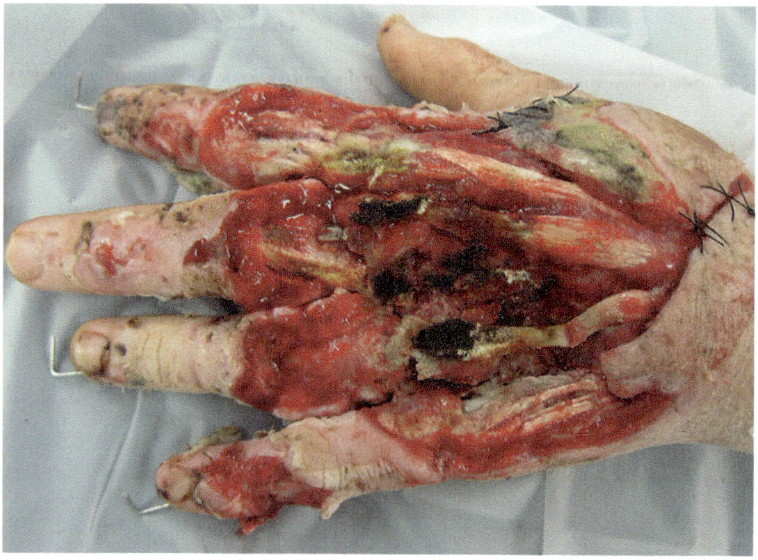

Fig. 15.7 Results of a porous sponge applied to tendons

fingers, if uninjured, need to be free to access perfusion. In the spirit of thinking ahead, position the elbow at 90° with the forearm in neutral rotation. If reconstruction is delayed or not possible, this is the position of maximal function for a stiff or immobile elbow.

A tip that is helpful for the accepting surgeon is to write the date and time of the last procedure and what was done on a wide piece of adhesive tape and place it on the dressing. Records can become misplaced during transit and this serves as a backup.

15.10 Future Considerations

Several recommendations have been made in this chapter with future considerations in mind. A review of those recommendations follows:

1. Preserve as much length as possible even if there is little or no soft tissue coverage. Advanced late reconstruction techniques are very successful at preserving length for prosthetic wear. An upper extremity with a preserved elbow joint is much more useful than an elbow disarticulation or a transhumeral amputation. The patient has one less mechanical joint to operate.
2. Preserve soft tissue attachments to bony fragments. Those flimsy pieces of soft tissue are the only blood supply to that fragment. Those fragments are very useful when piecing together a severely comminuted bone or joint such as the elbow.
3. Place external fixation pins under direct visualization in the distal humerus and the radius. This will help prevent iatrogenic nerve injury. If possible, place the pins outside the zone of injury.
4. Position the elbow at 90° and the forearm in neutral rotation. If reconstruction is delayed or not possible, this places the elbow in a position of greatest function.
5. Measure, tag, and document nerve injuries. This will aid the accepting surgeon when performing the definitive reconstruction. Avoid aggressive traction neurectomies.

15.11 Summary

Elbow injuries sustained on the battlefield are usually severe, involve multiple tissue planes, and are rarely isolated. Prompt resuscitation of the patient and early evaluation and treatment of these injuries are vital. Knowledge of the anatomy is essential to prevent further injury and adhering to proven extremity war trauma principles will ensure the patient has the best possible outcome.

Injuries to the elbow joint are notorious for causing long-term stiffness and loss of motion. Elbow injuries sustained in combat only serve to magnify this fact. Severe soft tissue and bony injuries and the protracted reconstruction and healing courses that accompany often lead to less than optimal function. Add to that the late occurrence of heterotopic ossification and results are even worse. Fortunately, we have achieved some very good intermediate-term results when the bony architecture of the elbow joint is preserved. Bone loss in the humerus, radius, and ulna can be successfully grafted but joint loss is poorly compensated for. Our best results have been achieved when there is a native joint to work with. After healing is complete and heterotopic ossification is mature, the joint can be released. With the aid of an indwelling regional catheter and continuous passive motion, range of motion can be restored to very functional levels. When the joint is destroyed, the patient is left with either an unstable interposition arthroplasty or an arthrodesis. Late allografting has met with dismal results thus far in our experience with the combat wounded.

Amputations about the elbow, when unilateral, are tolerated well and most of our patients accept and use their prosthetics. Much credit is due to our world-class prosthetic and rehabilitation departments but also to our patients. It does appear that patients with a preserved elbow joint, despite the length of the forearm, use their prosthetic more and have greater function. This confirms the statement made earlier that if possible the elbow joint should be preserved even if free tissue transfer is required to cover the injury.

Patients with transhumeral amputations wear their prosthetics less and use them less. They weigh more and are less functional due to the added powering of the elbow joint. Bilateral upper extremity amputees are less fortunate. They rely on their prosthetics for all activities and need as much function as possible. This again validates the fact that preservation of the elbow joint is very important.

The goal of each combat surgeon along the evacuation chain should be first to save lives, then to save quality of life. Following the recommendations outlined in this chapter will help ensure optimal function is restored after combat elbow trauma.

Arm and Shoulder Injuries

16

George P. Nanos III, David Dromsky, and Patricia L. McKay

It's not enough that we do our best; sometimes we have to do what is required

–Winston Churchill

Contents

BLUF (Bottom Line Up Front) Box

1. Rapid assessment for life-threatening hemorrhage and critical vascular injury is paramount to save life and limb.
2. The hallmark of initial treatment of war-related open humerus fractures and shoulder injuries remains prompt administration of antibiotics, provisional fracture stabilization, and debridement and irrigation of associated soft tissue injuries.
3. War-related shoulder injuries indicate significant energy transfer and mandate a thorough search for associated injuries, including vascular injury, pulmonary contusion, and spine fractures.
4. External fixation pins are generally placed anterolateral in the upper humerus, and direct lateral in the lower humerus. In the lower two thirds of the humerus, an open incision and careful dissection to the bone may prevent injury to the radial nerve. Spanning external fixation can be added to the shoulder and across the elbow as indicated.
5. Nerve injuries resulting from blast and high-energy penetrating injuries are rarely amenable to direct primary repair due to the extensive zone of injury and wound contamination.

G.P. Nanos III, MD (✉)
Department of Orthopaedic Surgery, Walter Reed National Military Medical Center, 8901 Wisconsin Ave., Bethesda, MD 20889, USA
e-mail: george.p.nanos.mil@health.mil

D. Dromsky, MC, USN
Department of Orthopaedic Surgery, Naval Medical Center San Diego, 34800 Bob Wilson Drive, San Diego, CA 92134, USA

P.L. McKay, MD, CAPT, MC, US Navy
Associate Professor of Surgery, F. Edward Hebert School of Medicine, Uniformed Services University of the Health Sciences, Bethesda, MD, USA
e-mail: patricia.mckay@usuhs.edu

L.B. Bone, C.N. Mamczak (eds.), *Front Line Extremity and Orthopaedic Surgery*, DOI 10.1007/978-3-642-45337-3_16, © Springer-Verlag Berlin Heidelberg 2014

6. Compartment syndrome of the arm is rare. If required, release of the anterior and posterior compartments of the arm may be performed via a medial or lateral incision.
7. In the absence of absolute indications for amputation, limb salvage should always be attempted if there is an expectation that hand prehension and sensation will be preserved.
8. A need for emergency flap coverage in the theater of conflict usually reflects severe destruction to other tissues and a large zone of injury, which likely contributes to the frequent failures. In such cases, deferring flap coverage or proceeding to amputation may be more advisable.
9. Transhumeral amputation prosthetic acceptance rates and ultimate functional outcomes are directly correlated to residual amputation length. Amputations should be performed within the zone of injury to maximize amputation length and outcomes.
10. Avoid overly aggressive traction neurectomy when performing amputation to optimize the patient for future reconstructive procedures such as targeted muscle reinnervation and hand allotransplantation.

16.1 Introduction

War-related injuries to the brachium and shoulder frequently involve penetrating injuries from gunshot wounds and blast fragments, as well as crush injuries from vehicular rollover and building collapse. Concomitant fractures, neurovascular injuries, defects in bone and soft tissues, and additional associated non-musculoskeletal injuries further complicate these challenging problems. A clear understanding of anatomy and a systematic approach to evaluation and management of the severely injured brachium and shoulder are essential to achieving the best result. A multidisciplinary approach will greatly assist the orthopedic surgeon, choosing interventions based on sound orthopedic principles while optimizing the physical and psychological health of the individual.

16.2 Anatomy

The humerus is joined to the shoulder proximally, and the elbow distally through complex muscular and ligamentous attachments. In brief, the shoulder includes the proximal humerus, scapula, and clavicle. Contributing to our understanding of shoulder biomechanics is the concept of the superior shoulder suspensory complex (SSSC), composed of a ring of bone and soft tissues at the superior aspect of the shoulder including the glenoid process, the coracoid process, the coracoclavicular ligament, the distal end of the clavicle, the acromioclavicular joint, the coracoacromial ligament, and the acromial process. The muscular connection of the upper limb to the trunk is via the axioappendicular muscles (anteriorly the pectoralis major and minor, subclavius and serratus anterior and posteriorly the trapezius, latissimus dorsi, levator scapulae, and rhomboids) which work in concert with the scapulohumeral muscles (deltoid, supraspinatus, infraspinatus, teres major and minor, and subscapularis) to position the arm in space through a tremendous range of motion. The critical neurovascular structures begin in a relatively protected deep medial location within the axilla. The axilla has a pyramidal shape which serves to protect the brachial plexus, axillary artery and vein, and lymphatics. The anterior axillary wall is comprised of the thick pectoralis muscles; the posterior wall is comprised of the scapula, subscapularis, teres major, and latissimus dorsi. Superiorly the apex of the axilla permits passage of the nerves and vessels via the cervicoaxillary canal protected by the first rib, clavicle, and superior aspect of the scapula. Medially the axilla is contained by the thorax from the first through fourth ribs and laterally by the narrow bony wall of the humerus at the intertubercular groove. In this region, penetrating injuries, fracture, dislocation, or scapulohumeral dissociation can be particularly devastating to the neurovascular structures of the arm and must be carefully evaluated and approached with a thorough understanding of the anatomical relationships.

Departing the axilla, the radial nerve and profunda brachii artery take a deep posterior course distal to the inferior border of the teres major tendon and follow the spiral groove to the inferolateral aspect of the humerus. The artery bifurcates into the middle and radial collateral branches proximal to the lateral epicondyle, while the radial nerve passes anteriorly through the lateral intermuscular septum approximately 10 cm proximal to the lateral epicondyle and continues inferiorly between the brachialis and brachioradialis muscles before splitting into superficial and deep branches. The median and ulnar nerves initially travel with the brachial artery along the medial intermuscular septum, with the ulnar nerve piercing the medial intermuscular septum with the superior ulnar collateral artery at mid-brachium and traveling posterior to the septum and medial epicondyle to the cubital tunnel and the median nerve and brachial artery traveling anterior to the septum and moving more anteriorly toward the midline as they approach the cubital fossa. The musculocutaneous nerve travels from the lateral cord, piercing the coracobrachialis and descending anteriorly, between the biceps and brachialis muscles, terminating in the lateral antebrachial cutaneous nerve as it emerges lateral to the biceps tendon in the cubital fossa.

16.3 Open Fractures

Initial treatment of combat-related open fractures of the humerus and shoulder girdle includes early administration of antibiotics, provisional fracture stabilization, and debridement and irrigation of all associated soft tissue wounds. Rapid assessment for hemorrhage and vascular control is critical on first presentation. Assessment for additional injuries is made, as well as documentation of a distal neurovascular examination. Fractures involving the superior shoulder suspensory complex (SSSC) should direct the surgeon to search for commonly associated injuries, to include injury to the chest wall, pulmonary contusion, skull fractures, cervical spine injuries, and brachial plexus and vascular injuries associated with the rare but life-threatening condition of scapulothoracic dissociation. Early fracture stabilization will minimize further injury to the soft tissues, assists in control of hemorrhage and minimizes pain caused by mobile fracture fragments.

Combat-related soft tissue wounds should be addressed in accordance with the same orthopedic principles applied to other regions. Debridement should be systematic, moving in concentric circles from the margins of the wound to the center. The skin should be sharply excised to smooth margins without devitalized flaps, and the subcutaneous tissues should also be excised to healthy margins. A careful assessment of the anatomy should precede excision of deep tissue to avoid inadvertent injury to vital neurovascular structures. Even traumatized neurovascular structures should be preserved, particularly if there is distal function. Devitalized muscle is sharply excised and organic material (dirt, rock, cloth, sand) should be excised or washed from the wounds. Metallic fragments may be too numerous and too deeply embedded for safe retrieval; they can be left behind and removed as needed if problems arise. It is common for numerous small wounds to be found following blast injury, and it may challenge the surgeon to determine those wounds requiring debridement and irrigation compared to those that can be treated expectantly with dressings. Our rule of thumb is to consider debridement of wounds greater than 2 cm, or those with clear penetration of underlying fascia. Following debridement, copious saline irrigation of all wounds is performed. Pulsatile lavage is no longer recommended in our practice due to concerns of increased tissue damage and deeper propagation of contamination.

Postoperative dressings can include negative pressure dressings when available, or wet to dry dressings, and may include a dilute Dakin's solution if frank contamination or evidence of early infection is present. Dermal substitutes may be considered if available to cover critical neurovascular structures and to avoid use of emergency flaps until the patient has reached a higher level of care. However, dermal substitutes are rarely available in a combat theater. Splinting of isolated large soft tissue wounds in the absence of fracture can facilitate healing through decreased tissue shear but is not always practical in the brachium.

16.4 Fracture Stabilization

The hallmark of treatment of closed humerus fractures and shoulder girdle injuries remains the use of coaptation splints, hanging casts, or cuff and collar constructs. The radial nerve remains the most commonly associated nerve injury with closed humerus fractures. It is prudent to observe all closed radial nerve injuries associated with humerus fracture for at least 6 months due to the high rate of recovery, and therefore, rarely is there an indication for exploration in the combat setting. Fracture stabilization with external fixation may be considered in the setting of polytrauma, fractures that will not maintain an acceptable reduction, or if medical evacuation and transport throughout the medical evacuation chain will be complicated by significant morbidity due to a splinted fracture.

Open fractures of the humerus are best treated with temporary external fixation to maximize hemorrhage control, reduce swelling, and provide optimal patient comfort. Pins are generally placed anterolateral in the upper humerus and direct lateral in the lower humerus. In the lower two thirds of the humerus, an open incision and careful dissection to the bone is made to prevent injury to the radial nerve. Typically, a two-pin construct per segment and two bar construct between segments are adequate to provide stable fixation and allow safe transport to a higher echelon of care. Additional spanning fixation can be added across the elbow or shoulder as indicated. Often, external fixation of shoulder girdle and proximal humerus fractures may not be practical. This would include most scapula fractures, including fractures of the glenoid, and clavicle fractures. In such cases, sling and swath immobilization may be appropriate for transportation or until definitive treatment can be accomplished.

Definitive fracture fixation with plate and screw constructs or intramedullary nails is not recommended in the combat setting unless the patient will not leave the theater of conflict. Appropriate staged debridement procedures should be performed every 24–72 h until wounds are considered clean, and fixation can occur at, or after, wound closure or coverage is obtained (Figs. 16.1a–e and 16.2a, b).

16.5 Vascular and Nerve Injury

It is true that vascular perfusion is the most important determinant of limb survival, and nerve status is the most important determinant of limb function. Vascular injuries are common following high velocity missile and blast injuries. When the surgeon is far forward without the benefit of a vascular or plastic surgeon, vascular shunting is immediately performed. The technique of placing and securing a shunt can be found in the chapter on treatment of vascular injury. Once vascular perfusion is reestablished, fracture treatment typically proceeds with external fixation, followed by debridement and irrigation of wounds, identification of associated soft tissue injuries, application of dressings, and immediate medical evacuation to a higher level of care. Serious consideration should be given to performing prophylactic fasciotomies to prevent compartment syndrome due to reperfusion injury in the forearm. Vascular reconstruction requires emergent transport to a higher echelon surgical hospital, and is usually performed by vascular surgeons or plastic surgeons.

Nerve injuries frequently occur from penetrating missile and blast injuries to the brachium. When lacerated nerve endings are encountered in the brachium or shoulder, they should be tagged with suture, and annotated in an operative note, to make identification easier at a higher level of care. Primary neurorrhaphy is rarely indicated in the frontline combat setting and almost never upon initial presentation. In general, only a clean, sharp laceration to a nerve would be suitable for early repair. Nerve injuries resulting from blast and high-energy penetrating injuries are usually not amenable to direct primary repair due to the extensive zone of injury and wound contamination. Primary neurorrhaphy or nerve reconstruction is never recommended unless the patient will remain in the theater of conflict (Fig. 16.3).

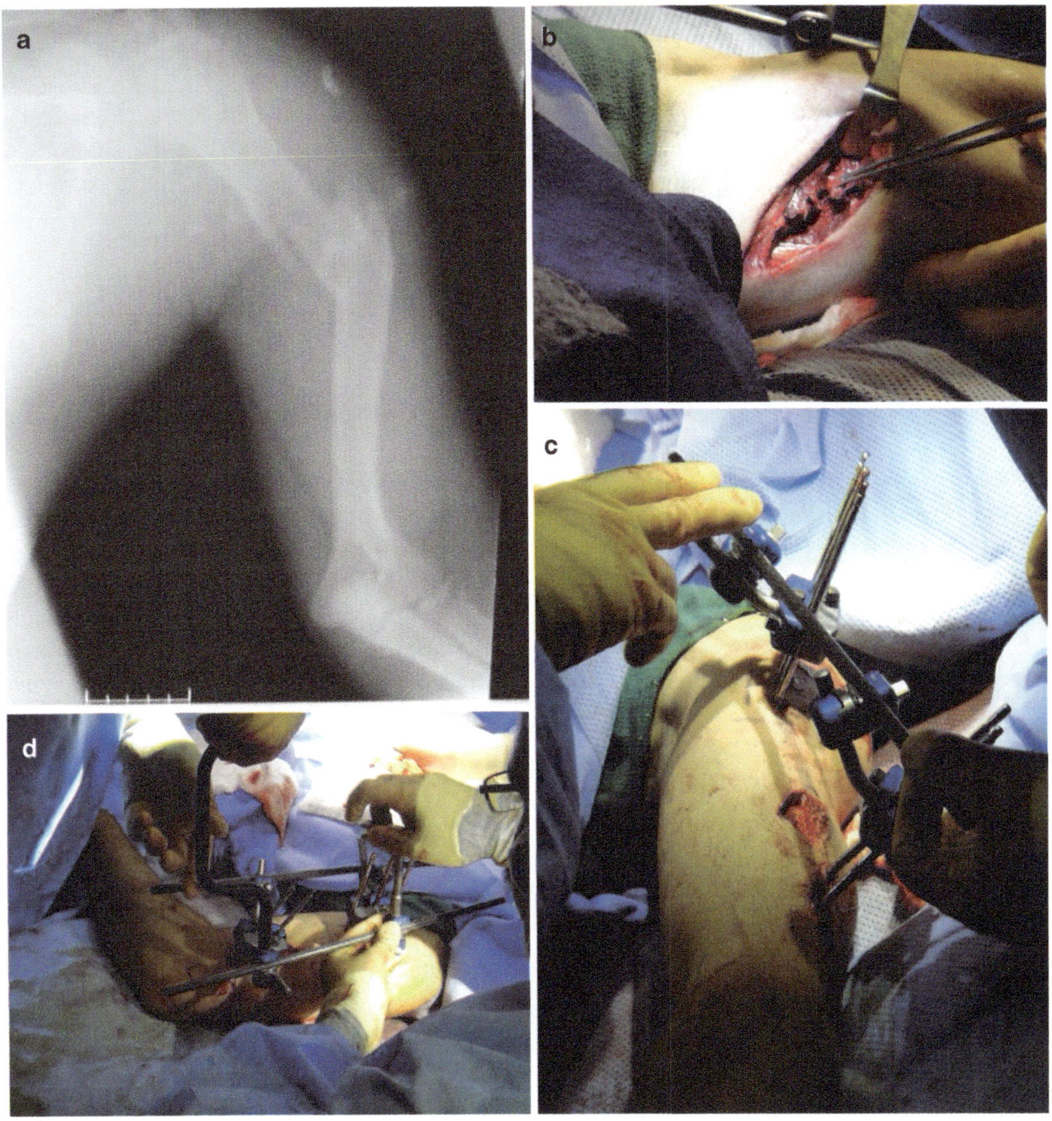

Fig. 16.1 (**a**) Comminuted humeral shaft fracture secondary to high velocity gunshot wounding seen at a forward surgical hospital, recorded with mobile expeditionary radiographic equipment. (**b**) Exit wound posteromedial arm. Distal extent of the radial nerve is identified and tagged with suture for later identification. (**c**) Surgical team assembling external fixation construct. Note entrance wound located on the lateral arm. (**d**) Surgical team completing the external fixation construct. Note use of two pins per fracture segment and two bars between fracture segments. (**e**) US Navy surgeons treat patient with open humerus fracture secondary to high velocity gunshot wounding mechanism

Fig. 16.1 (continued)

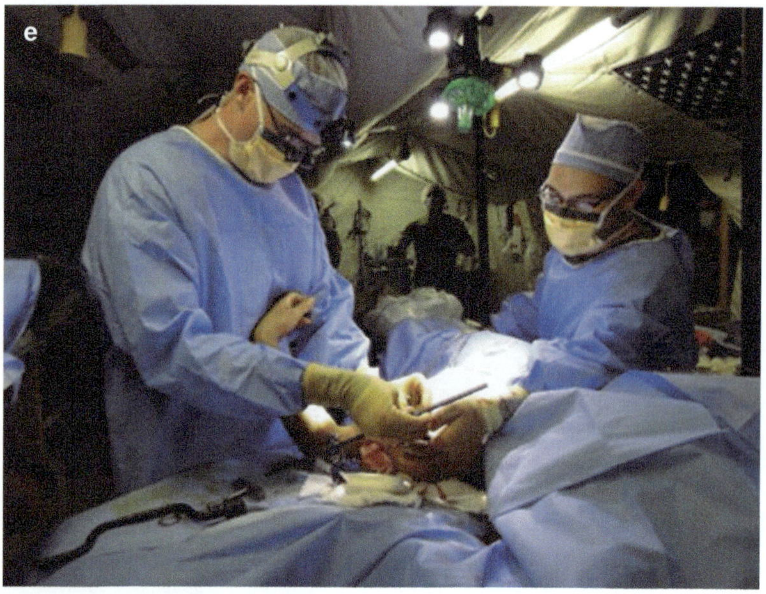

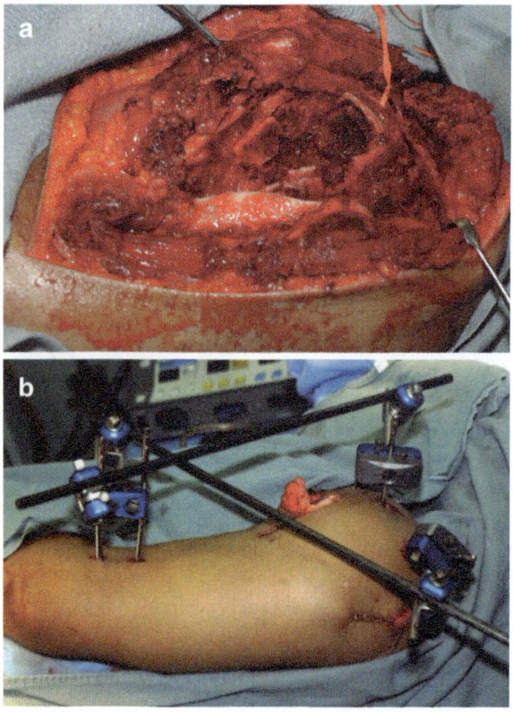

Fig. 16.2 (a) Proximal humerus fracture demonstrating severe comminution of the humeral head and shaft from high velocity projectile. The exit wound has been extended and devitalized bone and soft tissue debrided. (b) Placement of external fixator to stabilize bone and soft tissue. In this case, proximal pins were placed in the clavicle medially and the acromion laterally due to comminution of proximal humerus

16.6 Compartment Syndrome

The diagnosis of compartment syndrome is made by clinical evaluation. Specially designed pressure monitoring devices are rarely available in the forward surgical setting, or does time permit measurement of compartment pressures using alternate methods. The hallmark signs of compartment syndrome in the awake, cooperative patient are pain out of proportion to the injury, tense muscle compartments, and pain with passive stretch of muscle/tendon units. In the obtunded, sedated, or intubated patient, the need for fasciotomy is based on the presence of tense muscle compartments or a pattern of injury at risk for compartment syndrome such as crush, vascular disruption, and full-thickness burns.

The need to perform decompressive fasciotomies of the brachium is rare; fasciotomy of the forearm and hand is far more common. Release of the two compartments of the arm, the anterior compartment containing the biceps, the coracobrachialis and brachialis muscles, and the posterior compartment containing the triceps muscle can be performed via a one-or two-incision approach.

For release of arm compartment syndrome, we prefer the single incision technique,

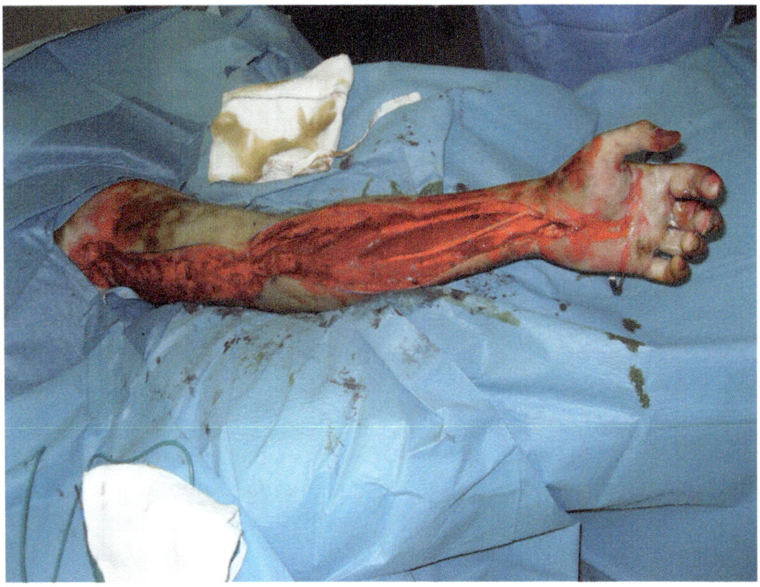

Fig. 16.3 Upper extremity fasciotomies performed for blast and burn injury. Note anterior and posterior compartment arm fasciotomies were performed via a medial approach

performed with an incision over the medial intermuscular septum, and simultaneous release of both the anterior and posterior compartments, or by a lateral approach with incision over the lateral intermuscular septum extending from the deltoid insertion to the lateral epicondyle. The median and ulnar nerves and the brachial artery are at risk and must be protected during the medial approach. Likewise, the radial nerve is at risk during the lateral approach. In our experience, secondary closure without need for skin grafting is more likely with a single incision approach.

Alternatively, a two-incision approach to arm fasciotomy may be employed. The anterior compartment is typically released through a single medial incision, and the posterior compartment is released through a posterolateral or direct posterior incision, allowing the surgeon to tailor the incision depending on additional exposure needs, such as for fractures.

Compartment syndrome of the shoulder or deltoid compartment is rarely reported. If suspected or encountered, the surgeon must remember the deltoid is a multipennate muscle, principally divided into three compartments of the deltoid muscle: the anterior and middle and posterior compartments. Decompression can be performed via a curvilinear type incision, or inverted "U," extending from anterior-inferior, decompressing the anterior compartment, coursing lateral and superior lateral to the acromion process, and then proceeding distal and posterior. Alternatively, separate incisions may be made, especially when associated wounds are present. Care must be made to ensure all fascial compartments of the multipennate muscle are released.

16.7 Limb Salvage Verses Amputation

The frontline surgeon will often be challenged with the grave decision to attempt limb salvage or to perform an amputation. In the upper extremity, the generally accepted absolute indication for amputation is a warm ischemia time greater than 6 h, although literature suggests this could extend to 8–10 h. The crushed extremity with arterial injury and the mangled extremity with the patient in extremis are also considered indications for amputation.

A major consideration for limb salvage versus amputation of the upper extremity is the dramatic difference in functional capability of modern prosthetic designs when compared to the normal hand. Despite dramatic improvements in prosthetic technology over the past decade, the numerous degrees of freedom of the human arm and the dexterity and sensory feedback of the hand are only partially replicated with current prosthetic technology. For this reason, the adage, "a bad hand is more functional than a good amputation," remains relevant today, and is likely the reason few patients request amputation following an initial limb salvage of the upper extremity. If there is an expectation that hand prehension and sensation can be preserved, then limb salvage should be attempted.

Rare is the indication for emergency flap coverage in a combat zone, and it has been fraught with frequent failure and subsequent amputation. The most common emergency flap for the brachium is the pedicled latissimus dorsi flap to cover vascular reconstructions that lack adequate soft tissue. A need for an emergency flap usually reflects severe destruction to other tissues and a large zone of injury, which likely contributes to the frequent failures. In such cases, amputation may be more advisable.

16.8 Amputation

When amputation has already occurred, or the indication exists to complete an injured extremity to an amputation, important principles must be considered to ensure the optimal outcome for the patient. The transhumeral amputation is the level with the least prosthetic acceptance rates in the upper extremity. Shoulder disarticulation essentially eliminates effective use of commercially available prosthetics in most cases. Maintenance of length, particularly the deltoid insertion, is directly related to prosthetic usage. In most cases, a transhumeral amputation with bone shorter than 5–7 cm will perform functionally as if it were a shoulder disarticulation. Therefore, guillotine amputations above the zone of injury are to be condemned. Careful debridement of devitalized bone and soft tissue within the zone of injury followed by repeat surgical debridement in 24–48 h should be performed. All viable skin flaps should be preserved to allow for future coverage. The surgeon should avoid aggressive traction neurectomies in the forward surgical setting, as newer techniques, such as targeted muscle reinnervation, are available to the transhumeral amputee. Furthermore, vascularized composite tissue allotransplantation, or hand transplantation, is growing in frequency and outcomes are improving.

In addition to standard postoperative dressings described previously, a light compression wrap helps to control edema. Splints may be used for additional protection during transport, but are not required for the acute traumatic transhumeral amputation (Fig. 16.4a–d).

16.9 Summary

War-related injuries to the brachium and shoulder are frequent, usually complex, and commonly occur in the polytrauma setting. Rapid recognition of hemorrhage and vascular injury is paramount to preserve life and limb. A strong understanding of the anatomy, adherence to sound orthopedic principles, and a systematic approach to evaluation and management of the severely injured brachium are also essential to achieving the best results. A multidisciplinary approach to the treatment of these severe injuries will ensure optimal functional outcomes for our patients.

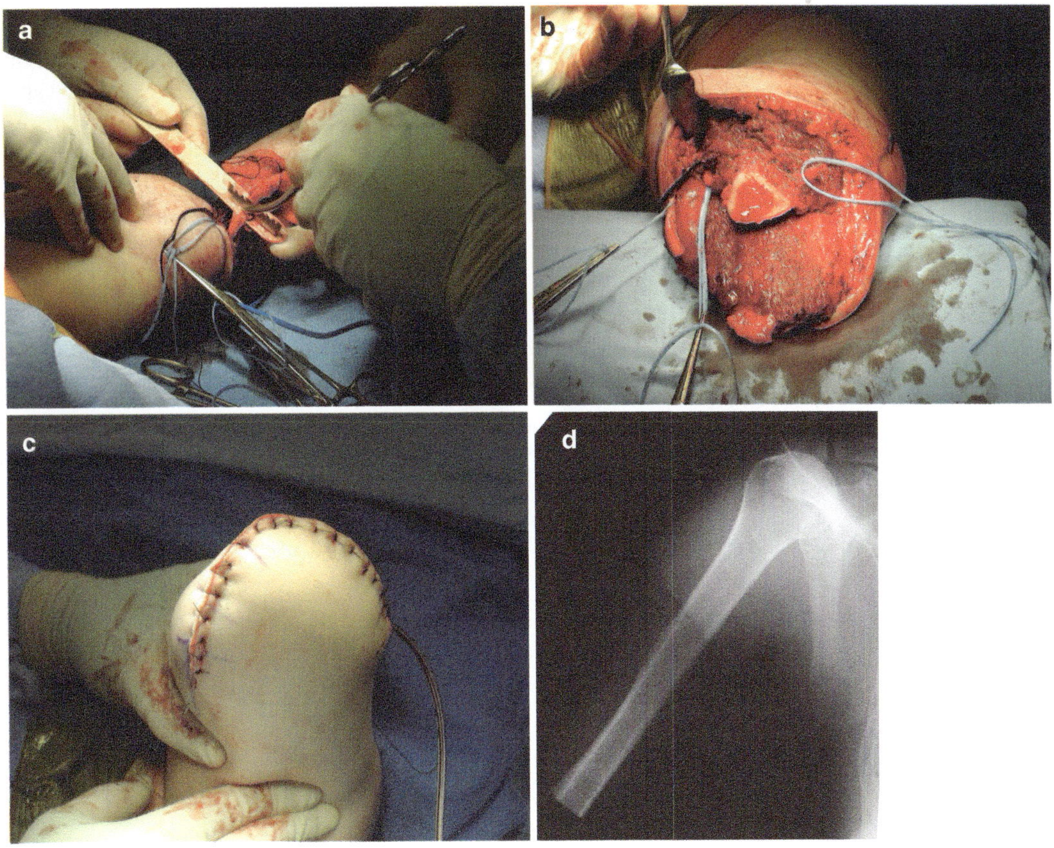

Fig. 16.4 (**a**) Transhumeral amputation, careful identification, and sharp transection of radial nerve without excessive traction. (**b**) Transhumeral amputation – ulnar, median, and radial nerves visible; residual humerus is smooth. A posterior flap is preserved for soft tissue coverage. Myodesis (muscle to bone) improves myoelectric control and reduces co-contraction found with myoplasty (biceps to triceps). (**c**) Transhumeral amputation – the incision is medial to lateral to minimize bulk and create smooth conical contour without marginal invaginations or "dog ears". (**d**) Transhumeral amputation radiograph, preservation of deltoid insertion improves prosthetic function and use

Upper Extremity Vascular Injuries

17

Mark E. Fleming, Jonathan J. Sexton, and David Whittaker

Contents

BLUF (Bottom Line Up Front) Box

1. Prehospital tourniquets should be liberally utilized.
2. Temporary shunting should be utilized at forward surgical sites with limited resources as a damage control measure.
3. Consider a sternotomy or thoracotomy for clamping of subclavian vessels for very proximal (junctional) axillary and subclavian vessel injuries.
4. Massive blood transfusion protocols should be anticipated to be required for upper extremity vessel injuries and repairs.
5. Liberal use of fasciotomies should be considered after revascularization procedures.
6. Expeditious external fixation application should be undertaken before the vascular repair.
7. Minimize the risk of the lethal triad (coagulopathy, hypothermia, acidosis).

M.E. Fleming, MC, USN (✉)
Department of Orthopaedics, Walter Reed National Military Medical Center, 8901 Wisconsin Ave, Bethesda, MD 20889, USA

Uniformed Services University of the Health Sciences, Bethesda, MD, USA
e-mail: mark.e.fleming.mil@health.mil

J.J. Sexton, MC, USA
Department of Surgery, Walter Reed National Military Medical Center, Bethesda, MD, USA

D. Whittaker, MC, USN
Department of Surgery, Vascular Surgery Service, Walter Reed National Military Medical Center, Bethesda, MD, USA

Uniformed Services University of the Health Sciences, Bethesda, MD, USA

L.B. Bone, C.N. Mamczak (eds.), *Front Line Extremity and Orthopaedic Surgery*,
DOI 10.1007/978-3-642-45337-3_17, © Springer-Verlag Berlin Heidelberg 2014

17.1 Overview

Upper extremity vascular traumas account for less than 2 % of all combat-related injuries [1]. While rare, these injuries are potentially devastating. In World War II, 24 % of upper extremity arterial injuries required amputation of the arm [2]. By the close of the Vietnam War, advancements in surgical technique and medical evacuation systems reduced this rate to 5 % [3]. Yet, the US military experience in Iraq suggests that the rate of arm amputation following combat-related arterial injury is on the rise [1, 4]. While similar to lower extremity vascular injuries, nuances in the diagnosis and management upper extremity vascular injuries must be recognized to maximize successful limb salvage.

17.2 Mechanism of Injury

In past and present armed conflicts, explosive devices and gunshots account for 60 and 30 %, respectively, of upper extremity vascular injuries [1]. Despite this consistency over time, 10 % of modern combat-related vascular traumas in the arm result in amputation. In comparison, only 5 % of these injuries led to amputation during the Vietnam War [1, 3]. The reason for this discrepancy remains unknown. During World War II, DeBakey noted that the type of arterial injury correlated with the rate of amputation (i.e., lacerations resulted in fewer amputations than thrombotic injuries). Blasts clearly cause greater injury to vessels than gunshots. However, the hallmark weapon of the modern battlefield – the improved explosive device – is no more destructive than standard military artillery. The likely explanation for the surge in arm amputations following vascular injury relates more to the use of body armor than the employed weapon. Modern combatants more often survive blast injuries and subsequently present to the trauma bay with devastating wounds of the upper extremity that in previous conflicts never reached the operating room. These wounds frequently carry a significant soft tissue component which disrupts collateral flow to and from tenuously viable limbs which predisposes to compartment syndrome and further places the limb at risk for amputation [5].

17.3 Diagnosis

17.3.1 Physical Exam

Clinical findings of peripheral vascular injury are classified into hard signs and soft signs. Hard signs include frank arterial bleeding, absent distal pulses, an expanding or pulsatile hematoma, a murmur or thrill, or manifestations of acute ischemia (pain, pallor, pulselessness, paresthesias, poikilothermy, paralysis). In simple penetrating injuries, hard signs are practically diagnostic of vascular trauma and necessitate operative exploration. Blunt and complex penetrating injuries to the extremities – which are common in trauma – often create soft tissue abnormalities that may mimic hard signs. In these scenarios, diagnostic imaging helps to confirm the presence and level of arterial injuries [6].

Soft signs of vascular injury include diminished pulses, stable hematomas, nerve deficits in anatomic proximity to major arteries, and general proximity injuries. Depending on the combination of soft signs, the rate of vascular injury may be up to 20 % [6]. However, these injuries are generally benign and require no intervention [7]. Axillary traumas are a clear exception to this rule as a rich collateral arterial system in this region may mask injury to axillary artery. In fact, only 68 % of injuries to the axillary artery display hard signs of vascular injury compared to >85 % for the rest of the arm [8]. Therefore, proximity injury alone in this region is an indication for further diagnostic imaging.

Measurement of the arterial pressure index (API) is a useful noninvasive method to identify clinically significant vascular injuries, especially in the presence of soft signs. The API is defined as the quotient of the Doppler arterial pressure distal to the injury divided by the Doppler arterial pressure in the unaffected extremity [9]. Routine duplex ultrasound of patients presenting with upper extremity penetrating trauma and an API $\geq$ 0.9 rarely demonstrates occult vascular injury requiring intervention [10]. As well, multiple studies demonstrate that an API < 0.9 detects clinically significant peripheral vascular injuries with 95 % sensitivity [11].

17.3.2 Imaging

Formal catheter-based angiography remains the gold standard method of diagnosing and characterizing vascular injury. However, computed tomography angiography (with 64-slice or greater scanner) and color-flow duplex are equally effective in evaluating most peripheral vascular injuries [12–14]. Most civilian penetrating arterial injuries will not require intraoperative angiography. The low energy mechanisms tend to cause focal injuries tracking along the path of the projectile. However, blunt and complex penetrating injuries are frequently associated with diffuse or multifocal arterial injuries due to high-energy cavitational effect or the fragmentation process itself [6]. Thus, when operative intervention is elected, a formal intraoperative angiography is indicated to define the extent of arterial injury prior to initiating repairs.

17.4 Operative Anatomy and Arterial Exposures

17.4.1 Axillary Artery

The axillary artery is an extension of the subclavian artery. It begins at the lateral border of the first rib, travels posterior to the pectoralis muscles, and transitions into the brachial artery at the inferior border of the teres major muscle in close proximity to the humerus. The cords of the brachial plexus weave about the axillary artery throughout its course. Anatomically, the axillary artery is divided into three segments by the pectoralis minor muscle. The first segment is medial to the muscle and is the origin of the superficial thoracic artery. The second segment is deep to the muscle and is the origin of the thoracoacromial and lateral thoracic arteries. The third segment is lateral to the muscle and is the origin of the subscapular artery and the anterior and posterior circumflex arteries [15, 16]. These arterial branches form an extensive collateral arterial network around the scapula that can actually maintain reasonable distal perfusion and pulses despite transection of the main axillary artery [17].

A deltopectoral incision achieves in-line exposure of all three parts of the axillary artery. This incision starts at the midpoint of the clavicle and extends 5–7 cm along the anterior border of the deltoid muscle. Medial retraction of the pectoralis major muscle and lateral retraction of the cephalic vein and deltoid muscle exposes the underlying clavicopectoral fascia and pectoralis minor muscle. The clavicopectoral fascia is then incised along the medial border of the coracobrachialis muscle to the coracoid process. This reveals the axillary sheath and contents – specifically the third segment of the axillary artery, the axillary vein, and components of the brachial plexus. Within the axillary sheath in this region, the junction of the medial and posterior cords of the brachial plexus lies superficial to the third segment of the axillary artery while the axillary vein lies superficial and inferior to the artery. Further medial exposure of the third segment of the axillary artery is achieved by transecting the insertion of the pectoralis major muscle. To expose the second and first segments of the axillary artery, the insertion of the pectoralis minor muscle is transected, and the skin incision may need to be extended medially under the clavicle (infraclavicular incision). In the trauma setting, proximal control of the medial axillary artery may be achieved with a supraclavicular exposure to control the subclavian artery [15–17].

17.4.2 Brachial Artery

The brachial artery is an extension of the axillary artery that anatomically begins as the axillary artery passes the inferior border of the teres major muscle. Accompanied posteriorly by the median nerve, the artery travels distally in the medial bicipital groove, courses anteriorly over the humerus, and continues over the neck of the radius where it terminally bifurcates into the vessels of the forearm. Along its route, the brachial artery gives off four named branches as well as numerous anonymous branches. The named branches, from proximal to distal, are the profunda brachii (deep brachial) artery, the humeral nutrient artery, and the superior and inferior collateral arteries. The deep brachial artery, in association with the radial nerve, courses posterior to the humerus in the radial groove and then terminally divides into the middle and radial collateral branches. These terminal vessels, as well as the superior and inferior collateral branches, collateralize around the elbow with the recurrent forearm arteries [15, 16].

The brachial artery has often been seen as the anatomic equivalent of the popliteal artery. However, the lower extremity lacks a true equivalent of the deep brachial artery. Neither the lateral geniculate nor the descending branch of the lateral femoral circumflex artery form significant periarticular collaterals. In contrast, the deep brachial artery forms hearty collaterals with the recurrent collaterals of the forearm arteries conferring to the forearm a relative tolerance to distal brachial artery injury [16, 17].

In-line exposure of the brachial artery is accomplished with an incision over the medial bicipital groove. Proximal extension or distal extension via a medial to lateral S-shaped incision across the antecubital fossa exposes, respectively, the axillary artery and terminal bifurcation of the brachial artery [15].

17.4.3 Radial and Ulnar Arteries

The radial artery is the smaller terminal branch of the brachial artery. It runs a course from the midpoint of the antecubital fossa to the medial aspect of the radial styloid process. The entire artery, with the exception of the most distal portion, runs entirely on muscle and deep only to the brachioradialis muscle. The ulnar artery is the larger terminal branch of the brachial artery. From its origin, it immediately dives deep to the pronator teres and flexor digitorum superficialis (FDS) muscles and runs toward the medial forearm. It then courses toward the wrist in the groove between the FDS and flexor digitorum profundus (FDP) muscles. There are several variations of the arterial anatomy of the forearm that are worth remembering [15, 16]. These are the high division of the brachial artery, the axillary origin of the radial artery, and superficial radial and ulnar arteries [16].

Proximally, in-line exposure of the forearm arteries requires an S-shaped incision over the antecubital fossa extending to the medial bicipital groove. Subsequent transection of the bicipital aponeurosis exposes the terminal bifurcation of the brachial artery. To expose the radial artery, this incision is carried toward the styloid process of the radius along the medial edge of the brachioradialis muscle. In-line exposure of the ulnar artery requires a separate incision beginning four fingerbreadths below the medial epicondyle of the humerus, extending from the medial epicondyle to the pisiform [15].

17.4.4 Shunts

In civilian trauma, definitive arterial repair is generally undertaken at the time of the initial operation. In the combat setting, a variety of factors may preclude immediate vascular repair (e.g., lack of resources, wound contamination, metabolic derangements, orthopedic injuries). In recent US military operations, up to 50 % of peripheral vascular injuries underwent initial assessment at forward surgical units designed for stabilization and transfer. Arterial shunts were placed in 25–35 % of these patients prior to arrival at combat support hospitals. More than 80 % of the shunts placed in proximal limb arteries remained patent. Distal to the brachial artery, only 10–20 % of arterial shunts maintain function through transport. Despite this difference, early limb salvage rates in both the proximal and distal extremities remain upward of 90 % [4, 16, 17, 18]. The ultimate difference in limb salvage between temporary arterial shunting and immediate definitive vascular remains unknown. However, preservation of distal flow via temporary arterial shunting makes intuitive sense and should be strongly considered for all proximal arm arterial injuries requiring transport from forward surgical units to combat support hospitals. In the forearm, the use of vascular shunts does not seem to provide any limb salvage benefit over ligation, and therefore, it should be reserved for cases of acute ischemia of the hand (e.g., double artery injury or single artery injury with disrupted palmar arch) [20].

17.4.5 External Fixation

The nature of combat wounds essentially mandates that bony fractures undergo initial stabilization with external fixation. Gross contamination and time constraints make open reduction with internal fixation (ORIF) less than ideal at the forward operating facility. However, despite the relative quickness of external fixation, in the setting of a vascular injury, even a small amount of time may be precious. Typically, vascular shunting takes priority to reduce overall ischemic time. The vascular surgeon then stands by while external fixation occurs to ensure shunt patency and eventually complete definitive vascular repair if appropriate.

17.4.6 Fasciotomies

Isolated upper extremity arterial injuries are known causes of acute compartment syndrome (ACS) of the upper extremity. However, most cases of ACS – which typically affect the forearm – arise in the setting of upper extremity polytrauma. This is especially true when the trauma is restricted to the forearm. Isolated radial or ulnar arterial injury leads to acute compartment syndrome in less than 4 % of cases [21]. The incidence of forearm ACS following brachial artery injury ranges from 2 to 29 %. Other than prolonged ischemia, known independent risk factors for the development of ACS include multilevel arterial injury and open fractures. Other commonly cited risk factors for the development of ACS in association with arterial injury include soft tissue and venous injury [5].

17.4.7 Concomitant Venous Injuries

The patient's overall condition is the most important consideration. In unstable patients, ligation should be performed without hesitation. In stable patients, we advocate repair of the venous injury. This intervention presumably reduces chronic complications without increasing the risk of immediate complications such as venous thromboembolism [22]. However, contrary to popular belief, venous repair does nothing to reduce the rate of upper extremity compartment syndrome or amputation [23].

17.4.8 Indications for Early Amputation

Vascular injuries in the upper extremity frequently occur in association with injury to bones or nerves. Nerve injury occurs in up to 85 % of arterial trauma to the upper arm. In the forearm, associated nerve injuries occur even more frequently. The rate of associated orthopedic injuries varies from 10 to 85 % [1, 24–28].

Almost 75 % of patients with arterial trauma of the arm and bone or nerve injury will recover with mild or no residual upper limb disability. In the setting of arterial trauma and concomitant injury to a bone and nerve, limb salvage may lead to severe disability in 42 % of patients and eventual arm amputation in 17 % of patients [29].

This implies that even damage to multiple systems of the arm can be salvaged in >80 % of cases. Therefore, attempt at limb salvage should be attempted in all cases unless the effort will threaten the life of the patient or the extent of the injury simply leaves no alternative to amputation.

17.5 Vascular Repair Techniques

The high-energy nature of combat weapons typically precludes primary repair of arterial injuries. Even in minor injuries (i.e., simple laceration, tangential injury, <2 cm gap), significant regional intimal damage lurks beyond the area of gross arterial trauma. In our experience, primary repair of these injuries frequently leads to stenosis, dissection, or occlusion. More often than not, the best management of combat-related arterial injury – simple or complex – will be either ligation or bypass.

17.5.1 Ligation

Ligation is the simplest method of controlling an injured artery. In the forearm, ligation of a single artery with an intact palmar arch rarely leads to ischemia of the hand. However, the rate of distal ischemia approaches 40 % when ligation is employed in the setting of trauma to both arteries of the forearm or a single artery with a disrupted palmar arch [2, 19, 20]. Clearly, these latter situations call for revascularization. Unfortunately, temporary vascular shunts in the forearm rarely remain patent, and nearly 50 % of interposition grafts will fail [20].

The upper arm does not forgive arterial ligation like the forearm. Nearly 55 % of patients that undergo ligation of the proximal brachial artery – which has few collaterals – will require amputation. In the axillary artery and distal brachial arteries, 45 and 25 % of patients, respectively, will require amputation of the arm [2]. With the exception of the most basic arterial injury in the forearm, arterial ligation in the arm should only be considered as a life-saving necessity.

17.5.2 Interposition/Bypass Grafts

Autogenous interposition and bypass vein grafts are the method of choice for definitive repair of extremity arterial trauma. Interposition grafts are placed as anatomic substitutes for injured vessels. In contrast, bypass grafts may be placed in multiple pathways and anastomotic configurations to restore arterial flow.

Each type of graft has its pros and cons. Interposition grafts are relatively easy to place and require shorter lengths. However, they must be placed in zones of combat-related trauma and therefore are exposed to inflammation and contamination. Bypass grafts may be placed around zones of injury and are useful when anticipating future lengthening procedures, but they typically require longer lengths of conduit. Ultimately, a sufficient length of venous conduit is required before either type of autogenous vein graft is employed. Blast injuries – especially IEDs – frequently cause lower extremity injuries that may destroy suitable venous conduits (e.g., the greater saphenous vein) or cause such severe lower extremity trauma that removal of the greater saphenous vein may unacceptably threaten a tenuously viable limb. A quick preharvest assessment of potential vein conduits with a duplex ultrasound is strongly recommended to confirm the vein is patent (easily compressible) and of adequate diameter (>3 mm). Alternatives to the greater saphenous vein – in order of preference – include the lesser saphenous vein, the cephalic vein, and the basilic vein. The superficial femoral vein may also be used as a last resort for autogenous vein. Also, it is important to recognize that both artery and vein from an amputated limb may be harvested for use.

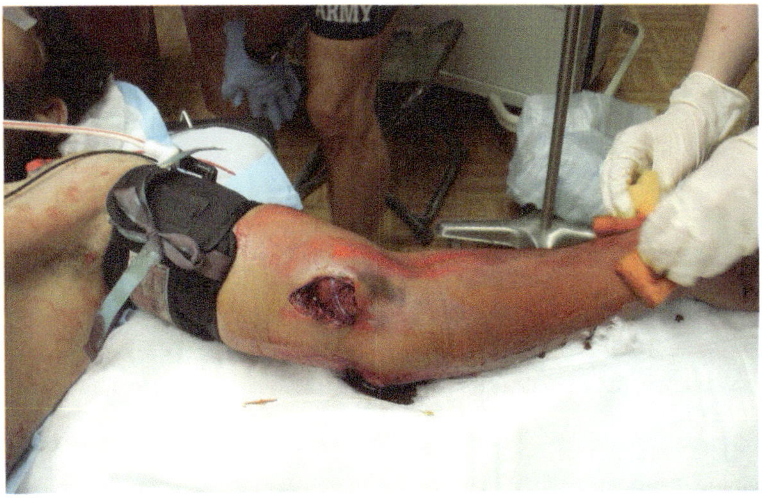

Fig. 17.1 Left upper extremity gunshot wound. Pneumatic tourniquet in place

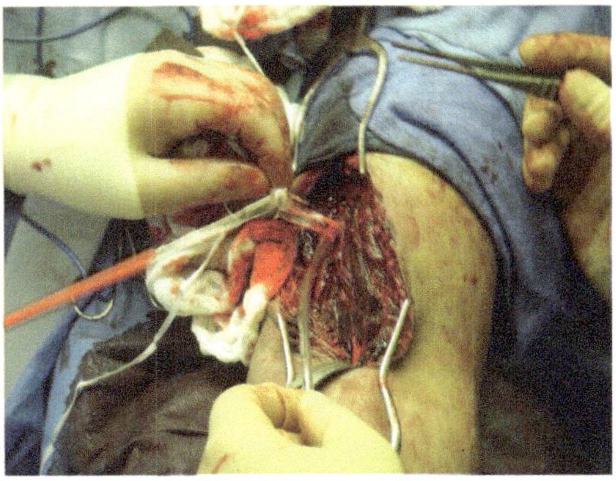

Fig. 17.2 After exposure, temporary intravascular shunt in the brachial artery

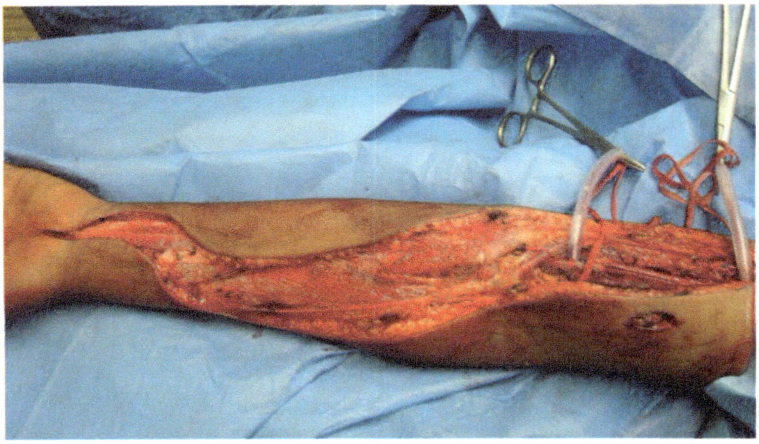

Fig. 17.3 Temporary intravascular shunt in the brachial artery. Use of liberal fasciotomies to minimize the risk of compartment syndrome and revascularization procedure

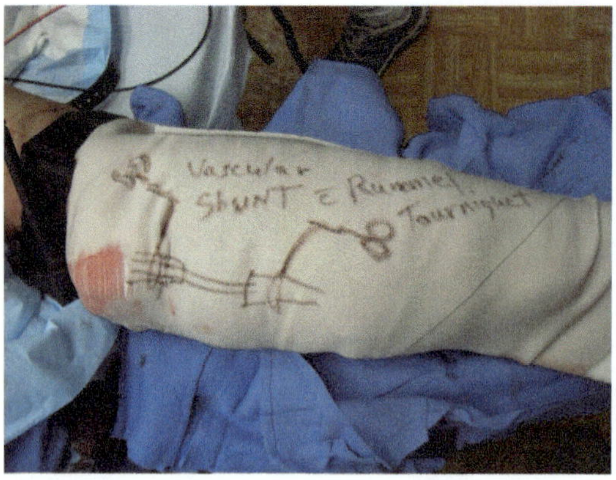

Fig. 17.4 Description of procedure well visible on dressing

In scenarios of limited vein conduit, prosthetic conduits (e.g., polyester or PTFE) are an alternative but undesirable option for definitive arterial repair. Recent wartime experience suggests that up to 80 % of prosthetic grafts placed for temporary or definitive repair of combat-related upper extremity arterial injury required replacement for thrombosis, ischemia, or exposure with presumed infection [30] (Figs. 17.1, 17.2, 17.3, and 17.4).

References

1. Clouse WD, Rasmussen TE, Perlstein J, Sutherland MJ, Peck MA, Eliason JL, et al. Upper extremity vascular injury: a current in-theater wartime report from Operation Iraqi Freedom. Ann Vasc Surg. 2006;20(4):429–34.
2. DeBakey ME, Simeone FA. Battle injuries of the arteries in World War II; an analysis of 2,471 cases. Ann Surg. 1946;123:534–79.
3. Rich NM, Baugh JH, Hughes CW. Acute arterial injuries in Vietnam: 1,000 cases. J Trauma. 1970; 10(5):359–69.
4. Clouse WD, Rasmussen TE, Peck MA, Eliason JL, Cox MW, Bowser AN, et al. In-theater management of vascular injury: 2 years of the Balad Vascular Registry. J Am Coll Surg. 2007;204(4):625–32.
5. Duckworth AD, Mitchell SE, Molyneux SG, White TO, Court-Brown CM, McQueen MM. Acute compartment syndrome of the forearm. J Bone Joint Surg Am. 2012;94(10):e63. May 16.
6. Feliciano DV, Mattox KL, Moore EE. Trauma, vol. xxxi. 6th ed. New York: McGraw-Hill Medical; 2008. 1430 p.
7. Applebaum R, Yellin AE, Weaver FA, Oberg J, Pentecost M. Role of routine arteriography in blunt lower-extremity trauma. Am J Surg. 1990;160(2):221–4. discussion 4–5.
8. Borman KR, Snyder WH, Weigelt JA. Civilian arterial trauma of the upper extremity. An 11 year experience in 267 patients. Am J Surg. 1984;148(6):796–9.
9. Feliciano DV. Management of peripheral arterial injury. Curr Opin Crit Care. 2010;16(6):602–8.
10. Mollberg NM, Wise SR, Banipal S, Sullivan R, Holevar M, Vafa A, et al. Color-flow duplex screening for upper extremity proximity injuries: a low-yield strategy for therapeutic intervention. Ann Vasc Surg. 2013;27:594–8.
11. Lynch K, Johansen K. Can Doppler pressure measurement replace "exclusion" arteriography in the diagnosis of occult extremity arterial trauma? Ann Surg. 1991;214(6):737–41.
12. Busquéts AR, Acosta JA, Colón E, Alejandro KV, Rodríguez P. Helical computed tomographic angiography for the diagnosis of traumatic arterial injuries of the extremities. J Trauma. 2004;56(3):625–8.
13. Knudson MM, Lewis FR, Atkinson K, Neuhaus A. The role of duplex ultrasound arterial imaging in patients with penetrating extremity trauma. Arch Surg. 1993;128(9):1033–7. discussion 7–8.
14. Fry WR, Smith RS, Sayers DV, Henderson VJ, Morabito DJ, Tsoi EK, et al. The success of duplex ultrasonographic scanning in diagnosis of extremity vascular proximity trauma. Arch Surg. 1993; 128(12):1368–72.
15. Wind GG, Valentine RJ. Anatomic exposures in vascular surgery, vol. xiv. Baltimore: Williams & Wilkins; 1991. 490 p.
16. Moore KL, Dalley AF, Agur AMR. Clinically oriented anatomy, vol. xxxiii. 5th ed. Philadelphia: Lippincott Williams & Wilkins; 2006. 1209 p.
17. Graham JM, Mattox KL, Feliciano DV, DeBakey ME. Vascular injuries of the axilla. Ann Surg. 1982;195(2): 232–8.
18. Taller J, Kamdar JP, Greene JA, Morgan RA, Blankenship CL, Dabrowski P, et al. Temporary vascular shunts as initial treatment of proximal extremity vascular injuries during combat operations: the new standard of care at Echelon II facilities? J Trauma. 2008;65(3):595–603.
19. Rasmussen TE, Clouse WD, Jenkins DH, Peck MA, Eliason JL, Smith DL. The use of temporary vascular shunts as a damage control adjunct in the management of wartime vascular injury. J Trauma. 2006;61(1):8–12.
20. Aftabuddin M, Islam N, Jafar MA, Haque E, Alimuzzaman M. Management of isolated radial or ulnar arteries at the forearm. J Trauma. 1995;38(1): 149–51.
21. Morin RJ, Swan KG, Tan V. Acute forearm compartment syndrome secondary to local arterial injury after penetrating trauma. J Trauma. 2009;66(4): 989–93.

22. Quan RW, Gillespie DL, Stuart RP, Chang AS, Whittaker DR, Fox CJ. The effect of vein repair on the risk of venous thromboembolic events: a review of more than 100 traumatic military venous injuries. J Vasc Surg. 2008;47(3):571–7.
23. Kim JY, Buck DW, Forte AJ, Subramanian VS, Birman MV, Schierle CF, et al. Risk factors for compartment syndrome in traumatic brachial artery injuries: an institutional experience in 139 patients. J Trauma. 2009;67(6):1339–44.
24. Nichols JS, Lillehei KO. Nerve injury associated with acute vascular trauma. Surg Clin North Am. 1988; 68(4):837–52.
25. Diamond S, Gaspard D, Katz S. Vascular injuries to the extremities in a suburban trauma center. Am Surg. 2003;69(10):848–51.
26. Cikrit DF, Dalsing MC, Bryant BJ, Lalka SG, Sawchuk AP, Schulz JE. An experience with upper-extremity vascular trauma. Am J Surg. 1990;160(2): 229–33.
27. Pillai L, Luchette FA, Romano KS, Ricotta JJ. Upper-extremity arterial injury. Am Surg. 1997;63(3):224–7.
28. Rozycki GS, Tremblay LN, Feliciano DV, McClelland WB. Blunt vascular trauma in the extremity: diagnosis, management, and outcome. J Trauma. 2003;55(5): 814–24.
29. Brown KR, Jean-Claude J, Seabrook GR, Towne JB, Cambria RA. Determinates of functional disability after complex upper extremity trauma. Ann Vasc Surg. 2001;15(1):43–8.
30. Vertrees A, Fox CJ, Quan RW, Cox MW, Adams ED, Gillespie DL. The use of prosthetic grafts in complex military vascular trauma: a limb salvage strategy for patients with severely limited autologous conduit. J Trauma. 2009;66(4):980–3.

Spine Injuries 18

Jason Zook, Dennis J. Rivet, and Melvin D. Helgeson

Contents

BLUF (Bottom Line Up Front) Box

1. Perform a thorough spine exam on every patient. The injuries are high-energy and missed fractures can be devastating.
2. Immobilize all known and suspected fractures to the best degree possible. If you don't have collars or braces, use what is available.
3. Communication is key; make sure everyone involved knows that your patient has a spine injury. This is especially important if you are not the last stop for your patient.
4. The most commonly missed spine fracture is the 2nd one. Don't forget to image the rest of the spinal column. This is easy to forget when there is a blatant C5/6 dislocation and their only complaint is neck pain.
5. Place a Foley catheter whenever a spinal cord injury is suspected.
6. If a patient has a spinal cord injury, maintain MAPs 80–90 (goal). This can prove a difficult proposition.
7. Don't forget the rectal exam! All spine-injured patients need perianal sensation and rectal examination and this is documented in the chart.
8. Frequent, periodic neurovascular checks! Document a thorough exam (date and time) in the chart. Follow

J. Zook, MD (✉)
Carolina Orthopaedic Specialists, 503 East Parker Road, Morganton, NC 28655, USA
e-mail: jasonzook@carolinaortho.com

D.J. Rivet, MD, FACSCDR, MC, USN
Department of Neurosurgery, Naval Medical Center Portsmouth, 620 John Paul Jones Circle, Portsmouth, VA 23708, USA
e-mail: rivetd@gmail.com

M.D. Helgeson, MD
Director of Orthopaedic Research,
Walter Reed National Military Medical Center, 8901 Rockville Pike, Bethesda, MD 20889, USA
e-mail: melvin.d.helgeson@health.mil

L.B. Bone, C.N. Mamczak (eds.), *Front Line Extremity and Orthopaedic Surgery*,
DOI 10.1007/978-3-642-45337-3_18,

ASIA exam or Combat Neuro exam guidelines. This allows for consistency of information and data collection.
9. If you are a spine-trained surgeon, don't be afraid to operate when indicated!

18.1 Introduction

As personal protective gear and multi-personnel armored vehicle technology has improved, we are seeing a greater number of casualties with previously non-survivable injuries. This, combined with the increasing force imparted via improvised explosive devices, results in a significant number of combat casualties with spine injuries. One of the common scenarios you will encounter is an MRAP (Mine-Resistant Ambush Protected) vehicle driving over or next to an IED, which will then often be thrown into the air or rolled over, commonly resulting in compression or burst fractures of the spinal column.

18.2 Initial Survey

The most important take-home principle is to *consider* the spine in every casualty you treat. Adherence to ATLS secondary survey principles will help you immensely. However, it is easy to forget about the spine when you are faced with a triple amputee whom is exsanguinating in front of you. Sometimes, due to necessity the secondary survey is delayed until after initial stabilizing surgery. Placement of cervical collar (if available) and initiation of logroll precautions in this situation are recommended until a more thorough examination can be performed. Keep in mind that the ATLS secondary survey is also only as good as the situation will allow; if the patient arrives intubated or with severe distracting injuries, you may yield limited information from palpation of the spine and rectal examination.

If you have time when initial X-rays are being taken in the trauma bay, be sure to image at a minimum the lateral cervical spine.

If you are fortunate enough to have a CT scanner at your facility, be sure to scan any areas of the spinal column of which you have any suspicion, often the entire neuraxis is scanned (Cervical, thoracic and lumbar spine). Don't forget that the presence of a compression or burst fracture imparts a significant risk of a secondary fracture, sometimes separated by several vertebral levels!

18.3 Clearing the Spine

If the patient is awake and alert, able to cooperate with the exam, and does not have any distracting injuries (open fracture, long bone fracture, penetrating abdominal or thoracic injury), then it is reasonable to clear the spine on a patient based on examination.

To clear the spine, the patient must be neurologically intact (see section on examination below), has no tenderness to palpation, and in the case of the cervical spine must be able to flex, extend, and rotate the neck without pain. If these criteria are met, you can discontinue the spine board and cervical collar, assuming these are even available or in place! The Joint Theater Trauma System has a flow sheet for clearance of cervical spine in awake and cooperative patients as well as those who are obtunded. See Figs. 18.1, 18.2, and 18.3.

18.4 Suspected Fracture

When you have a suspected fracture, be sure to maintain strict logroll precautions. If you are at a level 1 or 2 facility, you may not have access to either collars or braces. In this scenario, rolled towels, blankets, or IV bags (try to avoid the latter as you may need those fluids later!) can be used with silk tape to immobilize the head and torso. If you suspect the cervical spine, make a good effort to try and verify whether the patient has any pain in the thoracic and lumbar spine. It is always good to get someone off a spine board when possible, assuming the patient is on a board. Pressure sores can develop quickly in patients left on spine boards.

If you are in a location or situation without radiographic capability, and you have access to cervical collars (semirigid orthosis such as Aspen, Miami-J), there are certain situations in which it is prudent to immobilize the cervical spine. These include trauma resulting in loss of consciousness or even the question of loss of consciousness due to any form of head injury:

- Trauma resulting in loss of consciousness or temporary amnesia
- Vehicle rollover
- Fall from height (vs. fall from standing)
- Major explosive or blast injury
- Any high energy injury causing a direct blow or violent motion of the head, neck, or torso
- Injury mechanism that involved rapid acceleration/deceleration or lateral bending forces on the neck or trunk
- Ejection or fall from any motorized vehicle

Any patient complaining of neck pain, with or without neurologic complaint/compromise, should have their neck immobilized if time and situation permit.

18.5 Fractures/Dislocations

Spine-traumatized patients may be placed into one of four clinical categories: (1) patients with complete spinal cord syndromes, (2) patients with incomplete and progressive spinal cord syndromes, (3) patients with incomplete but nonprogressive spinal cord syndromes, and (4) patients with normal neurological function.

If you diagnose a fracture of the spinal column and do not have a spine surgeon or neurosurgeon at your facility, it is best to treat all fractures as potentially causing neurologic compromise. Strict spine precautions (logroll, maintain head of bed less than 30°) should be in place. These orders should be both verbally communicated and written down in a manner that does not leave

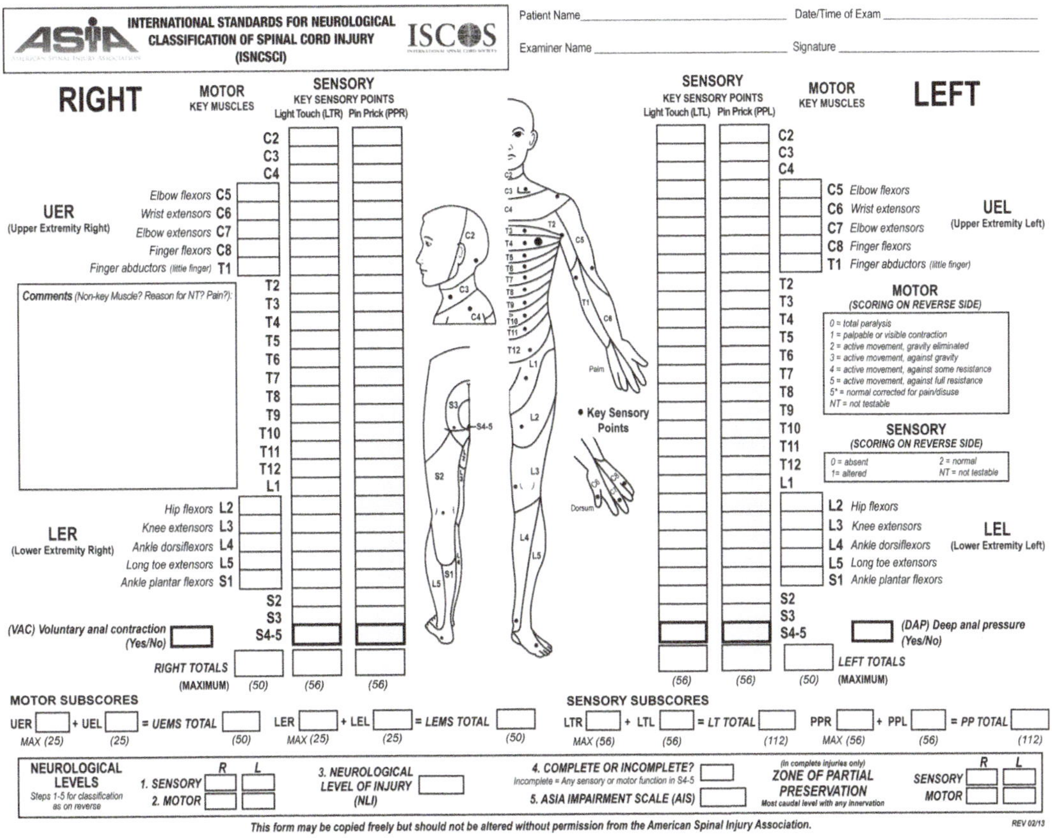

Fig. 18.1 Cervical spine clearance algorithm-reliable patient with no neurologic deficit

Muscle Function Grading

0 = total paralysis

1 = palpable or visible contraction

2 = active movement, full range of motion (ROM) with gravity eliminated

3 = active movement, full ROM against gravity

4 = active movement, full ROM against gravity and moderate resistance in a muscle specific position.

5 = (normal) active movement, full ROM against gravity and full resistance in a functional muscle position expected from an otherwise unimpaired person.

5* = (normal) active movement, full ROM against gravity and sufficient resistance to be considered normal if identified inhibiting factors (i.e. pain, disuse) were not present.

NT = not testable (i.e. due to immobilization, severe pain such that the patient cannot be graded, amputation of limb, or contracture of > 50% of the normal range of motion).

Sensory Grading

0 = Absent

1 = Altered, either decreased/impaired sensation or hypersensitivity

2 = Normal

NT = Not testable

Non Key Muscle Functions (optional)

May be used to assign a motor level to differentiate AIS B vs. C

Movement	Root level
Shoulder: Flexion, extension, abduction, adduction, internal and external rotation **Elbow:** Supination	**C5**
Elbow: Pronation **Wrist:** Flexion	**C6**
Finger: Flexion at proximal joint, extension. **Thumb:** Flexion, extension and abduction in plane of thumb	**C7**
Finger: Flexion at MCP joint **Thumb:** Opposition, adduction and abduction perpendicular to palm	**C8**
Finger: Abduction of the index finger	**T1**
Hip: Adduction	**L2**
Hip: External rotation	**L3**
Hip: Extension, abduction, internal rotation **Knee:** Flexion **Ankle:** Inversion and eversion **Toe:** MP and IP extension	**L4**
Hallux and Toe: DIP and PIP flexion and abduction	**L5**
Hallux: Adduction	**S1**

ASIA Impairment Scale (AIS)

A = Complete. No sensory or motor function is preserved in the sacral segments S4-5.

B = Sensory Incomplete. Sensory but not motor function is preserved below the neurological level and includes the sacral segments S4-5 (light touch or pin prick at S4-5 or deep anal pressure) AND no motor function is preserved more than three levels below the motor level on either side of the body.

C = Motor Incomplete. Motor function is preserved below the neurological level**, and more than half of key muscle functions below the neurological level of injury (NLI) have a muscle grade less than 3 (Grades 0-2).

D = Motor Incomplete. Motor function is preserved below the neurological level**, and at least half (half or more) of key muscle functions below the NLI have a muscle grade ≥ 3.

E = Normal. If sensation and motor function as tested with the ISNCSCI are graded as normal in all segments, and the patient had prior deficits, then the AIS grade is E. Someone without an initial SCI does not receive an AIS grade.

** For an individual to receive a grade of C or D, i.e. motor incomplete status, they must have either (1) voluntary anal sphincter contraction or (2) sacral sensory sparing with sparing of motor funtion more than three levels below the motor level for that side of the body. The International Standards at this time allows even non-key muscle function more than 3 levels below the motor level to be used in determining motor incomplete status (AIS B versus C).

NOTE: When assessing the extent of motor sparing below the level for distingusihing between AIS B and C, the ***motor level*** on each side is used; whereas to differentiate between AIS C and D (based on proportion of key muscle functions with strength grade 3 or greater) the ***neurological level of injury*** is used.

AMERICAN SPINAL INJURY ASSOCIATION

INTERNATIONAL STANDARDS FOR NEUROLOGICAL CLASSIFICATION OF SPINAL CORD INJURY

ISCOS

INTERNATIONAL SPINAL CORD SOCIETY

Steps in Classification

The following order is recommended for determining the classification of individuals with SCI.

1. Determine sensory levels for right and left sides.
The sensory level is the most caudal, intact dermatome for both pin prick and light touch sensation.

2. Determine motor levels for right and left sides.
Defined by the lowest key muscle function that has a grade of at least 3 (on supine testing), providing the key muscle functions represented by segments above that level are judged to be intact (graded as a 5).
Note: in regions where there is no myotome to test, the motor level is presumed to be the same as the sensory level, if testable motor function above that level is also normal.

3. Determine the neurological level of injury (NLI)
This refers to the most caudal segment of the cord with intact sensation and antigravity (3 or more) muscle function strength, provided that there is normal (intact) sensory and motor function rostrally respectively.
The NLI is the most cephalad of the sensory and motor levels determined in steps 1 and 2.

4. Determine whether the injury is Complete or Incomplete.
(i.e. absence or presence of sacral sparing)
*If voluntary anal contraction = **No** AND all S4-5 sensory scores = **0** AND deep anal pressure = **No,** then injury is **Complete.***
*Otherwise, injury is **Incomplete.***

5. Determine ASIA Impairment Scale (AIS) Grade:

Is injury Complete? **If YES, AIS=A** and can record ZPP (lowest dermatome or myotome on each side with some preservation)

NO ↓

Is injury Motor Complete? **If YES, AIS=B**

NO ↓ (No=voluntary anal contraction OR motor function more than three levels below the motor level on a given side, if the patient has sensory incomplete classification)

Are at least half (half or more) of the key muscles below the neurological level of injury graded 3 or better?

NO ↓ **AIS=C** **YES** ↓ **AIS=D**

If sensation and motor function is normal in all segments, AIS=E
Note: AIS E is used in follow-up testing when an individual with a documented SCI has recovered normal function. If at initial testing no deficits are found, the individual is neurologically intact; the ASIA Impairment Scale does not apply.

Fig. 18.1 (continued)

any confusion. It is important that the nursing staff that will be helping with medevac also know that there are spine precautions in place.

The vast majority of fractures will not require surgery, or if necessary can be delayed until the patient is at a level 3 facility or greater. Dislocations, fracture-dislocations, and injuries associated with neurologic compromise are considered reasons for immediate transport to a tertiary facility if patient status, current resources, and combat situation allow.

18.6 Spinal Cord Injury

If you suspect your patient has a spinal cord injury, several things must be done in order to give that person the best chance for survival and stabilization. First, a thorough examination must be performed. The ASIA (see Fig. 18.4) examination form is a validated exam tool that looks at motor and sensory exam for each neurologic level. Included is the assessment of perianal sensation, anal sphincter tone, and deep anal pressure. The form also has an instruction sheet that helps you to assess whether the patient is a complete or incomplete injury. A more abbreviated version adapted for the battlefield is the Combat Neuro exam (Fig. 18.5) which contains key components of the ASIA exam and can be utilized as well. Be sure to date and time all examinations, place them on separate sheets (if available), and document any changes.

With an incomplete injury (especially one with progressive neurologic deficit), the goal should be expeditious transport to a facility with neurosurgical/spine capability. Current recommendations are to place an arterial line and maintain MAP between 80 and 90. The rationale for this is to maximize perfusion to the spinal cord,

APPENDIX A, COMBAT NEURO EXAM WORKSHEET

- ❖ Need Safety Pin or Needle DATE:___________ TIME:____________
- ❖ Perform all elements for all patients with a fracture of the vertebral body (excludes stable isolated transverse or spinous process fractures) noted on CT scan.

Fractured Vertebrae: (circle all that apply)

C1 C2 C3 C4 C5 C6 C7

T1 T2 T3 T4 T5 T6 T7 T8 T9 T10 T11 T12

L1 L2 L3 L4 L5 Sacrum

MOI: [Vehicle vs. IED] [Dismounted IED] [Fall from Ht] [Aircraft Crash] [GSW] [OTHER]

Alertness at time of exam: [Intubated/Sedated] [Intubated/Alert/Compliant] [Extubated]

External Fixation: [RUE] [LUE] [RLE] [LLE] Splint: [RUE] [LUE] [RLE] [LLE]

Motor Strength:

Elbow Flexion (C5)
LEFT: [ ]No Motion] [ ]Motion against gravity] [ ]Normal] [ ][*] [ ]NT]
RIGHT: [ ]No Motion] [ ]Motion against gravity] [ ]Normal] [ ][*] [ ]NT]

Wrist Extension (C6)
LEFT: [ ]No Motion] [ ]Motion against gravity] [ ]Normal] [ ][*] [ ]NT]
RIGHT: [ ]No Motion] [ ]Motion against gravity] [ ]Normal] [ ][*] [ ]NT]

Elbow Extension (C7)
LEFT: [ ]No Motion] [ ]Motion against gravity] [ ]Normal] [ ][*] [ ]NT]
RIGHT: [ ]No Motion] [ ]Motion against gravity] [ ]Normal] [ ][*] [ ]NT]

MF DIP Flex (C8)
LEFT: [ ]No Motion] [ ]Motion against gravity] [ ]Normal] [ ][*] [ ]NT]
RIGHT: [ ]No Motion] [ ]Motion against gravity] [ ]Normal] [ ][*] [ ]NT]

SF Abduction (T1)
LEFT: [ ]No Motion] [ ]Motion against gravity] [ ]Normal] [ ][*] [ ]NT]
RIGHT: [ ]No Motion] [ ]Motion against gravity] [ ]Normal] [ ][*] [ ]NT]

Hip Flexion (L2)
LEFT: [ ]No Motion] [ ]Motion against gravity] [ ]Normal] [ ][*] [ ]NT]
RIGHT: [ ]No Motion] [ ]Motion against gravity] [ ]Normal] [ ][*] [ ]NT]

Knee Extension (L3)
LEFT: [ ]No Motion] [ ]Motion against gravity] [ ]Normal] [ ][*] [ ]NT]
RIGHT: [ ]No Motion] [ ]Motion against gravity] [ ]Normal] [ ][*] [ ]NT]

Ankle Dorsiflexion (L4)
LEFT: [ ]No Motion] [ ]Motion against gravity] [ ]Normal] [ ][*] [ ]NT]
RIGHT: [ ]No Motion] [ ]Motion against gravity] [ ]Normal] [ ][*] [ ]NT]

Great Toe Extension (L5)
LEFT: [ ]No Motion] [ ]Motion against gravity] [ ]Normal] [ ][*] [ ]NT]
RIGHT: [ ]No Motion] [ ]Motion against gravity] [ ]Normal] [ ][*] [ ]NT]

Fig. 18.2 Cervical spine clearance algorithm unreliable patient

Ankle Plantaflexion (S1)
LEFT: [ ]No Motion] [ ]Motion against gravity] [ ]Normal] [ ][*] [ ]NT]
RIGHT: [ ]No Motion] [ ]Motion against gravity] [ ]Normal] [ ][*] [ ]NT]

Rectal Exam:
Voluntary Anal Contraction [ ]None] [ ]Weak] [ ]Normal]
Tone [ ]None] [ ]Weak]
[ ]Normal]
Pinprick Anal Sensation (S4/5) [ ]Absent] [ ]Impaired] [ ]Normal]
Anal Wink [ ]Absent] [ ]Present]

Sensation:
Start at Clavicle and progress inferiorly until light touch sensation is abnormal. Then, test pin prick at this level and prick with sharp and then with dull surface at each dermatome. Check the LOWEST level where the patient had reliable detection of sharp and dull sensation. Indicate if levels are different on Left or Right side.

[ ]Clavicle (C3/4)
[ ]Lateral Elbow (C5)
[ ]Dorsal Thumb (C6)
[ ]Dorsal MF (C7)
[ ]Dorsal SF (C8)
[ ]Medial Elbow(T1)
[ ]Nipple Level (T4)
[ ]Xiphoid Level (T6)
[ ]Umbilicus (T10)
[ ]Mid-Inguinal Crease (T12)
[ ]Medial Thigh (Prox 1/3) (L1)
[ ]Medial Thigh (Mid Point) (L2)
[ ]Medial Knee (L3)
[ ]Medial Ankle (L4)
[ ]Dorsum Middle Toe (L5)

Reflexes:
Bulbocavernosis [ ]Absent] [ ]Present] [ ]Indeterminate] [ ]NT]
Patella LEFT: [ ]Absent] [ ]Present] RIGHT: [ ]Absent] [ ]Present]
Clonus LEFT: [ ]Absent] [ ]Present] RIGHT: [ ]Absent] [ ]Present]
Foley: [ ]Present] [ ]Voiding spontaneously without catheter]

ASIA Score: (circle score)
[A] COMPLETE (no motor/sensory function below level of injury)
[B] Pinprick sensation PRESENT at anus (S4/5) – NO Motor
[C] <½ the muscles below level of injury have motion against gravity
[D] >½ the muscles below level of injury have motion against gravity
[E] Normal

NEURO LEVEL: __________ (Lowest level with normal sense and at least antigravity strength)

Incomplete Syndrome: (SCI – Occ-T11 Fx) (Conus – T12-L2 Fx) (CES – L3-Sacrum)

MF = middle finger; SF = small finger; * Suspect NORMAL strength, but limited due to pain; NT = Not Tested

Fig. 18.2 (continued)

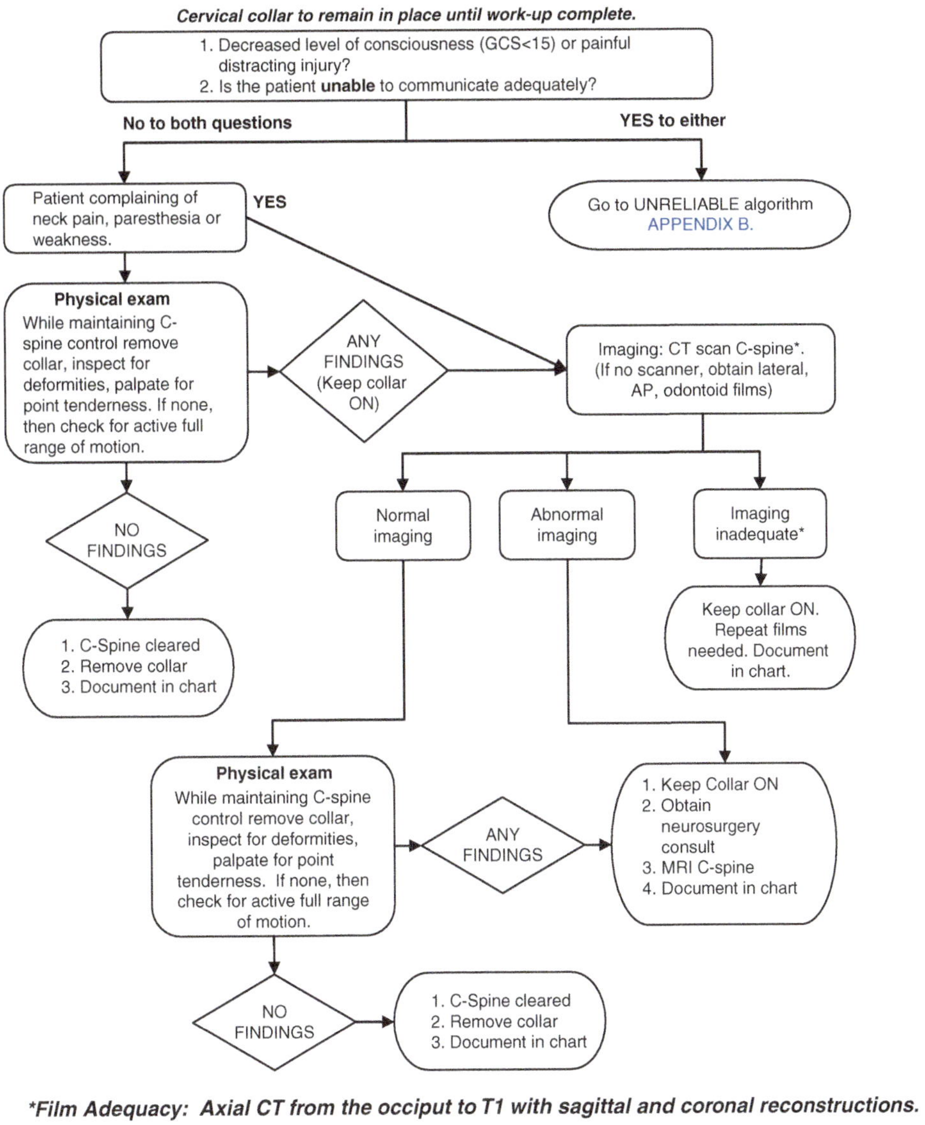

Fig. 18.3 JTTS cervical spine clearance form

though admittedly this data comes from animal models only. Maintenance of O_2 saturation >92 % is also recommended. A Foley catheter should be placed as well; urinary retention is common in spinal cord injury. Up to 30° reverse Trendelenburg of the bed is usually tolerated and logroll every 2 h should be instituted to prevent skin breakdown.

The use of corticosteroids is not supported by the literature and therefore is not recommended. DVT prophylaxis is highly recommended. Initially, placement of compression stockings (TED hose) and/or sequential compression devices (SCDs) can be performed, with supplementation of low molecular weight heparin within 72 h of injury or fixation/stabilization. Regular screening for DVT should be performed until the patient is transferred out. If DVT is identified, full anticoagulation should be performed, though consultation with an in-theater spine specialist is recommended.

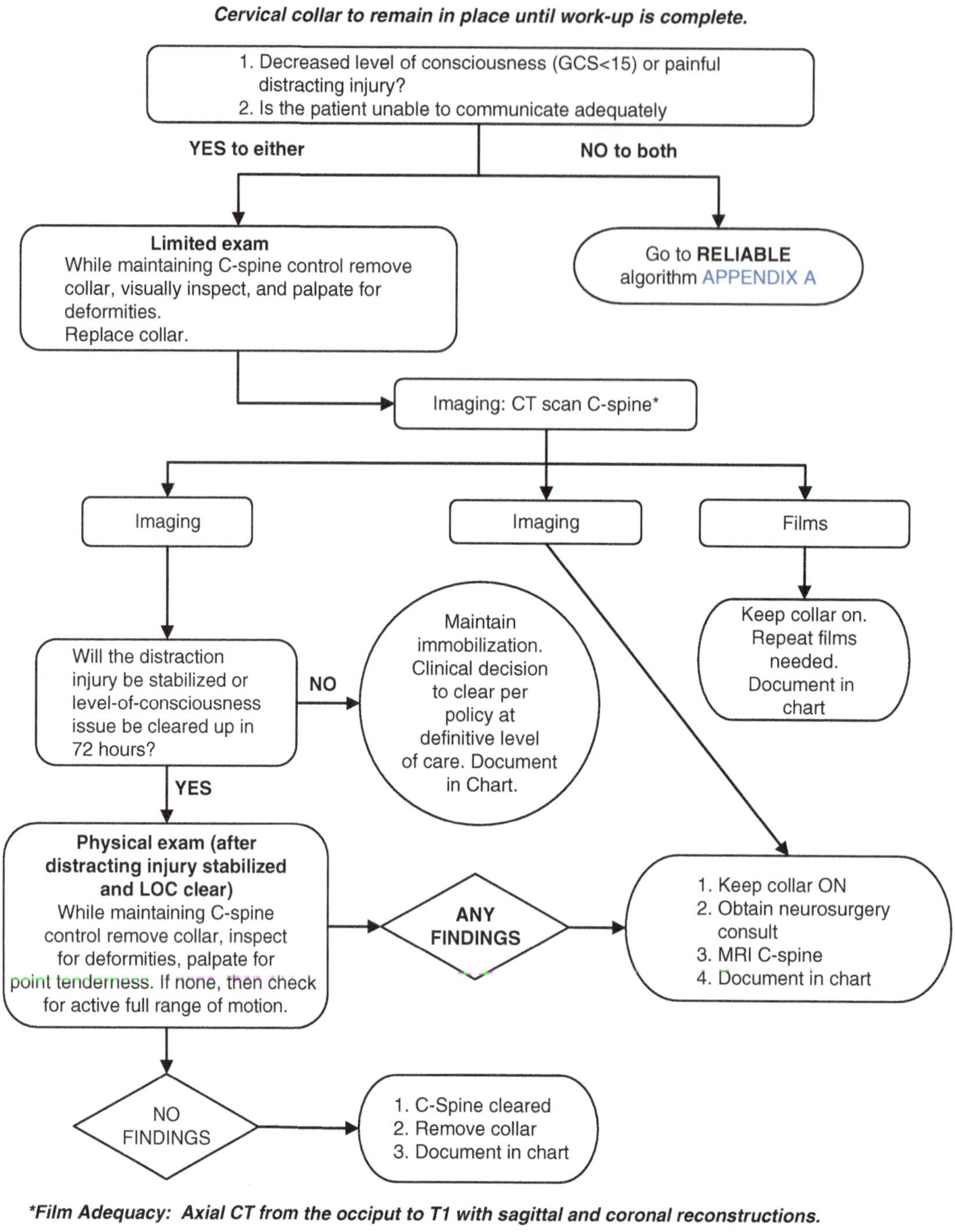

Fig. 18.4 ASIA exam pdf

Don't ever underestimate the power/energy imparted with IED blasts, even when the initial presentation to the trauma bay seems benign. After you get used to seeing multi-limb traumatic amputations, bowel eviscerations, etc. for a while, you will be tempted to let down your guard when a patient presents without field tourniquets in place. This is usually when disaster strikes. One of the authors (JDZ) personally witnessed a situation wherein a young army male was a back

JOINT THEATER TRAUMA SYSTEM - CERVICAL SPINE CLEARANCE STATUS

Mechanism: ☐ Explosive ☐ MVC ☐ Fall ☐ Other

Notes:____________________

Collar placed: ☐ Pre-hospital ☐ Hospital ☐ No Collar

Patient RELIABLE? ☐ Yes ☐ No Reason Unreliable: ☐ Altered Mental Status (GCS<15) ☐ Significant Distracting Injury

Notes:____________________

Patient Complaints ☐ None ☐ Neck Pain (where:____________________) ☐ Paresthesia

Notes:____________________

Physical Findings

Inspection: ☐ Normal ☐ Abnormal:____________________

Palpation: ☐ Normal ☐ Point Tenderness ☐ Deformity

Notes:____________________

Active Range of Motion: ☐ Full ☐ Limited:____________________

Notes:____________________

Imaging Studies [CT is Standard. Films acceptable only when CT is unavailable]

CT SCAN: ☐ Normal ☐ Abnormal:____________________

Notes:____________________

Lateral ☐ Normal ☐ Abnormal:____________________

AP ☐ Normal ☐ Abnormal:____________________

Odontoid ☐ Normal ☐ Abnormal:____________________

C L E A R A N C E

The Cervical Spine is:

☐ **CLEAR** of significant injury and instability on the basis of the following:
- ☐ Normal exam in completely reliable patient with no need for imaging.
- ☐ Normal imaging of full C-Spine and normal exam.

☐ **NOT CLEAR** on the basis of the following:
- ☐ Neurological complaint or abnormal physical exam finding
- ☐ Abnormal imaging
- ☐ Unreliable patient at time of evacuation /final disposition

Physician________________/________________ MTF:____________ Date/Time:____________

Print Name Signature

PATIENT'S IDENTIFICATION: (For typed or written entries give: Name – last, first, middle; ID No or SSN; Sex; Date of Birth; Rank/Grade)

JTTS Cervical Spine Clearance Note

Medical Record (Rev. May 2009)

Fig. 18.5 Combat Neuro exam from JTTS CPG cervical and thoracolumbar trauma

passenger in an MRAP, which was flipped by an IED. He presented to the trauma bay as part of a mass casualty. One of the other occupants had died of his wounds, several had open fractures. This particular individual complained only of mild to moderate back pain. He was completely neurologically intact, had no step-offs on ATLS survey, and his only finding was localized tenderness to palpation in the upper thoracic region. He was sent to the CT scanner and attention was turned to triaging the other casualties, which were arriving. By the time the patient returned from the CT scan, he was a T6 incomplete injury! It is unknown whether spine precautions were not strictly adhered to or whether this was part of the progression of his T5 and T6 burst fractures. The take-home point is that every patient with a high-energy mechanism should be treated with careful spine precautions until able to be cleared with imaging.

18.7 Cauda Equina Syndrome

Cauda equina syndrome is a condition wherein the distal nerve roots for leg, bowel, and bladder function become dysfunctional. This is usually secondary to a compressive lesion (herniated disc) but can also occur secondary to hematoma, infection, or fracture-dislocation. Patients typically complain of varying degrees of back and leg pain, altered sensation, numbness/tingling, and weakness in the legs. The hallmark complaint is saddle anesthesia (numbness in the areas of the groin and perineum that would touch a saddle on a horse). Though many people think that the bladder dysfunction is loss of control, this is in fact a late finding. Most people complain of hesitancy or inability to initiate micturition. MRI is the best study to demonstrate the level and location of the lesion, but unless you are at one of the three locations in theater with an MRI, you will have to rely on a myelogram. This involves the injection of nonionic contrast dye into the thecal sac and taking a plain X-ray (or performing CT scan if available).

If you have a radiologist willing to perform this and a surgeon who can perform the case (and of course proper instrumentation!), then proceed immediately. However, if you do not have the capability to perform the procedure, do not waste time confirming the level of compression.

Most literature supports recovery of bowel and bladder function if surgery can be performed within 24–48 h of the onset of symptoms (not when diagnosis is made). Therefore, expedient medevac should be your priority with a good sign out to the receiving physicians as to the situation. Depending on your location in the medevac transfer tree (Role 1->Role2->Role 3, etc.), this (and spinal cord injury) can be a case for direct transfer to Role 3 (Kandahar, Bagram, or Bastion). Kandahar and Bagram always have spine service available, but Bastion is variable so it is important to check first.

18.8 Penetrating Spine Injuries

With penetrating injuries, indications for surgery may include cauda equina injury, progressive neurologic deficit, incomplete deficit (particularly if a missile or fragment is still within the canal), or the presence of a CSF leak.

Cefazolin 2 g IV q 8 h for 24 h is sufficient for penetrating spine injuries without evidence of contamination. Fragments passing through enteric contents require extended-spectrum antimicrobial coverage for enteric organisms for a longer period of time because of increased risk of osteomyelitis.

18.9 Neurologic Examination

A good neurologic examination is essential to diagnosis as well as an important tool to help monitor progression or recovery of disease. The ASIA exam form (Fig. 18.4) has the key (and non-key) muscle functions listed as well as dermatomes for each neurologic level. The exam is designed for ease of performance and reproducibility.

If you stick to the key muscle functions on the page, you can perform a bilateral upper and lower extremity motor exam in less than a minute and a sensory exam with light touch and pinprick within a couple of minutes' more time.

Reflexes should be recorded and documented as well as clonus and Babinski test. Tests such as the bulbocavernosus test and anal wink are helpful at diagnosing spinal shock (these are absent in spinal shock and their return usually marks the end) and should be recorded.

In some settings such as mass casualties, there may not be time for an ASIA exam. In this setting, the combat spine exam (Fig. 18.5) can be utilized.

Until the patient is transported out, every effort should be made to make frequent examinations, with documentation of any deficits noted or changes in examination. Be sure to date and time the examination as well.

18.10 Transport of the Spine-Injured Patient

Patients with cervical spine injuries can usually be transported with a semirigid orthosis (Aspen, Miami-J). Traction is difficult to maintain appropriately with transportation and can prove problematic with air travel, especially with combat takeoff and landing maneuvers.

The following is from the Joint Theater Trauma System Clinical Practice Guideline (March 2012) for transport of thoracolumbar unstable injuries:

> If the patient has a thoracolumbar fracture that is unstable (3 column instability), then they should be transported by CCATT using a vacuum spine board (VSB). Use of a VSB is preferable to supine transport in a TLSO or other external brace. Prior to transport the theater spine surgeon and CCATT leader should agree upon suitability of VSB 'release of vacuum' and log-roll to reduce stress on pressure points. Log-rolling in a VSB without 'release of vacuum' does not significantly reduce skin pressure. Additionally, pre-transported skin integrity should be documented and care must be given to padding and pressure reduction maneuvers of the occiput and heels. Once cruising in smooth flight is accomplished, it would be reasonable to release the vacuum until either decent or turbulence is encountered. At a minimum, every two (2) hours the team should open the valve, release straps, +/- log-roll patient (holding patient in appropriate alignment) and provide adequate time for relief of pressure points as part of their normal turning schedule. The head of the bed should be elevated 30 degrees unless specifically told otherwise by the spine surgeon.

Burns and Extremity Injury: A Difficult Combination

19

Roman Hayda

Contents

BLUF (Bottom Line Up Front) Box

1. Burns occur in 5 % of combat casualties.
2. May be caused by routine-base operations such as trash burning or combat operations due to blasts.
3. Local nationals often sustain burns due to heating and cooking with open flames.
4. Initial evaluation is based on ATLS principles.
5. Beware of inhalation injury as marked by singed or burned perioral and nasal area.
6. Fluid resuscitation in the first 24 h is based on Parkland formula.
7. Rapid evacuation should be performed whenever possible to burn centers especially of burns involving greater than 30 % body surface area, face, or hands or those with inhalation injury.
8. Burned and fractured limbs may require prophylactic fasciotomy prior to evacuation due to swelling and large volume resuscitation.
9. When evacuation or transfer of local nationals is not possible, careful consideration of the resources required to treat should be taken into account.
10. Splinting can be performed on fractured limbs with burns in the short term, but external fixation should be considered in fracture of the lower extremities.

R. Hayda, MD
Department of Orthopaedic Surgery, Brown University Warren Alpert School of Medicine, Providence, RI, USA

Orthopaedic Trauma, Rhode Island Hospital, Providence, RI, USA
e-mail: roman_hayda@brown.edu

L.B. Bone, C.N. Mamczak (eds.), *Front Line Extremity and Orthopaedic Surgery*,
DOI 10.1007/978-3-642-45337-3_19, © Springer-Verlag Berlin Heidelberg 2014

On the front line, casualties with burns requiring care may be seen among warfighters as well as the local civilian population. Burns associated with fracture or other extremity injury can be very challenging to the orthopedic surgeon who gets limited exposure if any to burn patients during their training and practice. However, in the deployed setting or in humanitarian missions, the orthopedic surgeon may be required to treat these patients. Analysis of conflicts in the past century has shown that burn victims form about 5 % of war casualties on the modern battlefield. Similarly, burn injury is common in the developing world and conflict areas where cooking and heating needs are met with open flame devices exposing family members especially children to the potential of burns. For these reasons the orthopedic surgeon on the front line must be familiar in burn treatment principles.

As severe as some of these injuries may appear at initial presentation involving vast amounts of body surface areas and extremity fractures, appropriate initial care with subsequent referral to a burn center can result in survivors leading productive lives even in those with burns of the head and face and those with over 80 % surface area involvement. Although they may be disfigured and undergo treatment for several years, meaningful lives are resumed.

19.1 Causes of Burn Injury

Among combatants, burn casualties result from routine activities or from warfighting. In the deployed setting, personnel are required to maintain the base. Duties often include burning of trash and human waste to maintain hygiene. Despite safety efforts, these fires occasionally get out of control leading to burn injury. A more common scenario is of fire or explosion associated with fighting. Bombs, mines, and improvised explosive devices explode sending a variety of missiles causing injury but may also be associated with a fireball burning the casualties. These burns associated with blasts may also have significant open wounds and fractures from penetrating injury. Military vehicles may also be penetrated by munitions causing burn and other injury to its occupants. A final small but important subset of burn victims is caused by vehicles particularly aircraft that crash and explode. These are often fatal as extrication is difficult, but there are known survivors.

19.2 Burn Grades

Burn severity term is determined by its depth and amount of surface area covered. These are critical to assess accurately as it governs initial care. A first-degree burn is a very superficial involving the superficial layer of the epidermis akin to a sunburn. Although uncomfortable, this requires little treatment other than analgesia. A second-degree burn is partial thickness causing blistering associated with significant pain. A third degree burn is full thickness involving the full depth of the dermis, creating a thick inelastic leathery appearance. A fourth degree is a deep burn through the subcutaneous layer and as expected is very severe.

19.3 Initial Assessment

In a burn casualty as in any other trauma patient, basic ATLS principles are applied with evaluation and protection of the airway, breathing, and then circulation support. The obvious burn injury should not distract from the primary survey securing the airway, assuring breathing and circulation. In burn victims, the evaluation of the burn is an additional arm in initial evaluation. It is critical to assess the amount of surface area and degree of burn to guide initial fluid resuscitation. Otherwise the burn itself does not require any treatment in the first 24–48 h.

As in any trauma case, adherence to trauma and burn protocols is key. Burn victims may have an inhalation injury that may rapidly decompensate. Signs of inhalation injury may be burns or singed hair around the mouth and nose. Any sign of respiratory compromise to include stridor, hoarseness, carbonaceous sputum, or difficulty maintaining the airway requires intubation and respiratory support. In crash and blast victims with burns, added caution must be maintained for

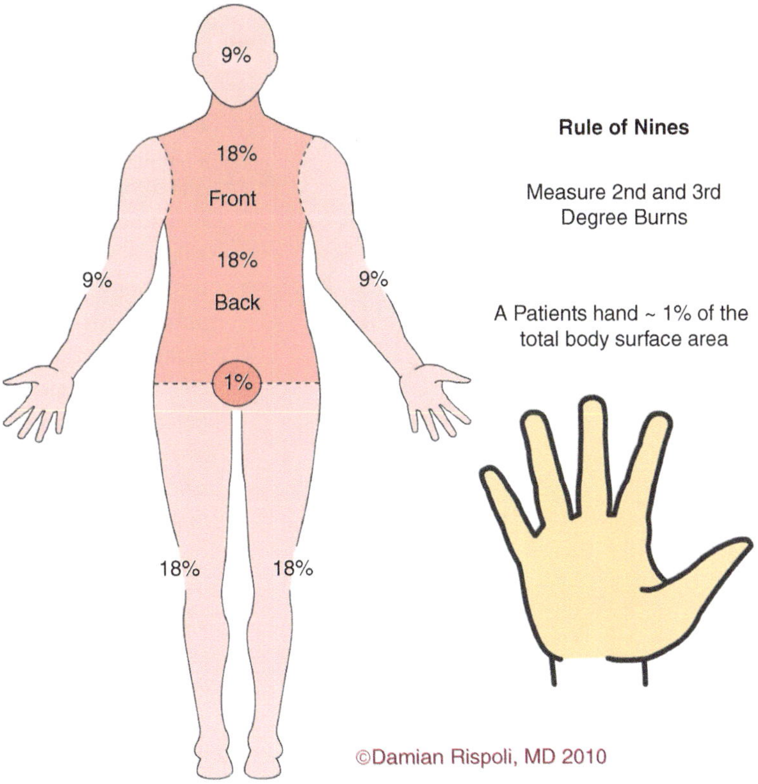

Fig. 19.1 Rule of nines diagram to illustrate total body surface area involved in Grade 2 and 3 burns: hand = 1 %, head 9 %, each arm 9 %, chest and abdomen 18 %, back 18 %, each lower extremity 18 %

the possibility of injury of the cervical spine. In these cases, spine protection with a rigid collar and evaluation is important.

The injury to the skin by the burn is typically obvious but may be covered by clothing or blankets and the like used by the rescuers to facilitate transport. The patient must be fully disrobed and inspected front and back to assess amount of surface area involved. Any circumferential clothing (boots, socks, belts) or jewelry (rings, bracelets, and necklaces) must also be removed. The rule of nines provides a rule of thumb to estimate the surface area involved by significant burns (greater than first degree) (Fig. 19.1). This will serve as a basis for initial fluid resuscitation.

19.4 Fluid Resuscitation

Due to the loss of skin caused by burns, patients lose a great deal of fluids, making fluid resuscitation critical. A common formula for resuscitation with LR is total volume = 2 cc × (%burn) × weight kg. Half of this volume should be administered in the first 8 h following burn. Due to volume shifts from trauma resuscitation and fluid losses through wounds, subsequent fluid needs are governed by vital signs and urine production as gauges of volume status. After 24 h D5W should substitute LR. In burns greater than 30 %, colloid solutions are used.

19.5 Escharotomy

Limb viability can be compromised by fully or near circumferential third degree burns that create inelastic bands on extremities compromising circulation. When the torso is involved, chest expansion is limited, compromising ventilation. This eschar may require urgent escharotomy consisting of longitudinal incisions in the coronal plane of limbs to include hands and digits as well as the chest wall to allow expansion (Fig. 19.2).

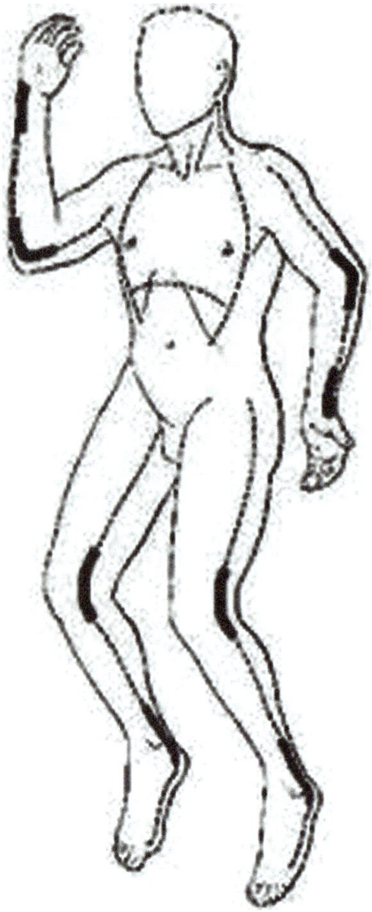

Fig. 19.2 Escharotomy incisions: note these cross joints in the coronal plane incising the skin only

These incisions are performed through the injured dermal layers to the subcutaneous fat and do not involve the fascia. In distinction with fasciotomy with which the orthopedic surgeon may be more familiar, escharotomy requires crossing of the joints if they are involved in the burn.

19.6 Fasciotomy

Limbs with underlying blunt or penetrating trauma may also develop compartment syndrome compromising the viability of muscle and nerve of involved compartment. Even limbs without evidence of injury may develop compartment syndrome during resuscitation and transport because of the large volumes of fluid required for resuscitation. Urgent fasciotomy should be done in limbs developing compartment syndrome. These incisions must not only incise the skin but release the underlying fascia of the involved compartment. Prophylactic fasciotomy should be considered in patients undergoing lengthy transport especially in the leg and forearm associated with fracture. A recent analysis of compartment syndrome in war casualties found that burn casualties are particularly prone to missed and delayed diagnosis of compartment syndrome. Diagnosis and treatment is difficult if not impossible in the course of transport potentially leading to extensive muscle necrosis and even amputation. These patients are often intubated making diagnosis difficult while large volume resuscitations increase the risk.

19.7 Initial Burn Management

Following casualty evaluation and initial stabilization, initial skin care should minimize further fluid losses and loss of thermoregulation. Grade 1 burn requires no dressing. Grade 2 burns with loss of superficial skin layers should be dressed with silvadene or other antibiotic creams and a loosely applied thin gauze or xeroform (Fig. 19.3). Thicker gauze pads or specific burn dressing sheets are applied over this to absorb fluids and retain heat. Grade 3 and 4 burns do not require a dressing per se in the initial period and can be left in place as a "biologic" dressing, but escharotomy wounds and transitional burn areas will require dressings.

19.8 Initial Fracture Care

During the initial evaluation and resuscitation phase after the vital functions of airway breathing and circulation are secured, the limbs are evaluated for musculoskeletal injury as in all trauma patients. Fractures and dislocations are reduced. Wounds are evaluated, gross debris may be removed, and initial cleansing performed as the patient condition allows. Splints and traction may be applied. Appropriate antibiotics for open fractures are also administered, while those not immunized may require tetanus prophylaxis or treatment. External fixation of femur fractures and complex tibia fractures even through burned areas assist with resuscitation and transport (Fig. 19.4).

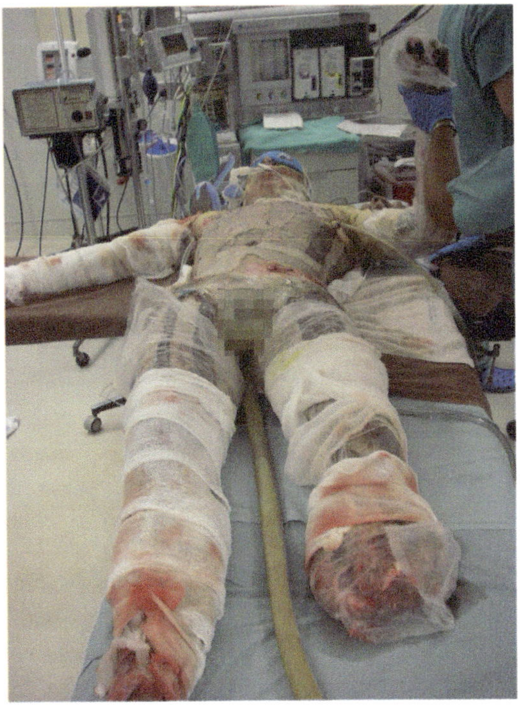

Fig. 19.3 Fine mesh and xeroform dressing applied on burn patient

Subsequent to evaluation and resuscitation, definitive care begins. In burn patients hypothermia is even a bigger problem than other trauma patients. The large fluid volumes and the large wounds associated with evaporative fluid losses compromise thermoregulation. These effects are magnified once tangential excision of burned skin is performed. It is imperative that these patients stay covered with blankets and their rooms may require warming to near core temperature levels. Burns of this magnitude cannot be managed short of the ICU setting and should be evacuated as soon as possible from typical austere environment settings.

19.9 Evacuation

Evacuation to specialized burn centers should be considered for any patient with burns of the face, hands, or feet or when over 30 % of body surface area is involved. If the casualty is critically ill, a burn critical care aeromedical evacuation team is mobilized to expedite transport to stateside burn facilities allowing movement from the battlefield to the US burn facility within 48 h. This coordination should be initiated as soon possible upon arrival to the initial treatment facility.

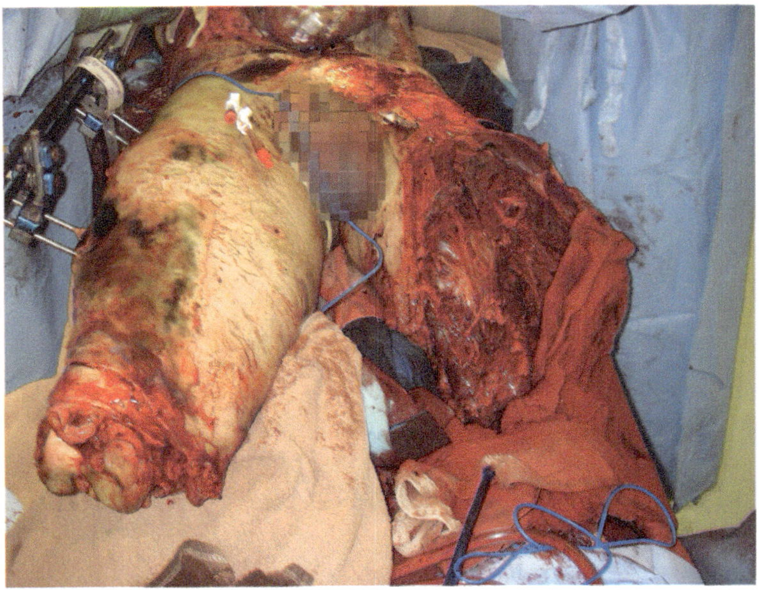

Fig. 19.4 Blast victim with burns, amputations, and fracture. Note external fixator on femur

In the event that evacuation is not possible which may occur in the indigenous population, the medical team may consider engaging in their definitive care. For those evacuated an understanding of subsequent treatment may be useful to guide initial care.

19.10 Burn Skin Treatment

Once the burn patients are stabilized, often in 48–96 h, consideration for definitive burn care may be done. Partial thickness burns are managed with supportive care and observed until healed. Full-thickness burns require tangential excision of the burn. All nonviable tissue must be excised. This may involve large areas and can cause considerable blood loss. In some cases immediate split thickness skin grafting is performed. A weck blade (Fig. 19.5) is a tool that may assist the surgeon in the excision of smaller burn areas as well as harvesting of skin graft when powered dermatomes are not available.

Wound care in the burn patient is critical to allow for healing of burns and avoiding infection. Second-degree burns should be managed with antibiotic cream. Silvadene is preferred. This dressing should be regularly changed as resources allow. It should be noted that this process is often painful requiring analgesia. Before and after skin grafts are applied, use of nonadherent dressing such as xeroform^{tm} protects the healing skin and maturing skin grafts. This material may be applied in sheets to protect the area. Wounds that become colonized with bacteria may require more advanced forms of care. Dakin's solution is particularly effective for pseudomonas colonization when applied in a daily damp to dry dressing. Silver-impregnated cloth applied to the wound can also control local wound colonization ultimately leading to healing.

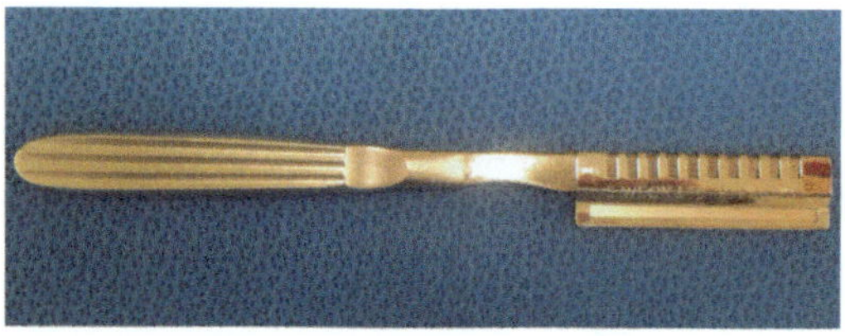

Fig. 19.5 Weck blades can be used to tangentially excise burned skin and to harvest skin graft

19.11 Contracture and Decubitus Prevention

Contractures in burned limbs are common. Healing skin and skin grafts contain myofibroblasts that can cause significant contractures (Fig. 19.6). Additionally the prolonged healing and limited use during the convalescence also contribute to the formation of contractures. In order to prevent contractures, limbs should undergo active and passive stretching as soon as is practicable regardless of whether they are involved in the burn. If prolonged recumbency is anticipated, ankles should b splinted in neutral (90°) position. If a patient is not able to use his hands, they should be splinted in an intrinsic plus position (wrist extended 30°, MCP at 70–90°, and IP extended). If the hand or foot is burned but salvageable, percutaneous K-wire pinning should be considered as splinting is difficult and contracture very powerful. In a leg with burns, external fixation to keep the ankle at neutral may also be useful not only to prevent contracture but to suspend the limb during skin grafting.

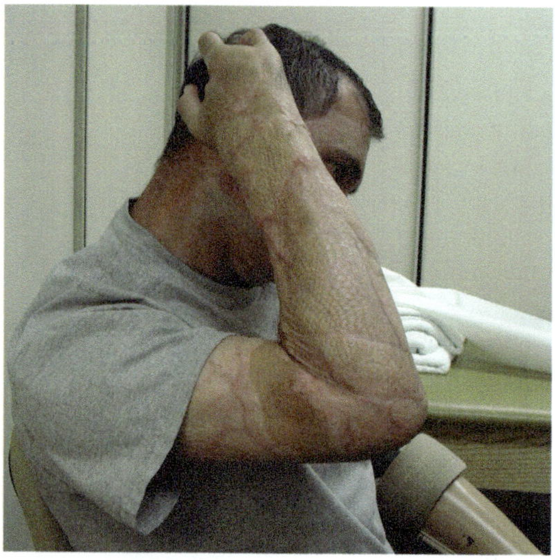

Fig. 19.6 Elbow contracture following burn treatment

Joints in burn victims are also prone to formation of heterotopic bone even in the absence of fracture or dislocation. The elbow is a common location. Early limb mobilization limits the risk but some may require excision. Excision may be undertaken as soon as 3 months when the bone appears radiographically mature, the skin condition allows for surgical approach, and the patient is able to participate in therapy.

Active measures should be instituted to avoid the development of decubitus ulcers. These patients are frequently immobile and malnourished placing them at increased risk for pressure sores in the sacrum, occiput, heels, and elbow. Patients and their providers must be taught to frequently turn and relieve pressure areas. Splints must be carefully applied to avoid this problem. Skin should be frequently inspected to avoid the development of full-thickness ulcers.

19.12 Fracture Care in Burn Casualties

Fracture care in the burn patient presents special challenges. Casting may not be feasible in the burned limb while operative management risks infection. Even in limbs not burned, splinting and casting is approached with caution in the acute phase due to potential large fluid shifts and compartment syndrome. When the fracture occurs in an unburned limb, standard forms of fracture treatment are carried out, although particular attention should be paid to the potential for compartment syndrome.

In the event a fracture occurs in the burned limb, the situation becomes more complex. Early on splinting and traction may be adequate but are often ineffective long-term methods of treatment as the burn treatment precludes most casting while internal fixation carries a high risk of infection. The limb should be carefully examined to see if the approach can be made through unburned areas. Intramedullary devices which can be placed antegrade or retrograde may allow for effective fracture fixation. Similarly percutaneous plating techniques may also avoid burned areas providing stable internal fixation. However, if no safe portal exists for internal fixation, external fixation with unilateral frames or circular frames should be utilized as it minimizes large implants prone to infection (Fig. 19.7). In cases where internal fixation is felt to be required such as a displaced intra-articular fracture with a burn, conventional internal fixation can be performed provided there is soft tissue coverage for the implant. The surgeon will have to be vigilant of infection and prepared to remove the implant should an infection develop. In cases treated in traction either definitively or temporarily, use of a thin tensioned wire with a Kirschner bow can limit the soft tissue irritation sometimes seen with the larger diameter Steinmann pins commonly used to apply traction. Such a method can also be used when suspending a limb to allow for skin graft on the posterior limb surface.

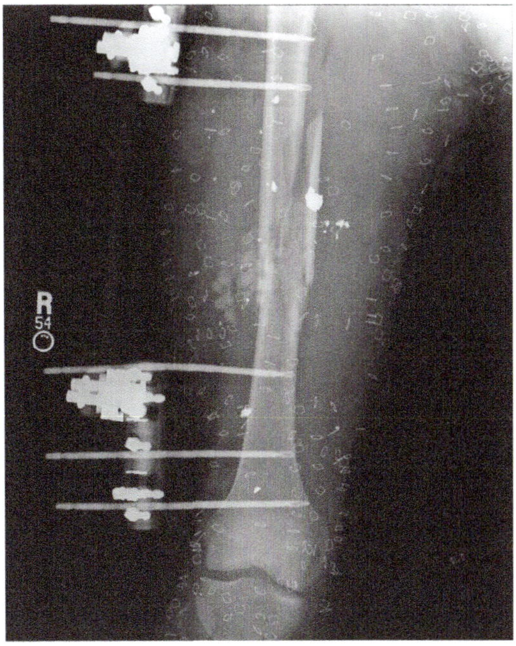

Fig. 19.7 Definitive fixation of the femur fracture

19.13 Amputation

Amputation in the burn patient may also be required. Indications include fourth-degree burns that leave bone, nerves, or vessels exposed or mummified limbs that cannot function.

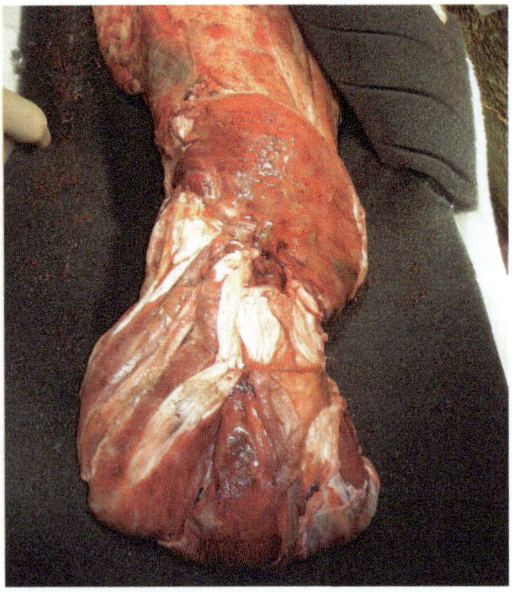

Fig. 19.8 Burn amputation with gastrocnemius flap covering residual tibia preserving the knee joint. It is temporarily covered with allograft skin

Complex fractures that require reconstruction which may not be feasible in that particular burn patient also require amputation as complex salvage attempts may not be tolerated either in the short term or long term. For casualties undergoing evacuation, the decision for salvage versus amputation can be delayed until they reach the definitive care facility particularly since viable parts in the amputated limb may be useful elsewhere.

In choosing amputation level, the most important criterion is soft tissue coverage of bone and other vital structures in order to preserve joint levels and limb length. In the leg, for instance, the entire gastrocnemius and soleus may be utilized to cover the tibia if it has been exposed by severe burns (Fig. 19.8). This muscle is then readily covered by skin graft preserving length. The plantar skin that may have escaped burn injury may also be useful if perfused through the posterior tibial vessels. Alternatively, atypical flaps may be considered when there are patches of unburned skin (Fig. 19.9a, b). When possible this patch of intact skin should be positioned in the area of highest stress and pressure as native skin is most resistant to breakdown in the prosthetic socket. In a transtibial amputation, the most critical area of coverage is the anterior distal corner of the residual limb. It is critical for the patient, their family, surgeon, prosthetist, and therapist to remember that in a burn patient, prosthetic use is possible but it may take months before the skin graft is mature enough to tolerate prosthetic use. Prosthetic use is likely to be more limited in burn victims compared to non-burned patients.

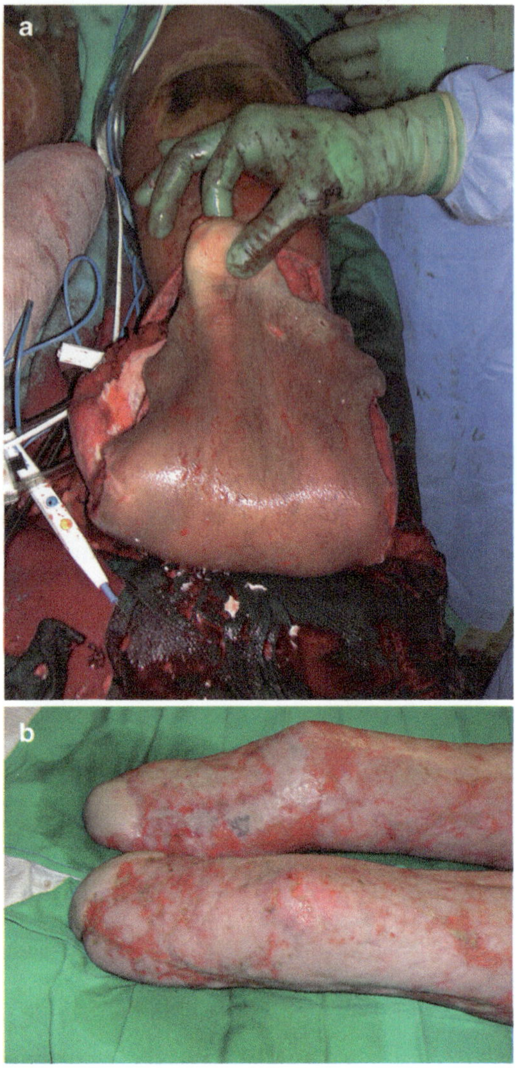

Fig. 19.9 (**a**) Burn amputation: note extra long posterior flap covers the critical anterior medial tibia. (**b**) Burn amputation with positioning of the intact skin in critical areas

19.14 Team Consideration in Burn Care

The team engaging in the care of a burn patient should realize that unlike many other injuries, prolonged recovery is the norm with slow healing wounds, revision surgery, infection, contracture, heterotopic bone, and other complications. Mortality and significant complications are common even in advanced burn centers particularly with high surface area burns. Age, comorbidities, and malnutrition which may exist in indigenous populations heighten these risks. Therefore, the medical team must maintain an awareness of the resources that it may expend on caring for these casualties. These burdens may also weigh significantly on the family and the communities of the victims. When possible early transfer to tertiary care facilities preferably those with burn teams can help to optimize outcomes. In select cases survival may be enhanced by performing amputations above the zone of injury.

If definitive care is taken on, a coordinated approach is highly useful. Surgeons, nurses, therapists, and nutritionists should strive to integrate their care and set realistic expectations. Pain management also becomes crucial in allowing for the often daily dressing changes that are required and therapy to prevent or correct contractures. Involvement of the family in this effort may also help to more easily transfer treatment to the outpatient setting particularly when the burn area is small. Patients and their families can be taught the basics of wound care and therapy.

19.15 Summary

The deployed orthopedic surgeon should be aware of the basic principles of caring for patient with burns. The basic principles of ATLS are followed with the addition of the amount of surface area burned directing the fluid resuscitation. The limbs may require urgent escharotomy or fasciotomy while the torso may require escharotomy to allow chest expansion for respiration. Casualties with burns to the face, hands, or feet or over 30 % body surface area should be considered for expeditious evacuation to specialized burn centers. When necessary a critical care burn team can effectively evacuate these casualties to US facilities within 48–72 h. Casualties undergoing evacuation should be liberally treated with prophylactic fasciotomy. Initial fracture care depends on closed reduction and splinting or external fixation when necessary. Following these principles, successful treatment can be rendered even in severely burned casualties with fractures (Fig. 19.10).

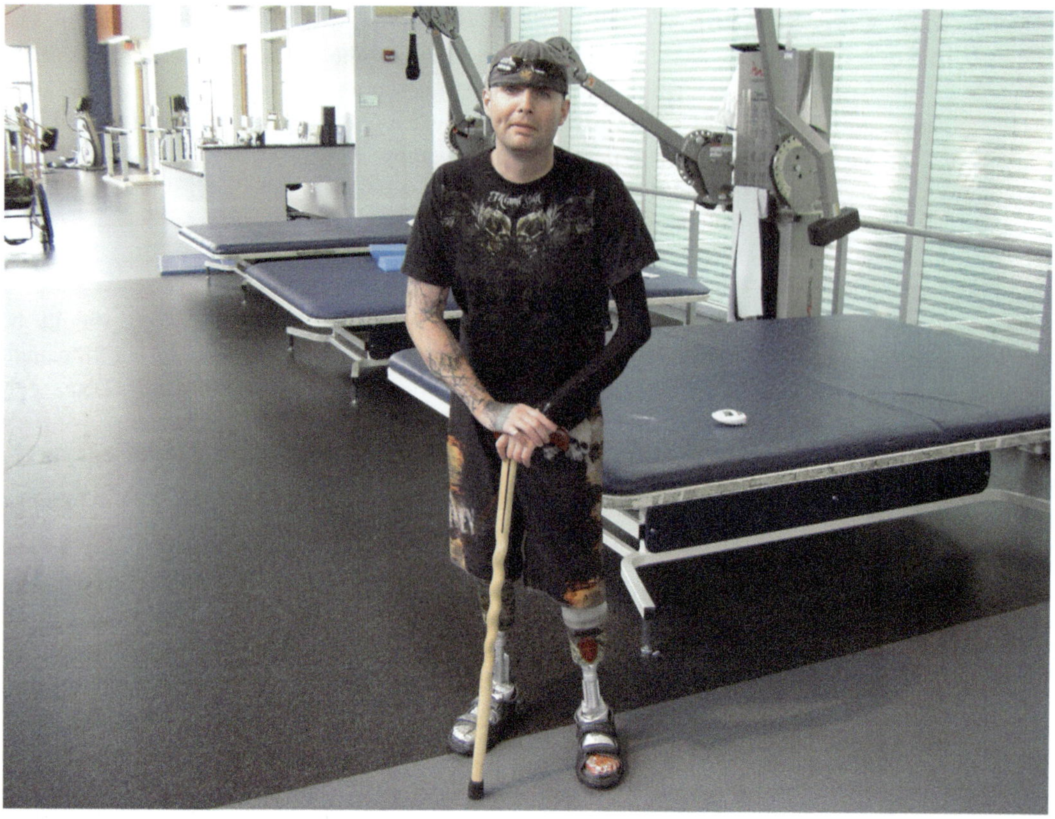

Fig. 19.10 Casualty with over 65 % body surface area, bilateral transtibial amputation, and open femur fracture treated with external fixation and excision of the femoral head and neck successfully ambulating following treatment

The Approach to the Complex Multiple Amputee

20

Joseph F. Alderete, Gregory A. Watson, and Garth A. Elias

Contents

BLUF (Bottom Line Up Front) Box

1. This patient is the most intensive and resource-degrading patient you will manage on the battlefield. Prepare, rehearse, and decisively engage to save this soldier's life.
2. Remember the 5 R's of Combat Trauma Triage: resources, rehearse, respond, route, and reset.
3. Identify your strongest lab NCO and have a plan for rapidly obtaining whole blood from the walking donor pool.
4. Trauma bay resuscitation is rapid and proceeds with momentum to the OR; this is where the true resuscitation will take place.
5. In combat trauma, C is simultaneously explored and managed with A and B: Aggressively control hemorrhage while securing the airway. Definitive control of both can happen in the OR suite. While this is happening "Make 'em naked, roll 'em over, CXR!"
6. Permissive hypotension should be the en route and trauma bay rule in this patient until definitive hemorrhage control can be obtained in the OR. Do not blow off the clot!
7. Decide upon early use of recombinant factor VIIa or TXATXA, 1 g over

J.F. Alderete, MD (✉)
Department of Orthopaedic Oncology, Orthopaedic Surgery Residency, San Antonio Military Medical Center, San Antonio, TX, USA
e-mail: snjalderete@gmail.com

G.A. Watson, MD, FACS • G.A. Elias, MD
Department of Critical Care Medicine, University of Pittsburgh, Pittsburgh, PA, USA

L.B. Bone, C.N. Mamczak (eds.), *Front Line Extremity and Orthopaedic Surgery*, DOI 10.1007/978-3-642-45337-3_20, © Springer-Verlag Berlin Heidelberg 2014

10 min, if time from injury is less than 3 h. Second dose of 1 g over 8 h beginning in OR. Consider use of recombinant factor VIIa.
8. Proceed to proximal vessel control immediately. Depending upon the patient condition and injury complex, this may be at the level of the proximal extremity, intra-abdominal iliac, and abdominal or thoracic aorta (trauma bay thoracotomy).
9. Do not delay rapid movement to the operating room for extremity films. These can be obtained with flat plates or using c-arm while the patient is being resuscitated and debrided.
10. Debride all nonviable tissue while maintaining the distal most possible amputation level. Remember, energy expenditure increases dramatically with prosthetic use as the amputation proceeds proximally.

20.1 Definition and Spectrum

The complex amputee is a spectrum of high energy injury that can be some of the most complex physiology encountered on the battlefield. With the advent of improved IOTV, or body armor, and the deployment and efficacy of combat tourniquet use, many more soldiers, airmen, sailors, and marines are surviving blast injury. These can be divided grossly into mounted and dismounted injuries, each with overlapping concerns but individual challenges.

They usually involve high (bilateral transfemoral or transtibial with contralateral transfemoral) amputations of the lower extremities with some form of protective upper extremity wound or wound complex (i.e., amputation or segmental fracture dislocation with severe soft tissue injury) as well as penetrating GU/GI injuries with blunt or penetrating truncal injuries.

20.2 Preparation

Caring for these complexes and challenging injuries begins at home. *Top Knife* (Mattox and Hirschberg, 2005) and *First to Cut* (available on the USAISR website) are two valuable resources which focus on the strategy and tactics found useful by these experienced trauma surgeons when confronted with severely traumatized patients. Developing a working knowledge of damage-control tactics will facilitate the team-oriented approach required for optimal care of these soldiers. The common language and thought framework will be especially important in the initial moments of encountering a patient with both legs blown off above the knee, genital and abdominal injury, and blunt or penetrating truncal trauma and to make it a really bad day, burns. Three other very useful articles to keep in one's digital deployment library are Tintle et al. *JBJS* (2010) Parts I and II covering Lower and Upper Extremity Amputations and Dr. Mamczak's Complex Dismounted IED Blast Injuries for a pre-deployment framework on what challenges face these patients (Figs. 20.1 and 20.2a, b).

The next step is identifying the team. There is no room in this ball field for ego. Identify the most competent medics, anesthesia providers, ICU nurses, and the surgical team for what will be "The Big Boy Bed." Roles should be decided and every task delineated before this patient is injured and rehearsed every day.

Once the team is identified and the roles set for managing the blast injury victim in extremis, one of the most important follow-on tasks will be the identification and management of the whole blood program. Borgman et al. in *J Trauma* (2007) described the evidence of the success of massive transfusion with fresh whole blood that many of us now take for granted. There should be no question that the risk to benefit ratio of whole blood transfusion favors its use in the austere environment when confronted with correcting the acidotic, hypothermic, and coagulopathic combat casualty over the use of component therapy. This usually starts with a dedicated and

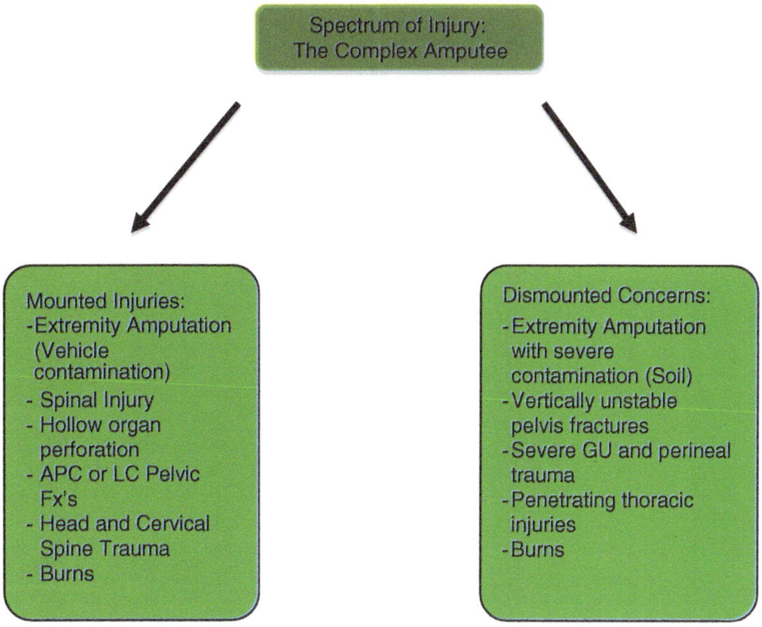

Fig. 20.1 Spectrum of injury: The complex amputee

aggressive lab NCOIC of the Charlie Medical Company in vicinity to a forward surgical team or indigenous to the Combat Support Hospital. The materials for the collection and transfusion of FWB are available to medical units through standard military supply channels before deployment. These include phlebotomy kits, collection and transfusion tubing, citrated blood bags, and reagents for blood typing. To eliminate the need for blood donor typing in the field, personnel are typed before deploying and a standard pool of blood type O donors are identified for FWB transfusions (Ketchum *JOT* 2006). A passionate and talented lab NCOIC who is familiar with transfusion practices can deliver the first unit of fresh whole blood in 13–17 min following delivery of the clot.

Finally, it's time to decide what parameters will trigger an expectant label and when the full court press will be pushed. This is the art of Combat Trauma Triage, and the complex amputee will put the system to the test.

Trauma Triage: Remember the 5 R's of Combat Trauma Triage: Resources, Rehearse, Respond, Route, and Reset. *The complex blast amputee will expend an average of 19 units of PRBCs with a 1:1:1 expenditure of FFP and platelets compared to six units of PRBCs in the single amputation subset.* Thus, as the trauma czar or triage commander, one has to seriously think about embarking on taking care of these patients especially if a MASCAL is expected.

Initial Evaluation: Make 'em naked, roll 'em over, CXR!!

As we discussed above, once the team has decided to expend resources on the complex amputee, every attempt is made to facilitate the rapid evaluation and progression to the operating room where the real resuscitation can begin. Identification and management of the airway proceed simultaneously with pressure application for ongoing hemorrhage. Ensure all tourniquets are tight and do not emit a finger underneath. Do not remove tourniquets in the trauma bay. Wait until definitive vascular control can be obtained in the operative suite. Often these patients have had a prolonged evacuation and *permissive hypotension should be the rule*. John Holcomb was once quoted as saying "anyone can resuscitate, but a true expert knows when to stop...." Once the A and C of the equation have been addressed or is in the process (patient is being

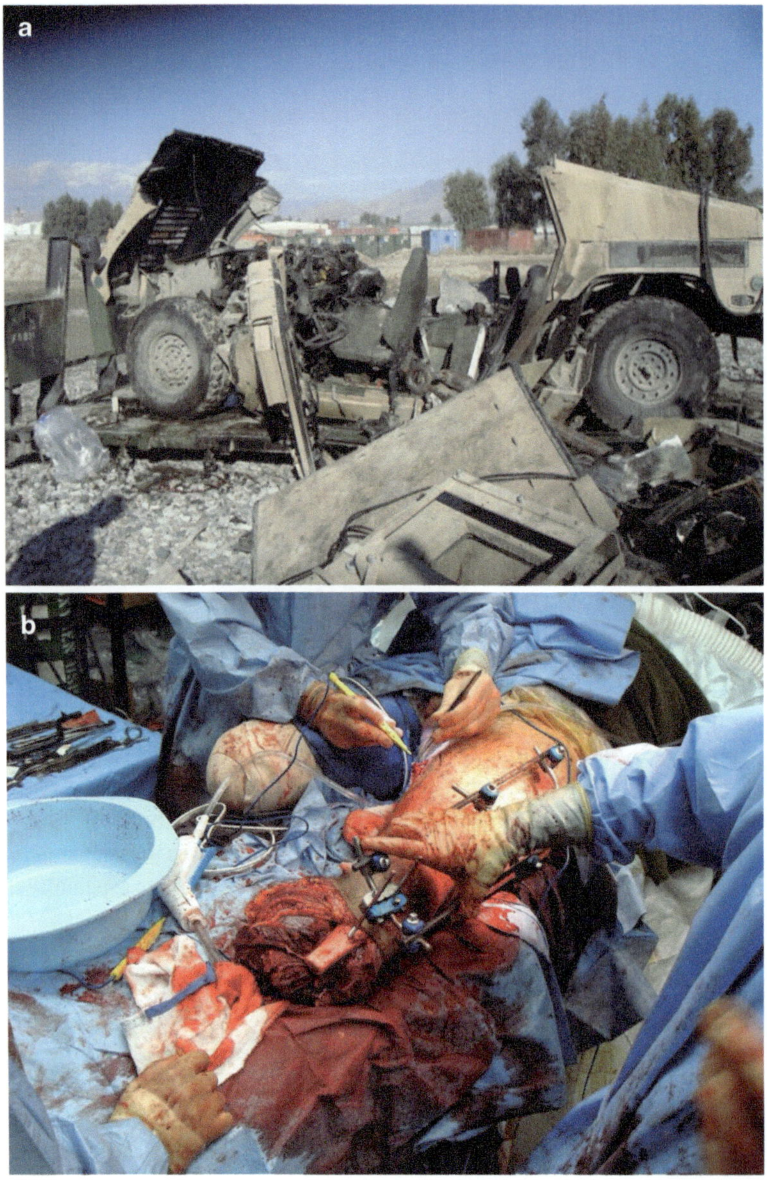

Fig. 20.2 (**a**, **b**) The complex multiple amputee is not a spectrum unique to the dismounted troop. This soldier was blown out of the turret of this up-armored vehicle sustaining bilateral LE amputations, thoracolumbar spine fractures, a small bowel perforation, and bilateral pneumothoraces

bagged en route to OR for intubation), within minutes IV access is addressed or readdressed. The orthopedic surgeon can assist his colleagues in the initial resuscitation by establishing intraosseous lines in the proximal humerus, sternum, or pelvis until definitive lines can be established. Finally, exposure and the CXR are rapidly obtained to facilitate identification of life-threatening thoracic trauma that would push a team's hand into ED thoracotomy to establish proximal control.

Damage-Control Surgery: 10–13 min!

The goal of damage-control surgery, simply stated, is to stop hemorrhage and control contamination in as expeditious a manner as possible. When confronted with the complex multiple amputee, one must consider several factors. How sick is the patient (stable, unstable, or in extremis), what level is/are the amputation(s), and what is the likelihood of associated truncal trauma? If the patient arrives in extremis and the decision has been made to attempt salvage, move rapidly (in the ATLS area) to left thoracotomy and empiric insertion of a right chest tube. This is the most expeditious way to obtain proximal vascular control (aortic crossclamp) and has the added advantages of allowing open-chest CPR and identification of any life-threatening intrathoracic injuries which can simultaneously be addressed. Resuscitation with blood components in a 1:1:1 ratio and the early use of FWB should be initiated, and TXA should be administered (if available) within the first 3 h of injury. If the patient's hemodynamics responds, one should move rapidly to the operating room to continue the resuscitation and address the injuries. As the patient's condition permits, the aortic crossclamp should be removed and proximal control obtained as close as is possible to the amputation level. The decision to perform laparotomy is dictated by the presence (or suspicion) of intra-abdominal injury, the need for control of the iliacs for proximal vascular control (i.e., high transfemoral amputations), or the presence of significant perineal trauma which will require GI and/or GU diversion. Even if none of these factors appear to be present, it is our contention that a patient with multiple amputations who arrives in extremis and has had intrathoracic injuries ruled out/addressed should undergo laparotomy as this is the best test available at forward echelons to rule out life-threatening abdominal injury.

The multiple amputee who arrives "stable" is almost unheard of, and likely is a patient with very distal amputations. Most of these patients will have proximal control obtained by the application of tourniquets, which should remain in place and prepped into the field in the OR. There is time to assess this patient in the ATLS area, and chest radiograph, pelvis XR, FAST exam, and necessary extremity radiographs should be performed. The need for chest tube insertion, thoracotomy, or laparotomy will be dictated by the results of those studies or the suspected trajectory of any penetrating projectiles. Proximal vascular control should be obtained as close to the amputation level as is possible.

The most challenging multiple amputee patient, in our opinion, is the one who arrives "unstable" but not in extremis. Rapid access and resuscitation should be instituted as outlined above. These patients present a "trap" to the novice, as the temptation may exist to spend excessive time in the ATLS area obtaining films or labs that may not be directly life threatening (especially if the patient's hemodynamics responds to resuscitation). DON'T DO IT!! Secure the airway, obtain access and initiate resuscitation, expose/examine the patient, and obtain chest/pelvis radiographs and perform a FAST quickly. There is no need to wait for the films to be developed, move quickly to the OR, and begin to prep while another member of the team reviews the radiographs; this can save valuable seconds! As described above, the need for chest tube insertion, thoracotomy, or laparotomy will be dictated by the results of those studies or the suspected trajectory of any penetrating projectiles. Proximal vascular control should be obtained as close to the amputated limb as is feasible. In the case of the high transfemoral amputee, this is often done by obtaining control of the iliac vessels. Though it is feasible to rapidly obtain control of these vessels via a retroperitoneal approach (incision medial to and paralleling the iliac crest), the high incidence of associated perineal and intra-abdominal trauma makes a standard laparotomy and transperitoneal exposure/control the more reasonable approach. Furthermore, the presence of a pelvic fracture and extraperitoneal hematoma would complicate an extraperitoneal approach to these vessels. We recommend beginning by making the laparotomy incision high, particularly if the patient is known to have a pelvic fracture. Identification of a large zone III hematoma will allow preperitoneal packing and guide one to obtain iliac control more proximally (just beyond the aortic bifurcation). Caring for these patients requires the ultimate team approach. While the trauma/general surgeon is obtaining proximal control and addressing the truncal injuries, the orthopedist may be stabilizing the pelvic fracture, completing extremity amputations, or beginning to debride wounds. Time is of the essence and only that which needs to be done to control hemorrhage and contamination should be undertaken at the initial operation.

20.3 Further Orthopedic Concerns

Debride, debride, debride! All nonviable tissue (no 4 C's of circulation, conductivity, medical, and consistency) should be debrided. That being said, all attempts should be made to facilitate the most distal level of amputation. These kids depend every day on inches of tissue for prosthetic fit and energy expenditure and you can make a significant difference in a patient's life just by going that extra step to save tissue in the "penumbra."

External fixation should be applied to facilitate soft tissue stability and preserve optimal amputation length. If there is viable tissue below a fracture, preserve it! The old dogma of amputation through fracture because of the zone of injury has no place in the OR suites of modern battlefield surgeons. Be aggressive but safe, think outside of the box, and apply external fixation to the most distal viable level (i.e., viable gastrocs in the patient in Fig. 20.2 from the HMVEE explosion resulted in a transtibial amputation salvage at the level of the extensor insertion, a huge win for this patient!).

Pelvic external fixation is designed to stabilize the clot. It does not have to make a pelvic injury perfect. The idea that closing down intrapelvic volume is an aid to resuscitation is a fallacy. All one is doing is stabilizing the fibrin clot in the dangerous pelvic sidewall veins that often serve as the source of ongoing high volume, slow flow blood loss. Therefore, do as one knows how! If you are accustomed to external fixation pins in the Iliac crest, then do not change this practice when confronted with the patient. AII pins, or so-called supra-acetabular pins, are very strong however and can control some very unstable hemi-pelvis where crest pins cannot. This practice does require fluoroscopy and should not be attempted in the role II without fluoro (Figs. 20.3a, b and 20.4a, b).

20.4 To Vac or Not to Vac!

Initially coming out of role II, a patient with this energy spectrum and degree of contamination should not have a vac on the extremities or perineum. We advocate the use of Dakin's solution versus SMAT (Silver Sulfamylon Amphotericin B) dressings where susceptible fungi are endemic. This can be poured into a basin and the Kerlix gauze sponges soaked in the solution until the patient can be dressed for transport. We give credit to Dr. Don Gajewski for one of the best dressing management/transport ideas I have seen which is the oversized OB/GYN sterile panty stapled shut to both extremities,

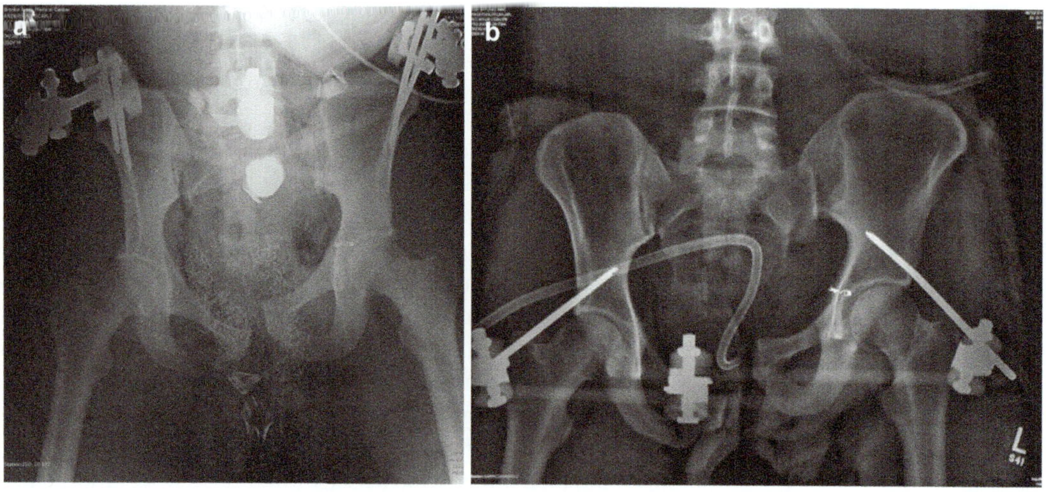

Fig. 20.3 (**a**, **b**) The supra-acetabular pin construct is an extremely powerful tool: however, no intra-theater construct will be perfect. Remember: stabilize the clot!

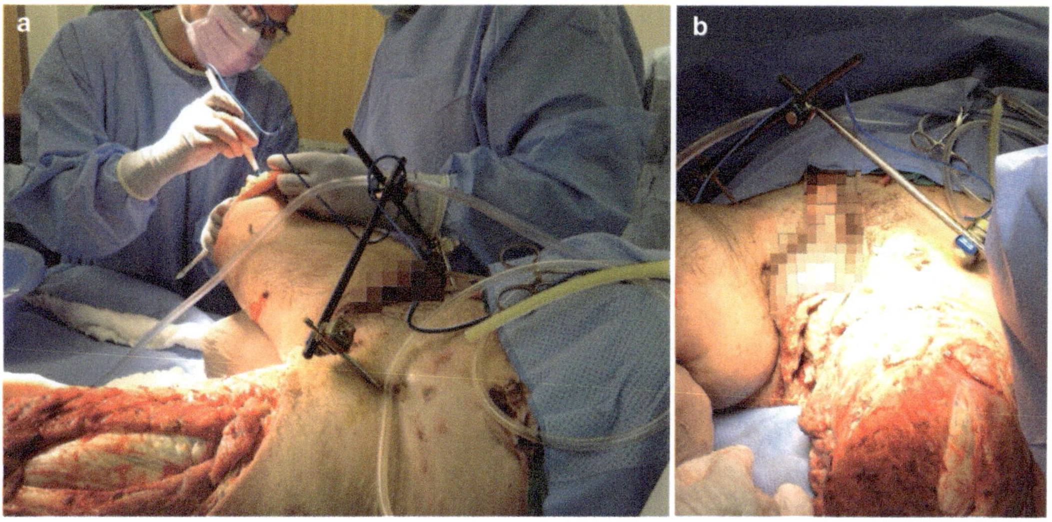

Fig. 20.4 (**a**, **b**) Once at the role III or higher, early consideration should be given to switching out crest pins for supra-acetabular pins. This allows your colleagues and the rest of the team to facilitation abdominal/perineal procedures without removing or loosening the fixator

facilitating compression of the Kerlix and upward pressure for soft tissues.

20.5 Antibiotic Choice

Most orthopedic injuries can be addressed from prophylaxis to *Staph. aureus*, even "routine" combat trauma open fractures. However, once one enters the realm of multiple amputations leading to massive transfusions and significant tissue contamination, one should consider a broad-spectrum antibiotic. Most of our patients are young and can handle the broad regimen of vancomycin and Zosyn.

Invasive fungi are an emerging trauma-related infectious spectrum that can lead to multiple wound revisions, revision amputation, multiorgan system failure, and death. "Early identification, using common characteristics of patient injury profile and tissue-based diagnosis, should be accompanied by aggressive surgical and antifungal therapy (liposomal amphotericin B and a broad-spectrum triazole pending mycology results) among patients with suspicious wounds" (Warkentien et al. *Clin Infect Dis* 2012). However, we are just now developing a CPG for the use of antifungal therapy and what dressing regimen should accompany the patient when a fungal infection is identified. It is our opinion that prophylactic liposomal amphotericin B be considered given the soil contamination and drastic immunocompromised patient that can lead to invasive fungal infection, which can be devastating. No one knows the duration of prophylaxis; however, most of these patients manifest infection by the time they reach Landstuhl; thus reasonable coverage is proposed to be 48–72 h.

Evacuation: Evacuation concerns for these patients center on patient pain control (so as to avoid bucking the vent on a medevac ride among other things) and prevention of further hemorrhage. Stapling the legs shut and stuffing ABD pads into an OB/GYN hospital mesh panty make a great high amputee dressing. Upper extremity wounds should be splinted appropriately and external fixation pins finally tightened. There is a great deal of data that support regional anesthesia in this population; thus when the dust settles and the patient is stable in the ICU, we would suggest using your regional CRNA/anesthesiologist gurus. Finally, we implore you to give a call to the surgeons receiving your patient as this can make all the difference in the world in avoiding repeat interventions or "neurovascular explorations" that can only lead to more hemorrhage.

Role III and IV Care: Role III to V care for the complex amputee focuses on stabilizing fractures, debriding nonviable tissue, and preventing infection. One should attempt to preserve length aggressively, as we can do a great deal with distal tissue to preserve a level if viable.

Areas for Improvement: Despite 12 years at war, there is still great disparity in treating patients like the complex amputee. Our first area for improvement is education and communication. We as surgeons preparing for combat must read the USAISR Clinical Practice Guidelines and expound upon them. We should attempt if at all possible to attend an Extremity War Surgery course and get to know people that can serve as later references. Our next step should be to improve data gathering. It has been very difficult to study the effects of ED thoracotomy and SIRS within the complex amputee population when the numbers we see recorded for lifesaving parameters mean little to nothing. Novel antihemorrhagic agents and so-called active dressings like the fibrin sealant gauze are especially hot topics in the face of catastrophic perineal and pelvic wounds. Finally, safe and effective antimicrobial therapy, especially antifungal, will be areas we can make a dramatic improvement on these patients lives.

Suggested Reading

Borgman MA, Spinella PC, Perkins JG, Grathwohl KW, Repine T, Beekley AC, Sebesta J, Jenkins D, Wade CE, Holcomb JB. The ratio of blood products transfused affects mortality in patients receiving massive transfusions at a combat support hospital. J Trauma. 2007;63:805–813. [PubMed].

Hess JR, Holcomb JB. Transfusion practice in military trauma. Transfus Med. 2008;18(3):143–50.

Ketchum L, Hess JR, Hiippala S. Indications for early fresh frozen plasma, cryoprecipitate, and platelet transfusion in trauma. J Trauma. 2006;60:S51–S58. [PubMed].

Mamczak CN, Elster EA. Complex dismounted IED blast injuries: the initial management of bilateral lower extremity amputations with and without pelvic and perineal involvement. J Surg Orthop Adv. 2012;21(1):8–14.

Tintle SM, Keeling JJ, Shawen SB, Forsberg JA, Potter BK. Traumatic and trauma-related amputations: part I: general principles and lower-extremity amputations and part II: upper extremity amputations. J Bone Joint Surg Am. 2010;92:17–18.

Hirshberg A, Maddox K. *Top Knife* and *First to Cut,* 2005 (available on the USAISR website)

Warkentien T, Rodriguez C, Lloyd B, Wells J, Weintrob A, Dunne JR, Ganesan A, Li P, Bradley W, Gaskins LJ, Seillier-Moiseiwitsch F, Murray CK, Millar EV, Keenan B, Paolino K, Fleming M, Hospenthal DR, Wortmann GW, Landrum ML, Kortepeter MG, Tribble DR, Infectious Disease Clinical Research Program Trauma Infectious Disease Outcomes Study Group. Invasive mold infections following combat-related injuries, Clin Infect Dis, vol. 11. 55th ed. Bethesda: Walter Reed National Military Medical Center; 2012. p. 1441–9.

Limb Salvage vs. Amputation

21

Rob Beer and Romney Andersen

Contents

BLUF (Bottom Line Up Front) Box

1. Field tourniquets should be swapped for pneumatic tourniquets in a controlled fashion in the operating room.
2. The zone of injury is more extensive than you think. Extend the wound and expose the tissue for the most effective debridement.
3. Consistency is generally the best guide to tissue viability.
4. Be aggressive with debridement of dead and contaminated tissue. Consider retaining questionable material if it would contribute to limb salvage at a lower level.
5. If you are uncertain about amputation in an otherwise stable patient, seek input from colleagues or stabilize and send off to next higher echelon of care.
6. Do not amputate at the level of a fracture just because there's a fracture. Preserve skeletal length and soft tissue for coverage.
7. Avoid guillotine amputations.
8. Begin with the end in mind: think about how the fracture will be definitively fixed and try to place your external fixation clear of any potential incisions and internal hardware.
9. If possible, salvage bone with significant pieces of articular cartilage.

R. Beer (✉) • R. Andersen
Department of Orthopaedics,
Walter Reed National Military Medical Center,
Bethesda, MD, USA
e-mail: rbeer90@gmail.com

L.B. Bone, C.N. Mamczak (eds.), *Front Line Extremity and Orthopaedic Surgery*,
DOI 10.1007/978-3-642-45337-3_21, © Springer-Verlag Berlin Heidelberg 2014

10. Don't close complex wounds or amputations, but return to the operating room frequently to reexamine and debride.
11. If you think a fasciotomy might be necessary, then do one.

21.1 Triage, Resuscitation, and Initial Assessment

There is no commonly seen parallel in the civilian trauma setting that can prepare one for the instant you see your first patient with traumatic amputations caused by an explosive device. Your ATLS training will serve as your backstop. The airway must be effectively secured, if it is not already. In a mature theater, it is likely that field medics have already taken several steps, to include endotracheal intubation and control of catastrophic hemorrhage with tourniquets. If this hasn't been done, apply a tourniquet to stop major hemorrhage immediately. Begin resuscitation with blood products the instant intravenous or intraosseous access is obtained. It is quite conceivable that as an orthopedic surgeon, you will be supervising the resuscitation. Know the transfusion protocols for your theater.

When the casualty arrives in the resuscitation bay, it is tempting to begin to remove tourniquets and begin assessing limb viability. Do not do this. If possible with a conscious patient, you can attempt a neurovascular exam, otherwise prepare to swap the field tourniquets with pneumatic surgical tourniquets in the operating room. In this controlled setting, the anesthesia team can better handle the systemic sequelae that might result from reperfusion and you are better situated to gain proximal and distal vascular control. Prep all involved extremities, including the tourniquets, into the sterile field and work in parallel if possible with teams addressing abdominal and thoracic injuries. Advise the anesthesiologist when you are removing field tourniquets. Assess for continued major hemorrhage and inflate the pneumatic tourniquet as needed. Repeat for each affected extremity. Because of effective training for first responders, tourniquets are applied almost automatically if extremities are involved. You shouldn't be surprised if you don't encounter major hemorrhage after removing the field tourniquets.

The decision to immediately amputate an extremity is driven by several factors. The first is the need to save the life of the patient. Historically, limbs mangled in warfare were preemptively amputated since sepsis was usually unavoidable. With modern tourniquets, antibiotics, and surgical techniques, it usually is not necessary to immediately amputate in order to keep the patient alive. Today, the decision to immediately amputate is normally driven by the condition of the soft tissue envelope, particularly the overlying musculature, which is insufficient for skeletal coverage. It is often the case that in blast injuries, the limb is either already amputated (traumatic) or has minimal soft tissue attachments, in which case the decision is relatively uncomplicated and the amputation (primary) is completed. Other considerations include a dysvascular limb that cannot be temporarily shunted or one that already has extensive myonecrosis. It is conceivable that delayed evacuation time may result in a limb that has sustained a warm ischemia time of greater than 12 h. Care should be taken in reperfusion of this extremity, as the systemic toxic sequelae can be fatal. Carefully examine the musculature and if there is nothing viable, primary amputation is indicated. If you are uncertain about primary amputation, consult a colleague if available, otherwise debride, stabilize, and transfer to the next echelon of care. It is often wise to delay amputation until after an initial debridement, since heavily contaminated wounds can look remarkably different after a meticulous cleaning. Also, consider retaining amputated parts to help salvage other extremities. Bone can be banked in the subcutaneous tissue. Retaining other parts, such as the great toe, requires microvascular surgical capabilities, but can help in reconstructing a thumb, for example.

The decision to amputate can be more vexing if the patient is a local national. There may be little in the way of national infrastructure to support rehabilitation and prosthetic fitting. Culturally and socially, the amputee will face numerous barriers and challenges. It is important to know the local attitudes towards amputations. At the same time, complex limb reconstruction is usually not an available option, given the lack of resources and specialty support it generally requires. The unfortunate fact is that many limbs may receive amputations that otherwise might have been salvaged in more modern medical systems. You should be familiar with what capability the host nation has locally and if any non-governmental organizations also operate programs to assist wounded local nationals (Fig. 21.1a–d).

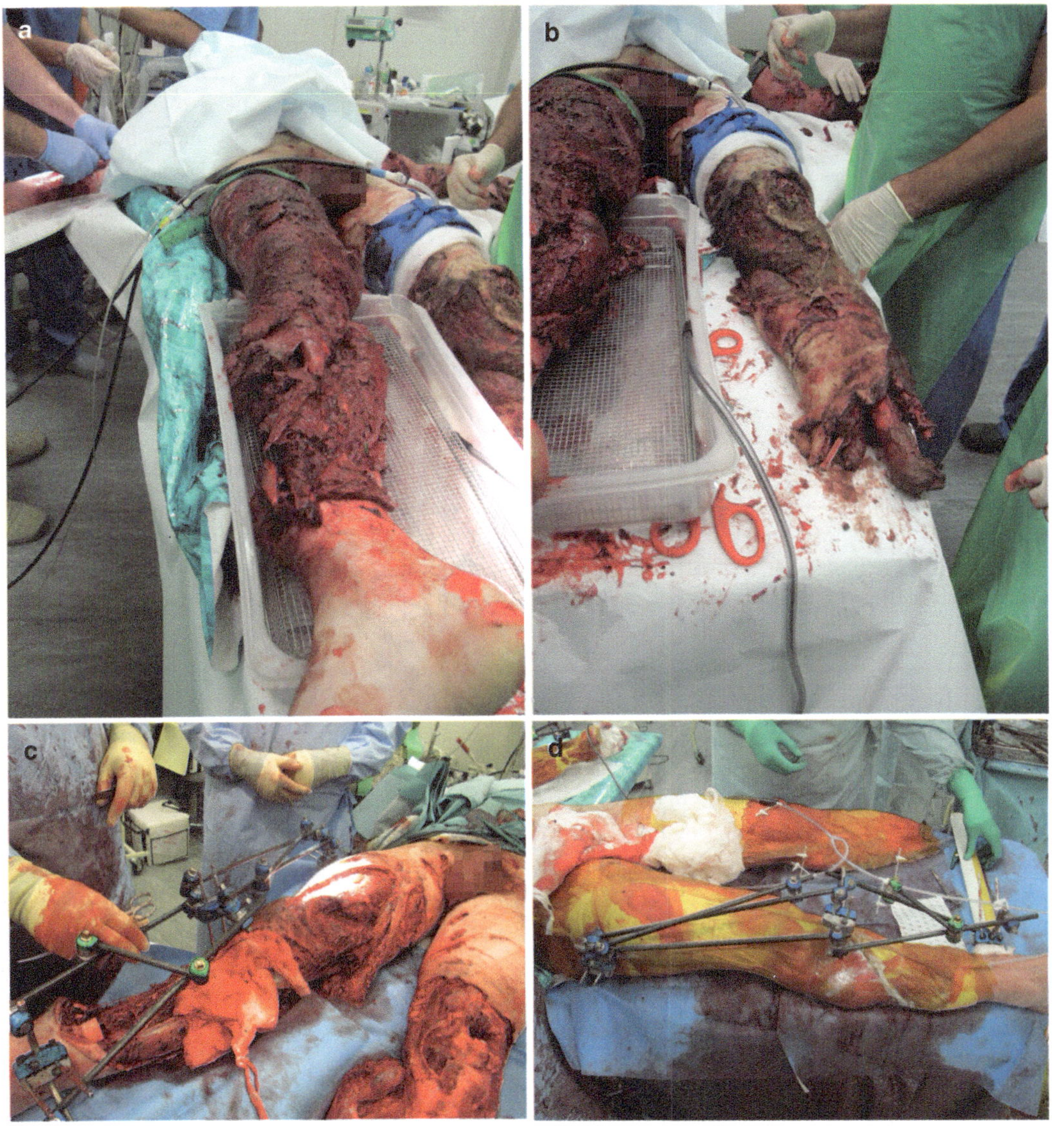

Fig. 21.1 (**a**) IED casualty with extensive lower extremity injuries being resuscitated in the operating room. Field tourniquets have been swapped out for OR pneumatic tourniquets. (**b**) IED casualty with left traumatic leg amputation. (**c**) IED casualty with open tibia fracture and extensive soft tissue injury after initial debridement and application of external fixation. (**d**) IED casualty with antibiotic beads and gauze in the wound bed and an impermeable dressing applied after the initial debridement and irrigation of wounds

21.2 Primary Amputation

If it is clear that primary amputation is required, there are several principles to remember. Chief among these is to preserve length, which usually means trying to keep bone and muscle to cover a below-knee amputation, or a long transfemoral. If you are uncertain about tissue viability for coverage, it should be preserved and the decision passed on to the next echelon, where there may be more limb reconstruction expertise. Do not necessarily amputate at the level of a fracture, as these can often be fixed to preserve a more functional amputation level. It is rare that a guillotine amputation is necessary and one should try to avoid them. A mangled foot that is amputated at the level of the ankle joint or just proximal is one instance where it is acceptable. Initially, these amputations should not be closed and like any other wound, inspected and cleaned in the operating room every 24 h or until evacuated to the next level of care. Use circumferential compression wraps or negative pressure wound therapy dressings for transport. A simple but effective means of communicating with the next level of care is to place a piece of silk tape with the date and time of the last dressing change and a short description of the underlying injury.

21.3 Debridement

Effective debridement is the most important step in the initial management of the mangled extremity. First and foremost, remember that the zone of injury is usually quite extensive and that liberal wound extension is mandatory to effectively inspect, debride, and clean these wounds. Sharp debridement of all devitalized tissue and removal of foreign bodies, organic material, and other gross contamination is paramount. Consistency of tissue is generally the best guide to viability, but debridement is still a skill that comes with experience. The amount of time you are able to spend on this important step is likely to be driven by the physiologic status of the patient and whether or not you need to hurry to get the patient ready for an available air evacuation. To the extent possible, be meticulous about hemostasis and perform a thorough debridement. For large and complex wounds, it's best to have a simple system of proceeding from the skin edges to the superficial muscle and then deep muscle tissue and bone. Lavage these wounds generously with saline. High pressure lavage should be avoided and simple gravity irrigation used, with castile soap if available. Potable water can be used as a last resort as well. Large extremity wounds require 9–12 l of fluid for adequate lavage. A daily return to the operating room is mandatory for these complex wounds until evacuated to the next higher echelon of care. These wounds should not be closed. Antibiotic beads, if available, can be placed in the wound and covered with gauze and an impermeable dressing to form a bead pouch. Alternatively, negative pressure wound therapy foam sponges can be used with a vacuum device. For severely contaminated wounds, consider Dakin's solution-soaked dressings (Fig. 21.2a, b).

21.4 Skeletal Stabilization

When applying an external fixation device for skeletal stabilization, it is important to remember several principles. The following factors increase the stiffness of an external fixation construct: (1) increasing pin diameter, (2) increasing the number of pins, (3) increasing the pin spread, (4) decreasing the distance of bar to bone, and (5) increasing the number of bars. In general, 5 mm pins of varying lengths are used in a uniplanar fashion to stabilize in the field. Field expedient kits are available that provide pins, clamps, bars, and a hand drill to construct a simple spanning ex-fix for the tibia and femur.

Stiffness of the construct is important, but other factors must be considered before placing the ex-fix. Obviously, try to avoid placing the pins through open wounds if possible. Think about how the fracture may ultimately be fixed and place your pins so as to avoid future incisions and hardware locations. Moreover, it can be difficult to load casualties into aircraft with external fixation devices that stick out too far to the side of the patient. If possible, cut excessive pin length and locate the pins to minimize

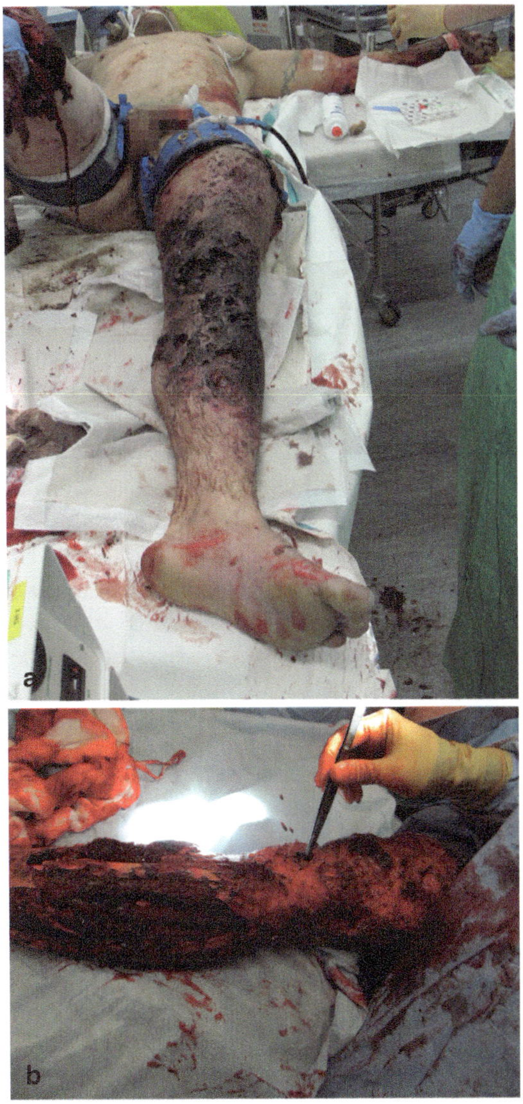

Fig. 21.2 (**a**) IED casualty with a left leg injury showing the effects of shrapnel. (**b**) IED casualty after the initial debridement demonstrating large underlying zone of injury of the soft tissues

this problem, i.e., anterolateral on the thigh and anteromedial on the tibia.

Without fluoroscopy to guide pin placement, placing the self-drilling pins relies on tactile feedback as the tip of the pin cuts through bone. Initial resistance lessens as the tip moves through the medullary canal and then increases again as it contacts the far cortex. Typically five half turns from this point ensures bicortical placement.

21.5 Fasciotomy

Severely injured extremities should continually be checked for signs of compartment syndrome. You will likely have to rely on objective findings and your gut, since the patients often are intubated on arrival and remain so until evacuated. Thus, clinical findings are not available. The two types of fasciotomies to consider are therapeutic and prophylactic. The decision to perform a therapeutic fasciotomy should be made based on the pattern and severity of injury as well as objective findings. Compartment pressures can be measured using an arterial pressure monitoring kit and fasciotomies performed if compartment pressures are within 20–30 mmHg of diastolic blood pressure. It is important to consider the time of injury before proceeding, particularly if there was a delay in evacuation and the casualty has sustained a warm ischemia time of more than 12 h to that extremity. In that case, there is no muscle left to save and the potential complications too catastrophic. Do not perform fasciotomies under that circumstance.

Because of the potential for prolonged evacuation times when the casualty is not under the direct observation of a surgeon, consideration should always be given to performing prophylactic fasciotomies. High altitude is not a concern and does not contribute to the development of compartment syndrome. However, it is possible that the vibratory effects of aircraft flight can contribute to the development of compartment syndrome. Strong consideration should be given to performing fasciotomies in the extremity that sustained a vascular injury and was reperfused either with a shunt or with a vein graft. In general, if you think an injury pattern is at risk for developing compartment syndrome, then perform fasciotomies after skeletal stabilization. In the event of severely burned extremities, however, avoid prophylactic fasciotomies. Wounds should be left open and dressed appropriately for transport and note the date and time of fasciotomies on overlying silk tape.

Correct surgical technique is critical to performing appropriate fasciotomies for traumatic injuries. Full length, two-incision fasciotomies on the leg should be performed. It is important to draw out both incisions prior to making the first cut. After the first cut is made, the skin retracts and can lead to a very narrow anterior skin bridge. On the thigh, the anterior and posterior compartments can be released through a single incision. The medial is released through a separate incision if needed. There is no consensus on performing foot fasciotomies. In the case of the leg, care should be taken to ensure that the septum dividing anterior and lateral compartments is properly identified, thus ensuring release of both compartments. Fascial incisions should be as long as the skin incisions. The usual pitfall to avoid when releasing the posterior and deep posterior compartments is failure to fully release the soleus leash from the tibia. Care should also be taken to avoid injury to the superficial peroneal nerve and saphenous vein. Moreover, releasing the deep posterior compartment should be done under direct visualization to avoid damage to the posterior neurovascular structures.

21.6 Summary

Mangled extremities present challenging decisions to the frontline surgeon. If you have any uncertainty about the potential for limb salvage, it is generally best to debride, lavage, stabilize, and evacuate to the next echelon of care. Be very cautious about undertaking local efforts at limb salvage in host nationals. Preserve tissue and skeletal length in order to provide the best chance at a more functional amputation level. Do not hesitate to perform fasciotomies, even prophylactic, if your clinical judgment thinks they might be needed.

Orthopedic Consultation

22

Christina Cawley

Contents

Bluff (Bottom Line Up Front) Box

1. Know where you are: Roles 1, 2, and 3.
2. Know what support you have available.
3. Know what the service member's job requirement and unit functions demand.
4. Establish what the service member's expectations are.

Orthopedic surgeons have been deployed to a variety of settings in the recent conflicts of Iraq and Afghanistan. Some are large, better staffed, and equipped than a community hospital, while others are very austere. The type of troops and units you support also vary widely. These factors will significantly affect your decision to keep and rehabilitate troops or to recommend evacuation to the rear.

22.1 Levels of Care

The "Role 1" is typically a battalion aid station consisting of medics and perhaps a physician assistant, maybe an ER, or family practice provider. Rarely are surgeons positioned at this level.

The next higher configuration is "Role 2" and has the most asset variability. By doctrine this is an FST (forward surgical team) or service equivalent, with 20 providers. Typically this is comprised of two general surgeons, one orthopedic surgeon, one or two anesthesia providers, an OR

C. Cawley, DO, MS PT, FAOAO
Department of Orthopedic, Walter Reed National Military Medical Center Surgery, Bethesda, MD, USA
e-mail: cawley.chris19@gmail.com

L.B. Bone, C.N. Mamczak (eds.), *Front Line Extremity and Orthopaedic Surgery*, DOI 10.1007/978-3-642-45337-3_22, nurse, an ICU nurse, and several medics. Many Role 2's are operationally split FST's comprised of one general surgeon, one orthopedic surgeon, and one anesthesia provider. Some are Role 2 "plus," which means that a "charley med" company is colocated with the FST. In this case there will be other physicians and physician assistants, and perhaps physical therapist or physical therapy technician. If there is a TBI clinic, you will have an occupational therapist and an occupational therapy technician who can make splints and do therapy for most upper extremity issues.

A "Role 3" is a military hospital with specialist surgical and medical capabilities, preventative medicine, and dentistry. In this situation there will be a therapy department and you will not need to be directly involved.

22.2 Type of Troops

The type of units your FOB supports will affect the types of injury you keep and rehabilitate rather than evacuate. War fighters and trigger pullers have less job flexibility than support troops. The physical demands on a field grade officer or NCO, who can remain effective in their job while in a splint or cast, are vastly different than an E2 turret gunner or a dog handler. A service member who works in the S2 shop can probably be kept in theater with a distal radius fracture, but not a helicopter pilot. Your decision process needs to account for job description and how the injury will impact the individual and unit's safety and function.

22.3 Injury's to Keep

People can be their own worst enemy on deployment. This includes soldiers of all ages who want to stay with their units after being injured. You will see any kind of overuse syndrome you can imagine. Soldiers with these injuries should take 2 weeks off and rest. Rest, NSAIDs, stretching, and gradual resumption of the offensive activity can cure most sprains, strains, and tendonitis you will see. Ice is usually one of our recommendations for these conditions, but it is not often readily available in theater.

The gym is especially dangerous territory for toes and fingers. Dropping heavy plates can result in crush and nail bed injuries. Technically they are open fractures; however, they can be successfully treated at all levels in theater. This requires vigilance for infection for the first several weeks. If infection does develop, prompt evacuation to role 3 for treatment often can result in return to duty.

Lumbar, thoracic, and cervical muscle pain is common place due to poor sleeping and working environments. Nothing in theater is ergonomically correct, and it all takes a toll. Identifying and correcting the culprit may be a challenge, but worth trying, while stretching and NSAID's are good options.

Closed non-displaced ankle, distal radius, ulnar shaft, and finger fractures are reasonable to consider for retaining in theater, especially if they can be treated in a cast or splint and not significantly hinder job performance. Another consideration is timing. For example, the unit just arrived in theater for a 12 month tour, a soldier breaks his ankle, and you expect that he will be good as new after 8 weeks on crutches. You may recommend keeping him because it will ultimately conserve that unit's fighting strength. They just started their tour, are bound to lose troops to more severe injuries, and he will be able to contribute to the cause for 10 months.

Clavicle fractures and distal bicep ruptures are special situations in my opinion. If a "mature" individual sustains a distal bicep rupture, fully understands the injury and its ramifications, and chooses nonoperative management, keep him in theater. The same injury in a young person should be evacuated in a timely fashion for surgical treatment. Low energy, minimally displaced clavicle fractures in noncombatant troops should be evaluated on a case by case basis. Many FOBs are blackout at night, and the terrain is uneven at best. A trip and fall that produces a simple clavicle fracture is a real possibility. However, even a simple clavicle fracture will make it difficult to wear body armor or bear arms. If you are on a large FOB with good and plentiful force protection, and the individual works strictly in the TOC, the risk benefit ratio may be favorable. Whereas, on a small FOB that gets hit often, the liability to the unit may require evacuation. If there are only 3 months left in the unit's tour, this soldier isn't going to be useful for carrying and loading things. They may not even be able to carry their own duffle on the way home, so evacuation may be best.

22.4 Management of Common Chronic Tendon Injuries

Achilles, patellar and rotator tendinopathy, in addition to lateral epicondylitis are common chronic tendon injuries that you will encounter in healthy active populations. Most of these conditions are attributable to overuse, and many patients will improve with rest, appropriate protection, and activity modification. However, patients with chronic symptoms lasting more than 6 weeks may need further care for full, pain-free return to function. In an austere environment you will not have access to prolotherapy, topical nitroglycerin, iontophoresis, phonophoresis, therapeutic ultrasound, extracorporeal shock wave therapy, or low level laser therapy. Evidence supports eccentric strengthening programs as a first-line option for treatment of these conditions, and with a bit of creativity, you can help your troops develop and implement a program of their own.

Achilles tendinopathy presents with pain during and after prolonged walking or running, in the area between the myotendinous junction and insertion onto the calcaneus. An intense eccentric strengthening program of the gastrocnemius/soleus complex can provide 60–90 % improvement in pain and function. This can be accomplished by standing on the balls of your feet with your heels hanging over the edge of a surface like a step. Rise up on both legs until you are standing on your toes. The ankle of the injured leg is lowered to full dorsiflexion and returned to the starting position. This same sequence is repeated with the knee in about 45° of flexion. Three sets of 15 exercises are performed daily. The first 1–2 weeks use only your body weight, then add weight using a loaded rucksack or protective vest with some of the plates removed. A typical regimen lasts 12 weeks.

Patellar tendinopathy or jumper's knee can be treated in a similar way. Find a "downhill" surface, like a wedge or ramp. Face "downhill" so that your knees are straight and your ankles are plantar flexed in the starting position. Slowly bend your knees to approximately 45° then return to starting position. The frequency, progression, and duration of the protocol are the same as those for Achilles tendinopathy.

Lateral epicondylitis, though not really an "itis," can be approached the same way. Performing slow steady wrist extension repetitions with increasing weight, while your wrist is suspended over a bolster, is one way to achieve this. There is no literature that demonstrates the relative effectiveness of any treatment for this malady.

Rotator cuff tendinopathy, evidenced by pain with lifting, pain with overhead motions, and discomfort at night, is common. Most often this is not caused by trauma, but has its root in provocative and repetitive activities. Treatment should be focused on achieving full range of motion, strengthening the rotator cuff muscles, and stabilizing the scapula. Shoulder internal and external rotation with a weight in your hand can be performed standing or laying on your back with the elbow bent to 90°. Start with the weight against your stomach and slowly rotate your arm away from your body, then return to your stomach. The supraspinatus can be isolated by standing with your arms at your sides, thumbs pointed toward the floor. Lean your trunk forward and lift your arms up and out from your sides, keeping the elbow straight. Lift them until they are level with your trunk, not higher. The regimen includes three sets of 15 exercises daily, increase the weight each 1–2 weeks, for a total of 12 weeks.

22.5 Things to Send

Conditions that merit evacuation include multi-ligament knee injury, repeat shoulder dislocations, and spine pain with history of even minor trauma or neurologic changes. Such knee and shoulder injuries are not fixable with return to duty in the time frame of a deployment. In the setting of seemingly minor trauma, cervical, thoracic, or lumbar spine pain that can be localized should be sent to a role 3 for imaging.

Injuries that should be evacuated include nerve injuries or palsies. I have seen radial and ulnar nerve palsy resulting from minor trauma or insidious onset that was delayed in presentation: "Hey Doc, my fingers keep getting stuck in the magazine when I reload." You examine their ulnar nerve and they have no sensation, intrinsic weakness, and may be starting to claw. At that point evacuation is necessary. They are a liability to themselves and the unit. If the ulnar nerve is entrapped and can be released, the individual has a good prognosis. If neglected or significantly delayed, intrinsic muscle damage may result in a permanently useless hand. I mention the ulnar nerve specifically because I have seen many troops, on both sides of the ocean, with compression syndromes. Contributing factors may include large forearm muscles from exercise and leaning an arm on the window sill of vehicles while training their weapon on potential targets. The devastating potential of this condition can be difficult to impress upon commanders or brigade surgeons. You have to be prepared to think outside the box.

Conclusion

Orthopedic injuries are a very common downrange. You will be consulted on any number on non-battlefield injuries. Their management and soldier disposition will depend on all of the factors mentioned. Maintaining troop strength is a goal, but the primary goal is what is best for the soldier, airman, or marine. When in doubt, consult with your higher as well as the higher of the injured soldier.

Index

L.B. Bone, C.N. Mamczak (eds.), *Front Line Extremity and Orthopaedic Surgery*,
DOI 10.1007/978-3-642-45337-3, © Springer-Verlag Berlin Heidelberg 2014

GPSR Compliance

The European Union's (EU) General Product Safety Regulation (GPSR) is a set of rules that requires consumer products to be safe and our obligations to ensure this.

If you have any concerns about our products, you can contact us on ProductSafety@springernature.com

In case Publisher is established outside the EU, the EU authorized representative is:

Springer Nature Customer Service Center GmbH
Europaplatz 3
69115 Heidelberg, Germany

Batch number: 10286956

Printed by Printforce, the Netherlands